ALCOHOL AND CARDIOVASCULAR DISEASES

The Novartis Foundation is an international scientific and educational charity (UK Registered Charity No. 313574). Known until September 1997 as the Ciba Foundation, it was established in 1947 by the CIBA company of Basle, which merged with Sandoz in 1996, to form Novartis. The Foundation operates independently in London under English trust law. It was formally opened on 22 June 1949.

The Foundation promotes the study and general knowledge of science and in particular encourages international co-operation in scientific research. To this end, it organizes internationally acclaimed meetings (typically eight symposia and allied open meetings, 15–20 discussion meetings, a public lecture and a public debate each year) and publishes eight books per year featuring the presented papers and discussions from the symposia. Although primarily an operational rather than a grant-making foundation, it awards bursaries to young scientists to attend the symposia and afterwards work for up to three months with one of the other participants.

The Foundation's headquarters at 41 Portland Place, London W1N 4BN, provide library facilities, open every weekday, to graduates in science and allied disciplines. The library is home to the Media Resource Service which offers journalists access to expertise on any scientific topic. Media relations are also strengthened by regular press conferences and book launches, and by articles prepared by the Foundation's Science Writer in Residence. The Foundation offers accommodation and meeting facilities to visiting scientists and their societies.

Information on all Foundation activities can be found at http://www.novartisfound.demon.co.uk

Novartis Foundation Symposium 216

ALCOHOL AND CARDIOVASCULAR DISEASES

1998

JOHN WILEY & SONS

Chichester · New York · Weinheim · Brisbane · Singapore · Toronto

Other Wiley Editorial Offices

John Wiley & Sons, Inc., 605 Third Avenue,
New York, NY 10158-0012, USA

WILEY-VCH Verlag GmbH, Pappelallee 3,
D-69469 Weinheim, Germany

Jacaranda Wiley Ltd, 33 Park Road, Milton,
Queensland 4064, Australia

John Wiley & Sons (Asia) Pte Ltd, 2 Clementi Loop #02-01,
Jin Xing Distripark, Singapore 129809

John Wiley & Sons (Canada) Ltd, 22 Worcester Road,
Rexdale, Ontario M9W 1L1, Canada

Novartis Foundation Symposium 216
viii+272 pages, 25 figures, 30 tables

Library of Congress Cataloging-in-Publication Data
Alcohol and cardiovascular diseases / [editors, Derek J. Chadwick
(organizer) and Jamie A. Goode].
        p.   cm.   – (Novartis Foundation symposium ; 216)
"Symposium on Alcohol and Cardiovascular Diseases, held at the
Novartis Foundation, London, 7–9 October 1997"–CIP intro.
        Includes bibliographical references and index.
        ISBN 0-471-97769-1 (hardcover : alk. paper)
        1. Heart–Pathophysiology–Congresses.   2. Alcohol–Physiological
effect–Congresses.   3. Alcohol–Pathophysiology–Congresses.
I. Chadwick, Derek.   II. Goode, Jamie.   III. Symposium on Alcohol
and Cardiovascular Diseases (1997 : London)   IV. Series.
        RC682.9.A42   1998   98-27198
        616.1'071–dc21   CIP

British Library Cataloguing in Publication Data

A catalogue record for this book is available from the British Library

ISBN 0 471 97769 1

Typeset in 10½ on 12½ pt Garamond by Dobbie Typesetting Limited, Tavistock, Devon.
Printed and bound in Great Britain by Biddles Ltd, Guildford and King's Lynn.
This book is printed on acid-free paper responsibly manufactured from sustainable forestry,
in which at least two trees are planted for each one used for paper production.

Contents

Participants

Peter Anderson   Lifestyles and Health Unit, World Health Organization, Regional Office for Europe, 8 Scherfigsvej, Copenhagen DK2100, Denmark

Susan J. Bondy (*Novartis Foundation Bursar*)   Addiction Research Foundation, 33 Russell Street, Toronto, Ontario, Canada M5S 2S1

Michael H. Criqui   University of California, San Diego, Department of Family & Preventive Medicine, Clinical Sciences Building, Rm 349, 9500 Gilman Drive, La Jolla, CA 92093-0607, USA

Gino Farchi   Laboratorio di Epidemiologia e Biostatistica, Istituto Superiore di Sanità, 00161 Rome, Italy

Michael Farrell   Addiction Resource Unit, 63–65 Denmark Hill, Camberwell, London SE5 8RS, UK

Kaye Fillmore   Department of Social and Behavioral Science, UCSF, Box 0646, Laurel Heights, San Francisco, CA 94143-0646, USA

J. Michael Gaziano   Veterans Affairs Medical Center, Harvard Medical School, 1440 VFW Parkway, West Roxbury, MA 02132, USA

Philip B. Gorelick   Center for Stroke Research, 1645 West Jackson Blvd, Suite 400, Chicago, IL 60612, USA

Morten Grønbæk   Copenhagen Center for Prospective Population Studies, Danish Epidemiology Science Centre at the Institute of Preventive Medicine, Copenhagen University Hospital, DK-1399 Copenhagen K, Denmark

Henk F. J. Hendriks   TNO Nutrition and Food Research Institute, P O Box 360, 3700 AJ Zeist, The Netherlands

Matti Hillbom   Department of Neurology, University of Oulu, University Central Hospital of Oulu, Kajaanintie 50, SF-90220 Oulu, Finland

John F. Keaney Jr.   Boston University School of Medicine, Whitaker Cardiovascular Institute, W507, 80E Concord Street, Boston, MA 02118, USA

Ulrich Keil   Institute of Epidemiology and Social Medicine, University of Münster, Domagkstr. 3, Münster, D-48129, Germany

Arthur L. Klatsky   Kaiser Permanente Medical Center, 280 West MacArthur Boulevard, Oakland, CA 94611, USA

Marrku Kupari   Division of Cardiology, Department of Medicine, Helsinki University Central Hospital, 00290 Helsinki, Finland

Michael G. Marmot   International Centre for Health and Society, University College London, 1–19 Torrington Place, London WC1E 6BT, UK

George Miller   MRC Epidemiology and Medical Care Unit, St Bartholomew's and The Royal London School of Medicine, Charterhouse Square, London EC1M 6BQ, UK

Timothy J. Peters *(Chairman)*   Department of Clinical Biochemistry, King's College School of Medicine & Dentistry, Bessemer Road, London SE5 9PJ, UK

Ian B. Puddey   Department of Medicine, University of Western Australia, Royal Perth Hospital, GPO Box X2213, Perth, Western Australia

Jürgen Rehm   Addiction Research Foundation, Clinical, Social and Evaluation Research Department, 33 Russell Street, Toronto, Ontario, Canada M5S 2S1

Serge Renaud   INSERM Unit 330, Université Bordeaux 2, 146 Rue Leo-Saignat, 33076 Bordeaux Cedex, France

Peter J. Richardson   Consultant Cardiologist, King's College Hospital, Denmark Hill, London SE5 9RS, UK

A. Gerry Shaper   Department of Primary Care and Population Sciences, Royal Free Hospital School of Medicine, Rowland Hill Street, London NW3 2PF, UK

Alvaro Urbano-Márquez   Alcohol Research Unit, Department of Medicine Hospital Clinic, University of Barcelona, Villarroel 170, Barcelona 08036, Spain

S. Goya Wannamethee   Department of Primary Care and Population Sciences, Royal Free Hospital School of Medicine, Rowland Hill Street, London NW3 2PF, UK

Chairman's introduction

Timothy J. Peters

Department of Clinical Biochemistry, King's College School of Medicine and Dentistry, Bessemer Road, London SE5 9PJ, UK

In most Western countries the production, purveying and pathology of alcohol beverages is a multibillion dollar business. We have vacillated between its beneficial and detrimental effects throughout the last century. Of recent interest is the apparent beneficial effect of modest alcohol consumption, one to three drinks per day, on mortality and morbidity rates, particularly relating to cardiovascular disease. The objectives of this symposium were to bring together speakers and discussants from a wide range of disciplines to evaluate the evidence for the so-called J-shaped curve and to seek a biological explanation for the apparent beneficial effects of low levels of consumption. The final aim was to discuss how the conclusions from the symposium might be translated into effective and acceptable public health measures.

The physical and intellectual objectives of the programme were clearly achieved: the participants and readers will clearly have a view as to whether worthwhile conclusions were reached.

Alcohol and cardiovascular diseases: a historical overview

Arthur L. Klatsky

Kaiser Permanente Medical Center, 280 West MacArthur Boulevard, Oakland, CA 94611, USA

Abstract. Evident disparities in relationships make it desirable to consider several disorders separately. (1) Alcoholic cardiomyopathy was perceived 150 years ago, but understanding was clouded by recognition of beriberi and of synergistic toxicity from alcohol with arsenic or cobalt. (2) A report of a link between heavy drinking and hypertension in WWI French soldiers was apparently ignored for >50 years. Epidemiological and intervention studies have now firmly established this association, but a mechanism remains elusive. (3) The 'holiday heart syndrome', an increased risk of supraventricular tachyarrhythmias in alcoholics, has been widely known to clinicians for 25 years; data remain sparse about the total role of heavier drinking in cardiac rhythm disturbances. (4) Failure of earlier studies to distinguish types of stroke impeded understanding; it now seems probable that alcohol drinking increases risk of haemorrhagic stroke but lowers risk of ischaemic stroke. (5) Heberden reported angina relief by alcohol in 1786, and an inverse alcohol–atherosclerosis association was observed by pathologists early in this century. Recent population studies and plausible mechanisms support a protective effect of alcohol against coronary disease. International comparisons dating back to 1819 suggest beverage choice as a factor, but this issue (the 'French Paradox') remains unresolved.

1998 Alcohol and cardiovascular diseases. Wiley, Chichester (Novartis Foundation Symposium 216) p 2–18

Those who cannot remember the past are condemned to repeat it.
  George Santayana, The Life of Reason, 1905

The effects of ethyl alcohol upon the cardiovascular system have excited the interest of clinicians and investigators for well over a century. While much has been learned, many areas of knowledge remain incomplete. Physiological, clinical and epidemiological evidence cannot yet be integrated into definitive general concepts. Past attempts to generalize and simplify have probably had the effect of slowing progress in understanding this area. Disparity in relations of alcohol drinking to various cardiovascular conditions (Klatsky 1995a) has become increasingly clear.

To this must be added the disparity between the effects of lighter and heavier drinking. The choice of topics for this book recognizes these differences. In this historical overview, each of the following will be considered separately: cardiomyopathy, arsenic and cobalt beer drinkers' disease, cardiovascular beri-beri, systemic hypertension, cardiac arrhythmias, cerebrovascular disease, atherosclerotic coronary heart disease (CHD), total mortality and definitions of safe drinking limits. Emphasis is on aspects less likely to be covered in detail by other papers in this book; the latter are only briefly summarized. Hopefully, some light will be cast upon previous mistakes, so that we can proceed less burdened by the condemnation of repeating them.

Alcoholic cardiomyopathy

Circumstantial evidence only raises a probability.
  Mr Justice Pollock, 1865

A number of famous nineteenth century physicians commented about an apparent relationship between chronic intake of large amounts of alcohol and heart disease (Friedreich 1861, Walsche 1873, Strumpell 1890, Steell 1893, Osler 1899). A German pathologist (Böllinger 1884) described cardiac dilatation and hypertrophy among Bavarian beer drinkers, which became known as the 'Munchener bierherz'. He reported an average yearly consumption of 432 litres of beer in Munich, compared with 82 litres in other parts of Germany.

In 1900, an epidemic of heart disease due to arsenic-contaminated beer occurred in Manchester, England. Before this event, Graham Steell (1893), in a report of 25 cases, stated 'not only do I recognize alcoholism as one of the causes of muscle failure of the heart but I find it a comparatively common one'. Following the arsenic beer episode Steell (1906) wrote in a textbook that 'in the production of the combined affection of the peripheral nerves and the heart met with in beer drinkers, arsenic has been shown to play a conspicuous part'. In his textbook *The Study of the Pulse* William MacKenzie (1902) described cases of heart failure attributed to alcohol and first used the term 'alcoholic heart disease'. Early in the 20th century, there was general doubt that alcohol had a direct role in producing heart muscle disease, although some (e.g. Vaquez 1921) took a strong view in favour of such a relationship.

After the detailed descriptions of cardiovascular beri-beri (Aalsmeer & Wenckebach 1929, Keefer 1930), the concept of 'beri-beri heart disease' dominated thinking about the effects of alcohol upon the heart for several decades. For the past 40 years or so, increasing interest has been evident in possible direct toxicity of alcohol upon the myocardial cells, independent of, or in addition to, deficiency states. The sheer volume of clinical observations, indirect evidence of decreased myocardial function in heavy chronic drinkers, and a few good controlled studies have now solidly established the concept of alcoholic cardiomyopathy. The absence of diagnostic tests remains a major impediment to epidemiological study, since the entity is indistinguishable from other forms of dilated cardiomyopathy. Most cases of dilated cardiomyopathy in 1997 are of unknown cause, with a post-viral autoimmune process the leading aetiologic hypothesis. The most convincing circumstantial evidence that alcohol can cause cardiomyopathy consists of extensive data, in animals and humans, of non-specific cardiac abnormalities related to alcohol. A landmark study (Urbano-Márquez et al 1989) showed a clear relation in alcoholics of lifetime alcohol consumption to structural and functional myocardial and skeletal muscle abnormalities. The amounts of alcohol were large — the equivalent of 120 grams alcohol/day for 20 years. Thus, Walshe's term 'cirrhosis of the heart' seems very appropriate.

In view of the history just cited, it seems noteworthy that there has been little work so far about possible cofactors or predisposing traits for alcoholic cardiomyopathy. In this context, it seems appropriate to consider further the arsenic and cobalt beer drinker episodes and thiamine (cocarboxylase) deficiency — or beri-beri heart disease.

Arsenic beer drinkers' disease

Synergy: (def.) combined action or operation.
    Webster's 7th Collegiate Dictionary

In 1900 an epidemic (6000+ cases with 70+ deaths) occurred in and near Manchester, England, which proved to be due to contamination of beer by arsenic. There were skin, neurological and gastrointestinal signs and symptoms, but cardiovascular manifestations, especially heart failure, were especially prominent. A superb clinical description (Reynolds 1901) included: (1) 'cases were associated with so much heart failure and so little pigmentation that they were diagnosed as beri-beri. . . .'; (2) 'so great has been the cardiac muscle failure that . . . the principal cause of death has been cardiac failure. . . .', and (3) 'at post-mortem examinations the only prominent signs were the interstitial nephritis and the dilated flabby heart . . .'.

Lively entries in *The Lancet* over the next few years included allusion to a possible earlier (by 12 years) outbreak in France due to contaminated wine, and the probable source as contaminated sulfuric acid used to treat cane sugar. It was determined that the affected beer had 2–4 parts per million of arsenic, not — in itself — an amount likely to cause serious toxicity. It was pointed out that some persons seemed to have a 'peculiar idiosyncrasy', that 'many persons became ill who drank less beer than others not affected', and that 'the amount of arsenic . . .was not sufficient to explain the poisoning'. One entry (Gowers 1901) mentioned that the author prescribed 10 times the amount of arsenic involved for epilepsy over long periods of time with no toxicity. An appointed committee report (Royal Commission 1903) suggested that 'alcohol predisposed people to arsenic poisoning'. As best one can determine, no one suggested the converse.

Cobalt beer drinkers' disease

History repeats itself.
        Thucydides; History, I, c. 410 B.C.

Recognized 65 years after the arsenic beer episode, this condition was similar in some respects. In the mid-1960s reports appeared of epidemics of heart failure among beer drinkers in Omaha and Minneapolis in the USA, Quebec, Canada, and Leuven, Belgium. The condition developed fairly abruptly in chronic heavy beer drinkers. The North American patients suffered a high mortality rate, but those who recovered did well despite return, by many, to previous beer habits. The Belgian cases were less acute in onset, longer in duration and had a lower mortality.

The explanation proved to be the addition of small amounts of cobalt chloride by certain breweries to improve the foaming qualities of beer. Widespread use of detergents (new at that time) in taverns had a depressant effect upon foaming. This aetiology was tracked down largely by Quebec investigators (Morin & Daniel 1967), and the condition became justly known as Quebec beer-drinkers' cardiomyopathy. The largest Quebec brewery had added cobalt to all beer — not only draught beer. Removal of the cobalt additive ended the epidemic in all locations.

In Belgium, where the cobalt concentrations were lower and the cardiac manifestations less severe, there were more of the usual findings of chronic cobalt use, such as polycythemia and goiter. However, even in Quebec, where cobalt doses were greatest, 12 litres of contaminated beer provided only about 8 mg cobalt, less than 20% of the dose sometimes used as a haematinic. The haematinic use had not been implicated as a cause of heart disease, whereas the first cases of this dramatic heart condition occurred 4–8 weeks after cobalt was added to beer.

Thus, both cobalt and substantial amounts of alcohol seemed needed to produce this condition. Most exposed persons did not develop the condition. Despite much speculation, biochemical mechanisms were not established. One observer (Alexander 1969) summed up the arsenic and cobalt episodes thus: 'This is the second known metal induced cardiotoxic syndrome produced by contaminated beer'.

The arsenic and cobalt episodes raise the possibility of other cofactors in alcoholic cardiomyopathy, such as cardiotropic viruses, drugs, selenium, copper and iron. Deficiencies of zinc, magnesium, protein and various vitamins have also been suggested as cofactors, but deficiency of thiamine is probably the only one with solid proof of cardiac malfunction.

Cardiovascular beriberi

Things are seldom what they seem.
W. S. Gilbert, HMS Pinafore, 1878

As already stated, for many years this condition dominated thinking about alcohol and cardiovascular disease. The classical description (Aalsmeer & Wenckebach 1929) defined high-output heart failure in Javanese polished-rice eaters, with decreased peripheral vascular resistance as the physiological basis. It became assumed that heart failure in heavy alcohol drinkers in the West was due to associated nutritional deficiency states. Although some heart failure cases in North American and European alcoholics fitted this clinical pattern, most did not. Many had low output heart failure, were well-nourished and responded poorly to thiamine. Some felt that these facts were due to the chronicity of the condition, which ultimately might become irreversible. However, Blacket & Palmer (1960) stated the following view: 'It (beriberi) responds completely to thiamine, but merges imperceptibly into another disease, called alcoholic cardiomyopathy, which doesn't respond to thiamine'. Modern physiological techniques have established that in beriberi there is generalized dilatation of peripheral arterioles, with creation of an effective large arteriovenous shunt with resultant high resting cardiac outputs. A few cases of complete recovery with thiamine within 1–2 weeks were documented.

It is evident that many cases earlier called 'cardiovascular beriberi' would now be called 'alcoholic heart disease'. Does chronic thiamine deficiency play a role in some cases of alcoholic cardiomyopathy? This currently unpopular thesis has not been proved or disproved.

Hypertension

There is nothing new save that which has been forgotten.
Mme. Bertin, milliner to Marie Antoinette, c. 1785

Epidemiological studies

A threshold relationship between heavy drinking and hypertension was reported in WWI middle-aged French servicemen (Lian 1915). Unless Dr Lian's French soldiers were exaggerating, they were prodigious drinkers: the hypertension threshold appeared at >2 litres of wine per day. It was almost 60 years before further attention was paid to this subject. Since the mid 1970s, dozens of cross-sectional and prospective epidemiological studies have solidly established an empirical alcohol–hypertension link (Beilin & Puddey 1992, Klatsky 1995b). Almost all studies show higher mean blood pressures and/or higher hypertension prevalence with increasing alcohol drinking. These studies involve both sexes and various ages and include North American, European, Australian and Japanese populations. The apparent threshold amount of drinking associated with higher blood pressure in the more modern studies is at approximately 3 drinks/day. The studies show independence of the link from adiposity, salt intake, education, cigarette smoking and several other potential confounders. Alcoholic beverage type (wine, liquor or beer) seems to be a minor factor. Most studies do not show any increase in blood pressure at lighter alcohol drinking; several show an unexplained J-shaped curve in women, with lowest pressures in lighter drinkers.

Intervention studies

The landmark study of Potter & Beevers (1984) showed in hospitalized hypertensive men that three to four days of drinking four pints of beer raised blood pressure and that a similar period of abstinence resulted in lower pressures. These changes occurred in several days to a week without evidence of withdrawal increases in pressure. Similar results were later seen in ambulatory normotensives and hypertensives (Beilin & Puddey 1992). Other interventional studies have shown that heavier alcohol intake interferes with drug treatment of hypertension and that moderation or avoidance of alcohol supplements or betters other non-pharmacological interventions such as weight reduction, exercise or sodium restriction (Beilin & Puddey 1992). Even in the absence of an established mechanism, the intervention studies strongly support a causal hypothesis. It now seems probable that alcohol restriction plays a major role in hypertension management and prevention.

Arrhythmias

If all the year were playing holidays,
To sport would be as tedious as to work.
*   Shakespeare; Henry IV, I, c. 1598*

An association of heavier alcohol consumption with atrial arrhythmias has been suspected for decades, with occurrence after a large meal accompanied with much alcohol. The concept of the 'holiday heart phenomenon' was popularized (Ettinger et al 1978) on the basis of the observation that supraventricular arrhythmias in alcoholics without overt cardiomyopathy were most likely to occur on Mondays or between Christmas and New Year's Day. Some have suggested that atrial flutter was especially likely to be so associated, but various atrial arrhythmias have been reported to be associated with spree drinking. Atrial fibrillation is the commonest manifestation. The problem typically resolves with abstinence, with or without specific treatment. A Kaiser Permanente study (Cohen et al 1988) compared atrial arrhythmias in 1322 persons reporting 6+ drinks per day to arrhythmias in 2644 light drinkers. The relative risk in the heavier drinkers was at least doubled for atrial fibrillation, atrial flutter, supraventricular tachycardia, and atrial premature complexes.

Stroke

The cautious seldom make mistakes.
Confucius: Analects, IV, c.500B.C.

Earlier studies of relationships of alcohol drinking to stroke were made difficult by imprecise diagnosis of stroke type before modern imaging techniques improved diagnostic accuracy. All studies of alcohol and stroke are greatly complicated by the disparate relationships of both stroke and alcohol to other cardiovascular conditions.

Several reports suggested that alcohol use, especially heavier drinking, was associated with higher risk of stroke (Van Gign et al 1993). Some studies examined only drinking sprees; some others did not differentiate between haemorrhagic and ischaemic strokes. The importance of these deficiencies is highlighted by several recent studies suggesting that regular lighter drinkers are at higher risk of haemorrhagic stroke types, but at lower risk of several types of ischaemic stroke (Van Gign et al 1993).

At this time there is no consensus about the relations of alcohol drinking to the various types of cerebrovascular disease and agreement only that more study of this important subject is needed.

Coronary heart disease

Wine and spiritous liquors — afford considerable relief.
William Heberden, 1786

After the classic description of angina pectoris (Heberden 1786), alcohol was widely presumed to be a coronary vasodilator (White 1931, Levine 1951). However, data from exercise ECG tests (Russek et al 1950, Orlando et al 1976) suggest that alcohol does not improve myocardial oxygen deficiency and that symptomatic benefit is subjective and, possibly, dangerously misleading. Few data suggest any major immediate effect of alcohol upon coronary blood flow (Renaud et al 1993, Klatsky 1994).

In the first half of this century there were reports of an apparent inverse relationship between alcohol consumption and atherosclerotic disease, including CHD (Cabot 1904, Hultgen 1910, Leary 1931, Wilens 1947). One explanation offered was that premature deaths in heavier drinkers precluded development of CHD (Ruebner et al 1961, Parrish & Eberly 1961). Since 1974 several dozen population and case-control studies have solidly established an inverse relationship between alcohol drinking and either fatal or non-fatal CHD. Data supporting plausible protective mechanisms have also appeared (Renaud et al 1993, Klatsky 1994). It now seems likely that alcohol drinking protects against CHD.

The cause is hidden, but the effect is known.
  Ovid; Metamorphoses, IV, c.5.

In 1819 Dr Samuel Black, an Irish physician with a great interest in angina pectoris and of considerable perception with respect to epidemiological aspects, wrote what is probably the first commentary pertinent to the 'French Paradox'. His anecdotal observation (Black 1819) was based upon lack of discussion of the condition in the French medical literature, but his interpretation is noteworthy. With respect to the disparity in CHD between Ireland and France, he attributed the low angina prevalence in the latter to 'the French habits and modes of living, coinciding with the benignity of their climate and the peculiar character of their moral affections'. It was to be 160 years before data were presented from the first international comparison study to suggest less CHD in wine drinking countries than in beer or liquor drinking countries (St Leger et al 1979). We now have several confirmatory international comparison studies as well as reports of non-alcohol antioxidant phenolic compounds or antithrombotic substances in wine, especially red wine (Renaud et al 1993, Klatsky 1994). However, prospective population studies show no consensus about the wine/liquor/beer issue (Rimm et al 1996, Klatsky et al 1997). This question remains unresolved at this time.

The J-shaped alcohol–mortality curve

There are more old wine drinkers than old doctors.
  German proverb

This scientifically unsound (no denominators) proverb suggests general scepticism about medical reports. There was one report of the J-curve alcohol–mortality phenomenon which preceded other population study reports by half a century. A Baltimore investigator (Pearl 1926) described this relationship in a study of 5248 tuberculosis patients and controls. 'Heavy/steady' drinkers had the highest mortality; 'abstainers' were next; and 'moderate' drinkers had the lowest mortality. His interpretation was cautious; he concluded that moderate drinking was 'not harmful'. Perhaps his major contribution was to realize the fallacy in comparing all drinkers to abstainers, which masks the J-curve.

The 'sensible drinking limit'

Drink not the third glass.
 George Herbert: The Temple, 1633

The medical risks of heavier drinking and the relative safety of lighter drinking have long been evident. Thus, attempts to define a safe limit are hardly new. Probably the most cited such limit has been known for more than 100 years as 'Anstie's Rule' (Anstie 1870), which advised an upper limit of approximately three standard drinks daily. Although his limit was intended to apply primarily to mature men, Sir Francis Anstie was a distinguished neurologist and public health activist who emphasized individual variability in the ability to handle alcohol. Individual risk/benefit considerations should be a major focus of any discussion and the primary consideration when a health practitioner advises his or her client. It is noteworthy that several contemporary data-based definitions are similar to Sir Francis Anstie's common-sense-based concept.

References

Aalsmeer WC, Wenckebach KF 1929 Herz und Kreislauf bei der Beri-Beri Krankheit. Wein Arch Inn Med 16:193–272
Alexander CS 1969 Cobalt and the heart. Ann Intern Med 70:411–413
Anstie FE 1870 On the uses of wines in health and disease. JS Redfield, New York, p 11–13
Beilin LJ, Puddey IB 1992 Alcohol and hypertension. Clin Exp Hypertens Theory Pract A14 (1 and 2):119–138
Black S 1819 Clinical and pathological reports. Alex Wilkinson, Newry, p 1–47
Blacket RB, Palmer A J 1960 Haemodynamic studies in high output beri-beri. Br Heart J 22:483–501
Böllinger O 1884 Ueber die Haussigkeit und Ursachen der idiopathischen Herzhypertrophie in München. Disch Med Wochenschr (Stuttgart) 10:180
Cabot RC 1904 The relation of alcohol to arteriosclerosis. J Am Med Assoc 43:774–775
Cohen EJ, Klatsky AL, Armstrong MA 1988 Alcohol use and supraventricular arrhythmia. Am J Cardiol 62:971–973
Ettinger PO, Wu CF, De La Cruz C, Weisse AB, Ahmed SS, Regan TJ 1978 Arrhythmias and the 'holiday heart': alcohol-associated cardiac rhythm disorders. Am Heart J 95:555–562
Friedreich N 1861 Handbuch der speziellen Pathologic und Therapie, 5th sect. Krankheiten des Herzens, Ferdinand Enke, Erlangen

Gowers WR 1901 Royal Medical and Chirurgical Society epidemic of arsenical poisoning in beer-drinkers in the north of England during the year 1900. Lancet i:98–100

Heberden W 1786 Some account of a disorder of the breast. Med Trans R Coll Physicians (London) 2:59–67

Hultgen J F 1910 Alcohol and nephritis: clinical study of 460 cases of chronic alcoholism. J Am Med Assoc 55:279–281

Keefer CS 1930 The beri-beri heart. Arch Intern Med 45:1–22

Klatsky AL 1994 Epidemiology of coronary heart disease — influence of alcohol. Alcohol Clin Exp Res 18:88–96

Klatsky AL 1995a Cardiovascular effects of alcohol. Sci Am Sci Med 2:28–37

Klatsky AL 1995b Blood pressure and alcohol intake. In: Laragh JH, Brenner BM (eds) Hypertension: pathophysiology, diagnosis, and management, 2nd edn. Raven Press Ltd, New York, p 2649–2667

Klatsky AL, Armstrong, MA, Friedman GD 1997 Red wine, white wine, liquor, beer, and risk for coronary artery disease hospitalization. Am J Cardiol 80:416–420

Leary T 1931 Therapeutic value of alcohol, with special consideration of relations of alcohol to cholesterol, and thus to diabetes, to arteriosclerosis, and to gallstones. N Engl J Med 205:231–242

Levine SA 1951 Clinical heart disease, 4th edn. Saunders, Philadelphia

Lian C 1915 L'alcoholisme cause d'hypertension artérielle. Bull Acad Méd (Paris) 74:525–528

MacKenzie J 1902 The study of the pulse. Y J Pentland, Edinburgh

Morin Y, Daniel P 1967 Quebec beer-drinkers' cardiomyopathy: etiologic considerations. Can Med Assoc J 97:926–928

Orlando J, Aronow WS, Cassidy J, Prakash R 1976 Effect of ethanol on angina pectoris. Ann Intern Med 84:652–655

Osler W 1899 The principles and practice of medicine, 3rd edn. Appleton, New York

Parrish HM, Eberly AL 1961 Negative association of coronary atherosclerosis with liver cirrhosis and chronic alcoholism — a statistical fallacy. J Indiana State Med Assoc 54:341–347

Pearl R 1926 Alcohol and longevity. Knopf, New York

Potter JF, Beevers DG 1984 Pressor effect of alcohol in hypertension. Lancet 1:119–122

Renaud S, Criqui MH, Farchi G, Veenstra J 1993 Alcohol drinking and coronary heart disease. In: Verschuren PM (ed) Health issues related to alcohol consumption. ILSI Press, Washington DC, p 81–123

Reynolds ES 1901 An account of the epidemic outbreak of arsenical poisoning occurring in beer drinkers in the North of England and the Midland Counties in 1900. Lancet i:166–170

Rimm EB, Klatsky AL, Grobbee D, Stampfer MJ 1996 Review of moderate alcohol consumption and reduced risk of coronary heart disease: is the effect due to beer, wine or spirits? Br Med J 312:731–736

Royal Commission 1903 Royal Commission appointed to inquire into arsenical poisoning from the consumption of beer and other articles of food or drink. Final report, part I. Wyman & Sons, London

Ruebner BH, Miyai K, Abbey H 1961 The low incidence of myocardial infarction in hepatic cirrhosis — a statistical artefact? Lancet ii:1435–1436

Russek HI, Naegele CF, Regan FD 1950 Alcohol in the treatment of angina pectoris. J Am Med Assoc 143:355–357

St Leger AS, Cochrane AL, Moore F 1979 Factors associated with cardiac mortality in developed countries with particular reference to the consumption of wine. Lancet 1:1017–1020

Steell G 1893 Heart failure as a result of chronic alcoholism. Med Chron Manchester 18:1–22

Steell G 1906 Textbook on diseases of the heart. Blakiston, Philadelphia

Strumpel A 1890 A textbook of medicine. Appleton, New York

Urbano-Márquez A, Estruch R, Novarro-Lopez F, Grau JM, Mont L, Rubin E 1989 The effects
of alcoholism on skeletal and cardiac muscle. N Engl J Med 329:409–415

Van Gign J, Stampfer M J, Wolfe C, Algra A 1993 The association between alcohol consumption
and stroke. In: Verschuren PM (ed) Health issues related to alcohol consumption. ILSI Press,
Washington DC, p 43–80

Vaquez H 1921 Maladies du coeur. Baillière et Fils, Paris

Walsche WH 1873 Diseases of the heart and great vessels, 4th edn. Smith Elder, London

White PD 1931 Heart disease. Macmillan, New York

Wilens SL 1947 The relationship of chronic alcoholism to atherosclerosis. J Am Med Assoc
135:1136–1139

DISCUSSION

Keil: You told us that the protective effect of alcohol on coronary heart disease
(CHD) was first shown in 1974 (Klatsky et al 1974). However, in a recent paper by
Seltzer (1997), he claimed that he had been the first to examine the alcohol–CHD
relationship with Framingham data. He produced a manuscript, but not a paper,
showing its protective effects, which he submitted to the National Institutes of
Health (NIH). Dr Zukel from NIH said that this was scientifically and socially
unacceptable, and that Dr Seltzer should instead produce a paper showing a
detrimental effect of alcohol. In this area we are obviously continually dealing
with questions that have both scientific and moral aspects.

Klatsky: I didn't know Dr Seltzer, but when we presented the first report about
the inverse relation between alcohol drinking and CHD at a medical meeting,
somebody else from the Framingham study came up to me and told me that they
had found this association in the Framingham data, but they didn't know what to
make of it. It was barely statistically significant, and so they didn't publish it. When
one looks over the various earlier reports on alcohol and coronary disease, it's hard
to come to any firm conclusions from the Framingham cohort data. It is a
wonderful landmark study in many respects, but they didn't have enough
information about alcohol — and, in particular, they didn't have enough people
who reported heavy drinking — to clearly show the relationship between alcohol
and CHD. I think they also failed to separate lifelong abstainers from past drinkers.
So, everything considered, I think that Dr Seltzer's memory of the remote past is
probably only partially correct: there must have been political pressures involved,
but I also don't think the data would have been solid enough to make a statement
on a subject that seemed so controversial and difficult to present. When we
published our first study, we faced a real dilemma about how to present the
findings. In the original article we actually tried to attack the protective
hypothesis, because it seemed on one level to be a frightening conclusion.

Keil: In an editorial in the *Journal of the American Medical Association* in 1979 a
comment was made: 'This is a message for which this country is not yet ready'

(Castelli 1979) — another statement showing that people were initially hesitant about the conclusions.

Shaper: It's interesting how the pendulum has swung. We have now reached the stage where it is difficult to get results suggesting that alcohol is not protective through to the public!

Peters: You mentioned that for a long time alcoholic cardiomyopathy was misattributed to thiamine deficiency. Why did cardiologists have that 50 year hiatus, when they ignored the effects of alcohol? In a similar manner, alcoholic liver disease was thought for a long time to be nutritional in origin.

Klatsky: I think one sees what one knows. If one knows that thiamine deficiency can cause heart failure, even if it's clear that acute thiamine deficiency responds to acute administration of thiamine, it's a logical jump to assume that if there is an acute syndrome, there's also a chronic syndrome. That must have been the thinking at the time. I was taught at the Boston City Hospital to try administering thiamine, but not to expect it always to work when the heart failure becomes chronic.

Marmot: With regard to the current Russian scene, more than half of the excess mortality in Russia is attributed to cardiovascular disease. Some would attribute the roughly six-year decline in life expectancy of males over the last five years to alcohol. Is this at all credible?

Klatsky: There is no question that heavier drinking, however one wants to define it, is associated with increased mortality for a number of reasons. If a large proportion of a population drinks heavily, an increase in mortality will be seen, particularly among young people, in whom the relationship between heavier drinking and mortality is especially clear. I don't know whether alcohol is more lethal to young people or whether the people who drink heavily and survive to old age are those who are resistant to cirrhosis and other alcohol-related illnesses. But in Russia there is a high prevalence of very heavy drinking in a binge drinking pattern, which may be particularly unfavourable. As a consequence there likely is no J- or U-shaped alcohol–risk curve in Russia. Thus it's very probable that a lot of the excess mortality is due to alcohol. However, there may well be many unfavourable lifestyle traits among younger and middle-aged Russian men, such as cigarette smoking, unfavourable diet and lack of exercise. Consequently, it may be hard to sort out what proportion of mortality is attributable to each of these risk traits.

Marmot: My question is not whether alcohol can kill people, because clearly it can: rather, it concerns the magnitude of the effect. If one tried to do an estimate of the relative risk of cardiac death from heavy drinking, what would the prevalence of heavy drinking and relative risk of death have to be in order to account for a six year decline in life expectancy in men in the space of five years?

Klatsky: I don't know what the prevalence of cardiomyopathy is. It is probably lower than cirrhosis. Lelbach (1974) in Germany was interested in the proportion of heavy drinkers that would develop cirrhosis: I think he said that the figure was 18–20%. The decline of life expectancy is related to not only the prevalence of the conditions, but also the age at which people die. If people die young of accidents, suicide or cirrhosis, this will reduce overall life expectancy a lot more than if people are dying older.

Marmot: But most of the excess mortality is in middle-aged men.

Shaper: It is the temporal relationship that is important. When the Russian authorities clamped down on alcohol drinking some years ago, the mortality rate seemed to be steady or falling. Later, when alcohol became cheaply and freely available, the mortality rate rose rapidly: the excess mortality developed in only a few years. Therefore we are dealing with something that is not a chronic phenomenon but may have to do with large intakes of alcohol in young people, possibly with resulting myocardial instability.

Anderson: If you look at the trends in premature mortality in Russia from 1980 to present (Fig. 2 on page 242), the striking feature is the rapid increase in cardiovascular disease deaths. This is what we need to account for. We have been looking at this, and although it is clear that some are due to misclassification (some of the deaths are from direct alcohol poisoning rather than cardiovascular disease deaths), it is very important to try to unravel the mechanism behind this trend.

Rehm: It is not possible to simulate the increased mortality due to alcohol in Russia with the normal relative risks. However, it is possible if you take into account the specific pattern of drinking in Russia, which involves binge-drinking. The majority of epidemiological studies do not take this into account. The large cohorts, such as Framingham or the Nurses' health study, do not include people who habitually binge drink. Without taking drinking pattern into account we won't be able to explain the Russian excess mortality data.

Keil: An interesting point is raised by the meta-analysis published by Maclure (1993) and covering over 50 studies. The Finnish studies show an increased risk for coronary heart disease, which could well be a consequence of binge drinking. In Scandinavia, even in the higher social classes, a common pattern of drinking is for people to get drunk at the weekend, whereas in Central Europe drinking is more likely to be spread through the week. Many studies don't pick up these different drinking patterns.

Criqui: In the last two months there has been an analysis of this mortality pattern and an accompanying editorial in *The Lancet* (Leon et al 1997, Kromhout et al 1997). The conclusion is that much of this excess is due to alcohol *per se*. There is one discrepancy that's not addressed too often in population studies: everybody agrees that there is a U-shaped curve with total mortality increasing above about three drinks a day, but in some studies the risk of coronary disease goes up sharply after three drinks a day, whereas in other studies it stays down to up to six or seven drinks a day. It is interesting that this dichotomy exists.

Atherosclerotic disease is one issue, but sudden cardiac death is perhaps a separate cause of death that could be occurring in the former Soviet Union. In the early 1980s there was a program established in the USA, the Lipid Research Clinics Program, looking at blood lipids in 10 US populations, a population in Israel and two clinics in what was then the Soviet Union. When we looked at the first mortality data, it was very clear that high-density lipoprotein (HDL) cholesterol was very protective in all US populations and in Israel, but in the two Russian populations it was not: there was this clear anomaly where the higher the HDL cholesterol the higher the death rate, even then suggesting that perhaps the very heavy drinking produced an anomalous relationship between lipids and coronary disease.

Farrell: The issue of measurement of drinking is likely to be at the core of much of the discussion at this meeting. It is clear that in the future we are going to have to be more refined in our measurement of drinking, not just discriminating between binge and continuous drinking, but also tackling the problem of the assumption of stability of drinking patterns across years. We don't really have a good population understanding of fluctuations in patterns of drinking.

Farchi: Some unpublished results (G. Farchi, A. Menotti) obtained from the analysis of data collected on the Italian rural cohorts of the Seven Countries Study, may partially answer the question raised by Michael Marmot about alcohol consumption and survival. Men aged 45–64 in 1965 were followed for 30 years, until 1995. The maximum mean survival, 21.6 years, was experienced by men drinking between 49 g and 84 g of alcohol every day; above this threshold one year of life is lost for every 30 g/day alcohol.

Shaper: Is there really any significant difference between any of the figures?

Farchi: Differences between any of the figures are not statistically significant, but if a model is used, the coefficient of the quadratic terms is statistically different from zero, so highlighting a U-shaped significant trend.

Shaper: Arthur Klatsky, I'm delighted that you referred to Raymond Pearl. His book (*Alcohol and longevity*) has recently been reprinted (Pearl 1981), and one cannot but feel affectionate towards a man who dedicates his book 'To my friends of the Saturday Night Club'!

Pearl looked at an interesting group of people: he was studying tuberculosis and in order to get a control group, the non-tuberculous individuals were taken at random either from those persons who had committed some trivial offence (such as playing baseball in a vacant lot!) or from patients registered at the general dispensary of the Johns Hopkins Hospital. Interestingly, the group included many younger people: 50% of them were under 40. Pearl was also was interested in a relatively small group of people in whom he found change in alcohol consumption: those people who either increased their alcohol intake or who became abstainers. Thus, even at that very early stage there was interest in the question that Dr Farrell has raised of changing alcohol patterns. Finally, in his summary of the work, Pearl trod very cautiously, saying that moderate drinking of alcohol did not shorten life but, on the contrary, moderate steady drinkers exhibited somewhat lower rates of mortality and greater expectation of life than abstainers. He concluded that this superiority was not great in the male moderate drinkers and may not be significant.

Peters: The arsenic and cobalt poisoning episodes you described in your paper raise the question of individual susceptibility factors. Did the authors of these reports speculate as to what these might be?

Klatsky: They did not do so specifically. Particularly interesting in this respect, however, are the letters that were published in *The Lancet* at the turn of the century: they made it clear that some people who drank less beer got ill and died, as compared with others who drank substantially more. Incidentally, in both of these poisoning epidemics, the beer drinkers involved were big-time drinkers — they were not drinking just two or three pints a day!

In general, the study of cofactors for alcohol-induced toxicity is rather neglected. Some analogy can be drawn here with alcoholic cirrhosis. There are references in the older literature to previous or ongoing viral infection as a susceptibility factor in alcoholic cirrhosis. In the modern literature there are suggestions that ongoing low-level post-viral infection factors could be involved in myocardial toxicity to alcohol.

With regard to Dr Shaper's reference to Raymond Pearl, I believe that in his book he also talks about the possible 'constitutional weakness' of the abstainers. This is an interesting point.

Shaper: Yes. Pearl was very concerned with what he calls 'racial aspects': he started with 'racial' studies of alcohol and poultry. It is my understanding that by 'racial' he was referring to genetic differences, and he was concerned with the fact some poultry and some people might be more susceptible to alcohol.

Fillmore: On this issue, I would like to add a footnote to the observations regarding the former Soviet Union (Korolenko et al 1994, White 1996, Tarchys 1993). There is currently a real need for epidemiological work in that country. There is tremendous illicit alcohol production, and we don't really know what else might be present in the alcohol that is consumed: this brings us back to the cobalt and arsenic observations Dr Klatsky made. Does anyone here know of any analysis of what is going on there with respect to additives? The critical question here concerns the degree to which these deaths are attributable to alcohol.

Shaper: I attended a meeting recently with some of the Russians who were involved with this work, and they were saying that there is a tremendous amount of illicit brewing and distilling going on. It is almost like the prohibition days in the USA.

Gaziano: As I was listening to Dr Klatsky's talk, it dawned on me that from an epidemiological standpoint alcohol is a unique factor. Compared with other risk factors that we follow, which typically have an effect that is qualitatively in one direction, alcohol has so many competing effects on many diseases with multiple mechanisms that it's one of the few risk factors that I know that takes a qualitative turn from beneficial to harmful. Aside from the social and political aspects, this may well contribute to the difficulty of studying this risk factor.

Klatsky: I think you're absolutely right: not only are there competing effects, but I think there's a fairly consistent difference in the relationships even within coronary disease studies of the two major endpoints: non-fatal events (usually hospitalization for infarction) and fatal coronary disease. Most studies of fatal coronary disease show a U-curve, whereas most studies of non-fatal events show a levelling off: heavier drinkers also seem to have a lower death rate. There could be real difference in terms of the effects of heavier drinking on non-fatal and fatal coronary disease, because of the possibility of arrhythmias or other factors. There is also the classification problem in terms of the correctness of the diagnosis of coronary disease in heavier drinkers who are found dead.

Keil: You mentioned cobalt and arsenic, but you could also include lead. When we made our studies in the Augsburg area and were looking for blood lead, we found out that most of it comes from beer and wine (Hense et al 1994). Is it present at harmful levels?

Klatsky: I imagine that it could be. There is some older literature about lead-contaminated wine, and there's a fair amount of literature about congeners in distilled spirit as factors for toxicity, but there's more interest in them as factors in causing hangovers than in organ toxicity.

Puddey: I want to comment on the emerging concept, championed by some, that alcohol-related hypertension may be a benign phenomenon. I guess this has had its genesis in the J-shaped relationship described for alcohol and coronary disease, and alcohol and ischaemic stroke, the two major endpoints of hypertension *per se*. I was quite struck in Arthur Klatsky's presentation by the congestive cardiomyopathy caused by alcohol. In three of the earliest cases that he described, cardiac hypertrophy was the major feature of the pathology. To what extent is that a unique feature of alcoholic congestive cardiomyopathy, or could it be dictated by alcohol-related hypertension?

Klatsky: That's impossible to say. Obviously, hypertension is probably one of the major factors in left-ventricular hypertrophy of any sort. It is not unusual in idiopathic dilated cardiomyopathy for there to be hypertrophy along with the dilatation and the flabby weak heart. I think a pattern of hypertrophy on the cardiogram and total increased left ventricular mass is not uncommon in idiopathic dilated cardiomyopathy, which I think cannot be distinguished clinically from alcoholic cardiomyopathy without knowledge of the alcohol history of the patient. I would be interested to hear more about the benignity of alcohol induced hypertension: it is an unresolved issue.

References

Castelli WP 1979 How many drinks a day? (editorial) JAMA 242:2000

Hense HW, Filipiak B, Keil U 1994 Alcohol consumption as a modifier of the relation between blood lead and blood pressure. Epidemiology 5:120–123

Klatsky AL, Friedman GD, Siegelaub AB 1974 Alcohol consumption before myocardial infarction. Results from the Kaiser-Permanente epidemiologic study of myocardial infarction. Ann Intern Med 81:294–301

Korolenko C, Minevich V, Segal B 1994 Politicization of alcohol in the USSR and its impact on the study and treatment of alcoholism. Int J Addict 29:1269–1285

Kromhout D, Bloemberg B, Doornbos G 1997 Reversibility of rise in Russian mortality rates. Lancet 350:379–380

Lelbach WK 1974 Organic pathology related to volume and pattern of alcohol use. In: Gibbius RJ et al (eds) Research advances in alcohol problems. Wiley, New York, p 93–108

Leon DA, Chenet L, Shkolnikov VM et al 1997 Huge variation in Russian mortality rates 1984–94: artefact, alcohol or what? Lancet 350:383–388

Maclure M 1993 Demonstration of deductive meta-analysis: ethanol intake and risk of myocardial infarction. Epidemiol Rev 15:328–351

Pearl R 1981 Alcohol and longevity. ARNO Press, New York

Tarchys D 1993 The success of a failure: Gorbachev's alcohol policy 1985–1988. Europe–Asia Studies 45:7–25

Seltzer CC 1997 'Conflicts of interest' and political science'. J Clin Epidemiol 50:627–629

White S 1996 Russia goes dry. Cambridge University Press, Cambridge

Metabolic consequences of alcohol ingestion

T. J. Peters and V. R. Preedy

Department of Clinical Biochemistry, King's College School of Medicine and Dentistry, Bessemer Road, London SE5 9PJ, UK

Abstract. Many of the pathophysiological effects of alcohol ingestion relate to the pathways of ethanol metabolism. However, some of the acute and chronic effects of ethanol use are also attributable to the direct effects of ethanol, e.g. on membrane fluidity. Oxidation of ethanol to acetaldehyde is catalysed by alcohol dehydrogenase (ADH). There are at least six classes of ADH, some of which show inter-individual variation, i.e. genetic polymorphism, that influences the rate of ethanol oxidation. A consequence of ethanol oxidation is an increase in the NADH/NAD redox potential within the cytosol and mitochondria with subsequent alteration in several tissue metabolites. The popular hypothesis that most, if not all, of the consequences of chronic alcohol ingestion can be explained by these redox changes is still unproven. This should be considered in the context that most metabolic pathways of the liver are affected by alcohol, as are several endocrine axes in the whole body. In fact most, if not all, tissues and organs are deleteriously affected by chronic ingestion. Acetaldehyde, the product of ethanol oxidation, is chemically highly reactive, toxic and immunogenic. However, the concentrations achieved *in vivo* usually fall short of those used to produce these toxic effects in experimental situations. Oxidation of acetaldehyde is also coupled to redox changes, although primarily affecting the intra-mitochondrial redox. In addition, further oxidative pathways of ethanol metabolism can lead to the formation of fatty acid ethyl esters, hydroxyethyl free radicals and reactive oxygen species via the ethanol-specific cytochrome P_{450}-2E1 system. There is no conclusive evidence that nutrient supplementation has beneficial effects on overall ethanol-mediated tissue damage.

1998 Alcohol and cardiovascular diseases. Wiley, Chichester (Novartis Foundation Symposium 216) p 19–34

All the effects of alcohol ingestion, beneficial or detrimental, are directly or indirectly related to the metabolic consequences of ethanol. The claims during the 1940s and 1950s of Best, Daft and Himsworth amongst others that the toxic effects of chronic alcohol misuse relate to associated nutritional impairment were decisively disproven by the seminal studies of Charles Lieber during the 1960s. A caveat, however, remains that specific vitamin deficiency syndromes, such as

19

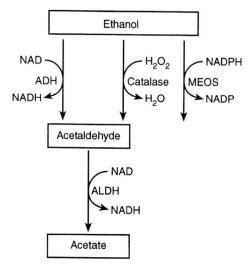

FIG. 1. Principal pathways of ethanol oxidation. MEOS, microsomal ethanol oxidizing system; ADH, alcohol dehydrogenase; ALDH, acetaldehyde dehydrogenase.

Wernicke–Korsakoff psychosis, niacin deficiency encephalopathy and alcohol–tobacco vitamin B_{12} amblyopia, may complement this toxicity, especially affecting the nervous system.

The basic pathway of alcohol metabolism (Fig. 1) is straightforward, with the progressive oxidation of ethanol to acetate via acetaldehyde. The major site of this oxidation is the liver parenchymal cells but other potential sites include the gastrointestinal tract (including colonic bacteria), vascular tissue and brain. The initial oxidation is catalysed by a cytosolic NAD-linked alcohol dehydrogenase (ADH). It is now clear that there are at least six classes of ADH. The hepatic enzymes form the class 1 enzymes and exhibit genetic polymorphism, and there are significant racial and ethnic variations in the enzyme types. This polymorphism may contribute to inter-individual variations in rates of ethanol metabolism.

The primary product of ethanol oxidation is acetaldehyde, a highly reactive intermediate which has potent vasoactive properties. It has also been implicated, directly and indirectly, in several aspects of the alcohol misuse syndrome ranging from alcohol dependency via the formation of opioid-like isoquinolines, to tissue damage by direct toxicity (particularly to thiol groups via reactive oxygen species formation), to the formation of acetaldehyde adducts and immunological reactions (Table 1). The further oxidation of acetaldehyde to acetate is catalysed by acetaldehyde dehydrogenase, predominantly the low K_m mitochondrial enzyme. Aldehyde dehydrogenases are widely distributed and thus the plasma levels of

TABLE 1   Metabolic and toxic effects of acetaldehyde

1. Alteration of biogenic amine metabolism
2. Formation of proaddictive isoquinoline opioid-like substances
3. Inhibition of mitochondrial oxidative phosphorylation
4. Inhibition of protein synthesis
5. Formation of adducts with thiol and amine groups in amino acids and peptides
6. Formation of autoantibodies to acetaldehyde neoantigen adducts
7. Generation of free radicals and reactive oxygen species
8. Lipid peroxidation
9. Microtubule disruption
10. Impaired vitamin metabolism

acetaldehyde are in the 1–2 μM range, compared with millimolar levels of ethanol and acetate. An exception occurs in Oriental subjects who have a genetic defect in their mitochondrial acetaldehyde dehydrogenase, rendering the enzyme almost completely inactive. These individuals metabolize ethanol at normal rates but show very reduced rates of acetaldehyde oxidation. After a relatively small dose of ethanol they have very high levels of acetaldehyde with toxic and aversive consequences particularly affecting the cardiovascular and gastrointestinal systems.

An important consequence of ethanol and acetaldehyde oxidation is the increase in both cytosolic and mitochondrial NADH/NAD ratios (Fig. 2). Many of the metabolic consequences of alcohol ingestion are a result of this redox change (Table 2). Thus the increase in cytosolic NADH/NAD ratio causes an increase in the lactate/pyruvate ratio mediated via lactate dehydrogenase. This increase in lactate has been implicated in such alterations as hyperuricaemia, collagen deposition, impaired gluconeogenesis and, via an increased NADPH/NADP ratio, increased fatty acid synthesis (Lieber 1985). The increased NADH/NAD ratio in mitochondria increases the β-hydroxy butyrate/acetoacetate ratio with development of ketoacidosis, impaired citric acid cycle activity and decreased fatty acid oxidation. Attractive as the redox hypothesis is, it may have been

CYTOSOL   MITOCHONDRIA

$\uparrow \dfrac{\text{NADH}}{\text{NAD}} \rightleftharpoons \dfrac{\text{Lactate}}{\text{Pyruvate}}$ $\uparrow \dfrac{\text{NADH}}{\text{NAD}} \rightleftharpoons \dfrac{\beta\text{Hydroxybutyrate}}{\text{Acetoacetate}}$

FIG. 2.   Redox consequences of ethanol and acetaldehyde oxidation.

TABLE 2   Redox consequences of ethanol- and acetaldehyde-induced redox changes

---

1. Enhanced triglyceride synthesis

2. Inhibition of Krebs cycle activity

3. Enhanced amino acid catabolism

4. Lactic acidosis

5. Ketoacidosis

6. Hyperuricaemia

7. Disturbances of cortisol and androgen metabolism

8. Enhanced fibrogenesis

---

overemphasized. Thus pre-treatment of rats with methylene blue, which dissipates the increased NADH/NAD ratio, does not prevent hepatic lipid accumulation when these rats are then fed alcohol (Ryle et al 1985, Ryle 1986). Similarly, direct measurement of human hepatic fatty acid synthesis *in vitro* shows no effect of ethanol on synthesis rates: tissue from alcoholics show base line rates of fatty acid synthesis below that of normal tissue with no change on the addition of ethanol (Venkatesan et al 1986, Simpson et al 1994).

Although alcohol dehydrogenase is the major catalyst of acetaldehyde formation, alternate pathways are variably important. The peroxidative activity of catalase, a cytosolic and a peroxisomal enzyme, can lead to the formation of acetaldehyde. However, the rate is small and is limited by the supply of H_2O_2, and probably accounts for no more than 5% of the ethanol oxidation by the body, although recent studies suggest this mechanism may be important in the brain (Smith et al 1997).

A more important non-ADH pathway is MEOS (microsomal ethanol oxidizing system), located predominantly in the smooth endoplasmic reticulum. This cytochrome P_{450}-2E1 has several important characteristics: a higher K_m for ethanol than ADH, its induction by chronic ethanol ingestion and other enzyme-inducing drugs, the concomitant oxidation of NADPH, and the generation of free radicals during its activity. Its contribution to overall ethanol oxidation is small at low blood ethanol levels (about 10%), but increases with increasing blood ethanol levels, particularly in chronic alcoholics where the MEOS system may contribute up to 50% of the ethanol oxidation rate. The adaptive responses to chronic ethanol oxidation — including induction of MEOS and mitochondrial, endoplasmic reticulum and peroxisomal proliferation — all contribute to the hepatomegaly of chronic alcoholics, who overall show a twofold increase in ethanol oxidation rates.

TABLE 3   Metabolic consequences of alcohol ingestion

1. Direct cellular effects

2. Increased membrane fluidity

3. Indirect effects of membrane fluidity changes, including alterations in properties of extrinsic and intrinsic proteins

4. Formation of fatty acid ethyl esters

5. Endocrine responses, including increased adrenal activity

It should, however, be noted that these enhanced oxidation rates all lead to increased rates of acetaldehyde formation.

The metabolic consequences of ethanol ingestion may also relate to the ethanol itself (Table 3). High levels of ethanol have a fluidizing effect on cell membranes, and this has direct effects on intrinsic membrane proteins including enzymes, receptors and cytoskeletal elements. The fluidizing effects of exposure to ethanol are counteracted by compensatory changes in membrane lipid components: increased cholesterol content and a higher proportion of more-saturated fatty acids in the phospholipid components oppose the fluidizing effects of chronic ethanol exposure, thus stabilizing the membranes in the presence of alcohol.

A relatively recent series of studies (see Laposta 1998) have highlighted the possible role of fatty acid ethyl esters in ethanol-induced organ damage. This includes toxic effects on cardiac mitochondria (Lange & Sobel 1983), pancreatic lysosomes (Haber et al 1993) and altered neuronal functions (Zhen & Hungund 1998). As well as mediating cellular damage, these fatty acid ethyl esters may form useful markers of chronic ethanol abuse.

In conclusion, it is clear that there are many possible metabolic consequences of ethanol ingestion, both local and systemic, direct and indirect. These include ethanol oxidation and esterification, redox (NADH/NAD) changes, acetaldehyde and acetate formation, free radical and reactive oxygen species formation and enzyme induction and inhibition. The relative contributions of these various effects are determined by the ethanol load, chronicity of intake, concomitant drug ingestion, nutritional status and the genetic make up of the individual. The relative importance of these individual effects still remain to be determined in specific individuals in spite of the increasing research efforts over the past 30 years.

References

Haber PS, Wilson JS, Apte MV, Pirola RC 1993 Fatty acid ethyl esters increase rat pancreatic lysosomal fragility. J Lab Clin Med 121:759–764

Lange LG, Sobel BE 1983 Mitochondrial dysfunction induced by fatty and ethyl esters: myocardial metabolites of ethanol. J Clin Invest 72:724–731

Laposta M 1998 Fatty acid ethyl esters: non-oxidative metabolites of ethanol. Addict Biol
    3:5–14
Lieber CS 1985 Alcohol and the liver: metabolism of ethanol, metabolic effects and pathogenesis
    of injury. Acta Med Scand Suppl 703:11–55
Ryle PR 1986 Hepatic redox state alterations as a mechanism of fatty liver production after
    ethanol: fact or fiction. Alcohol Alcohol 21:131–135
Ryle PR, Chakraborty J, Thomson AD 1985 The effect of methylene blue on the hepatocellular
    redox state and liver lipid content during chronic ethanol feeding in the rat. Biochem J
    232:877–882
Simpson K J, Venkatesan S, Peters TJ 1994 Fatty acid synthesis by rat liver after chronic alcohol
    feeding with a low fat diet. Clin Sci 87:441–446
Smith BR, Aragon CMG, Amit Z 1997 Catalase and the production of brain acetaldehyde:
    a possible mediator of the psychopharmacological effects of ethanol. Addict Biol 2:277–
    289
Venkatesan S, Leung NWY, Peters TJ 1986 Fatty acid synthesis *in vitro* by liver tissue from
    control subjects and patients with alcoholic liver disease. Clin Sci 71:723–728
Zhen G, Hungund BL 1998 Effects of acute and chronic ethanol exposure on fatty acid ethyl ester
    synthesis in mouse cerebellar membranes. Addict Biol 3:85–90

DISCUSSION

Puddey: The studies of Norman Palmer's on the effects of alcohol on insulin sensitivity are obviously of particular relevance to alcohol and cardiovascular disease (Xu et al 1996a,b, Peters et al 1996). These herald the underexplored area of the extent to which alcohol is responsible either for protection against or induction of diabetes. Norman Palmer really just looked at the acute effects of alcohol: I wonder whether the chronic homeostatic response to those acute changes in cellular insulin sensitivity is actually one of an increase in insulin sensitivity. Certainly, the epidemiological studies would suggest a decrease in the incidence of non-insulin-dependent diabetes with regular mild to moderate alcohol use.

Peters: Norman Palmer has recently found the same results after chronic ethanol administration.

Puddey: His recent unreported work suggests that in long-term animal feeding experiments you do get this improvement (T. N. Palmer, personal communication).

Peters: Yes, but when they're challenged acutely, even the chronic-fed animals do show this effect. It has been known for a long time in humans that chronic alcoholics have insulin resistance: the so-called 'alcoholic diabetes'. It has always been assumed that this was due to the liver disease, but even in the presence of very mild liver disease there is evidence of insulin resistance.

Criqui: I think it also depends on the dose per kg. In the epidemiological studies carried out in California there were measures of fasting insulin and post-challenge insulin throughout the range of individuals, not just diabetics or non-diabetics (Mayer et al 1993). There was a strong inverse relationship between mild/ moderate alcohol consumption and insulin resistance: that is, drinkers have greater insulin sensitivity. This was not true, interestingly, for fasting glucose. It is quite a marked effect. There is some evidence from epidemiological studies that individuals who have insulin resistance may particularly benefit from the effects of moderate alcohol consumption in terms of the incidence of cardiovascular disease.

Urbano-Márquez: With regard to the effect of alcohol on insulin resistance, in our experience heavy drinkers have insulin values higher than controls. But interestingly, after one month of stopping drinking their insulin values are similar to controls. The level of glucose also reduces to a value similar to controls after one month, whereas at the beginning the glucose value is higher than in the controls.

Klatsky: There is, of course, great interest in the differential effects of different major beverage types. Independent of the action of food, is there an important difference in the rate of absorption and peak blood alcohol levels between distilled spirits, wine and beer? Do the relative concentrations of the different beverage types matter in terms of the rate of absorption and the peak alcohol levels, given the same net volume of alcohol taken?

Peters: I don't know the data well, but certainly the effects of spirits versus beer on gastric function are strikingly different, so I wouldn't be surprised if there aren't differences in the rate of absorption.

Hendriks: Yes, there are differences in peak alcohol concentration. Spirits yield slightly higher peak alcohol concentrations as opposed to beer or wine after moderate alcohol consumption (Hendriks et al 1994).

Shaper: There is a paper by Boyland (1989) which advocates the drinking of water with spirits, and he makes this point: that the more dilute the alcohol the lower the blood concentration reached.

Peters: There is currently quite an interest in a gastric alcohol dehydrogenase that requires a high concentration of ethanol to be effective. Thus you would expect a greater proportion of spirits than more dilute beverages to be metabolized by the stomach. However, the actual role of gastric alcohol dehydrogenase is controversial: Charles Lieber and his colleagues, for example, believes it is responsible for 20–30% of ethanol metabolism (Lieber 1991), whereas others believe that it is only responsible for 1 or 2%.

Puddey: I was interested in two recent reports that suggest that alcohol dehydrogenase—and particularly the $\beta1\beta1$ subtype—is expressed in the endothelium of veins and arteries (Allai-Hassani et al 1997, Bello et al 1994). It has been suggested that it plays a role in the metabolism of aldehydes from lipid peroxidation. The theory has been proposed that alcohol will induce vascular alcohol dehydrogenase, and this induction may lead to further protection from lipid peroxidation at the level of the vessel wall. Others have suggested that too much alcohol will swamp the vascular alcohol dehydrogenase and that high levels may have potential for pro-atherosclerotic effects. Given the extensive surface area of the vascular endothelium, from the point of view of cardiovascular diseases, this is a mechanism that will bear further investigation and consideration.

Keil: I always used to tell my audiences that smoking and alcohol are doing opposite things with regard to coronary heart disease: smoking decreases HDL and peroxidizes LDL, whereas alcohol increases HDL and now I learn that it also peroxidizes LDL. Is this an established theory?

Peters: I think there's good evidence that acetaldehyde is a pro-oxidant. The question concerns how much antioxidant activity it induces.

Puddey: It depends on the endpoint that you are talking about, and it is probably also a dose-dependent relationship.

Shaper: You have shown us a long list of all the mechanisms and pathways that alcohol can be involved in. In any of these, is there any evidence of a J- or U-shaped curve? In other words, is there any point at which the lack of alcohol in a system or process appears to be deleterious?

Peters: I don't know of any. There are strains of mice that lack alcohol dehydrogenase, but I don't think they have increased susceptibility to hypertension or coronary heart disease. Part of the evidence that Charles Leiber's MEOS system is functionally important is from studies in deer mice which are believed to lack alcohol dehydrogenase. However, I'm not aware of any pharmacological or physiological studies on their cardiovascular system.

Keaney: What is the proposed mechanism by which acetaldehyde produces free radicals?

Peters: It serves as a substrate for xanthine oxidase to produce superoxide, but I'm not actually aware of a particular system that produces free radicals directly from acetaldehyde.

Puddey: Some investigators have suggested aldehyde oxidase as a free-radical-generating mechanism during alcohol metabolism (Mira et al 1995). Acetaldehyde also binds glutathione and may lead to glutathione depletion (Morton & Mitchell 1985).

Keaney: However, glutathione occurs at millimolar concentrations inside the cell, whereas acetaldehyde never reaches these concentrations.

Peters: Of course, another pro-oxidant effect is acetaldehyde adduct inducing an inflammatory response.

Renaud: Another cell type which you didn't mention in your presentation but which is directly influenced by alcohol and lipid peroxidation is the platelet. Platelets are directly involved in coronary heart disease. One drop of alcohol over platelets *in vitro* dramatically reduces their aggregation. Within 5 min in humans after an alcoholic drink there is a decrease in platelet activity. There is a second phenomenon that occurs later and is known as the rebound phenomenon, which is connected with lipid peroxidation. Red wine contains polyphenols that protect the membranes of platelets from being peroxidized and consequently it protects against the rebound effect. This is part of the reason for the superior protection from wine compared with other alcoholic beverages, because wine, at least in animal studies and *in vitro*, doesn't induce this lipid peroxidation, of course at moderate intake levels.

Peters: Going back to acetaldehyde, one of the problems is that many of the studies have used superphysiological concentrations. Blood levels are normally $1–2\,\mu M$, with tissue levels as high as $20\,\mu M$, but many of the studies have used $300–400\,\mu M$, so we need to interpret these results with caution.

Keaney: It is interesting that you mentioned the Oriental populations with a deficiency in metabolizing acetaldehyde. Even though they have a lower incidence of developing alcohol abuse than western populations, do those affected in this way but who still abuse alcohol develop more deleterious effects than those who abuse in western populations? If you hypothesize that acetaldehyde is a major mediator of the deleterious effects of alcohol, you would have to also assume that those people who have a defect in acetaldehyde metabolism should develop a higher incidence of these effects.

Peters: There is some evidence that the heterozygotes are more likely to develop alcoholic liver disease at lower net alcohol doses than western-type homozygotes. There are also certain individuals who potentiate the effect of alcohol by taking small amounts of disulfiram.

Keaney: Is there more cirrhosis or more liver damage in Orientals with the defect who consume alcohol than in western populations?

Peters: I don't know.

Klatsky: In the Orient, post-viral disease is by far the dominant cause of cirrhosis.

Keaney: This does, however, present an interesting experimental system in which you could address the hypothesis.

Puddey: This may prove impractical, because the person who has the defect develops such a tachycardia and dramatic nausea that they may keep away from alcohol.

Gaziano: But there are some heavy drinkers in this group. It would be interesting to look at them not only with respect to liver disease, but also other diseases, to see whether it is the acetaldehyde that is causing the problem.

Peters: The proportion of heavy drinkers in this group may be increasing, because antihistamines can prevent many of the acetaldehyde effects.

Klatsky: I've talked about flushing with a number of Asian flushers: they tell me it's a sort of all-or-none phenomenon. They get it, and it doesn't get worse if they then carry on drinking. I've often wondered whether anyone has studied the proportion of those who have the enzyme defect and yet go on to become alcoholics, to see whether there's anything about them that might cast light upon the traits that predispose to alcoholism. Here's a group that is to some degree protected against alcoholism and yet still become alcoholics.

Rehm: There's a large study by the NIAAA in the USA which has a specific subsample on this (COGA; Collaborative Study on the Genetics of Alcoholism), so it is being studied within a genetic framework.

Klatsky: Do you know anything about what they're looking for?

Rehm: No.

Marmot: Is acetaldehyde in any way involved in the HDL story?

Peters: There may be effects on LDL secretion, but I don't know of any direct effect on HDL metabolism.

Marmot: Do you know why alcohol raises HDL?

Keil: I had a long debate recently with colleague in Münster when I presented our alcohol CHD data. He didn't believe my results. The discussion then turned to HDL and I asked him whether it made any difference whether HDL was raised by exercise or by alcohol. He seemed to think that there was, but he didn't give me any detailed mechanism.

Criqui: The exact mechanism is not known. However, in challenge experiments where HDL is raised by alcohol, you can subfraction HDL. The simplest way to do this is to split it into HDL_2 and HDL_3 . HDL_2 is the component of HDL which is regularly higher in women, those who exercise regularly and thinner people. HDL_3 doesn't differ as much in these groups and thus the early belief was that HDL_2 cholesterol was the protective component of the total HDL. In addition, some years ago Bill Haskell did a challenge experiment where he gave volunteers an alcohol challenge and measured acute changes in lipoproteins (Haskell et al 1984). They found that only HDL_3 increased after the alcoholic challenge and that HDL_2 levels didn't change. He concluded from this that it was unlikely that the benefit due to alcohol occurred through the HDL increase. In fact, the wealth of the data now show that even though HDL_3 increases more than HDL_2, both components increase with alcohol consumption in most populations. Recent studies show that in some databases HDL_3 is equally or more protective than HDL_2 in terms of cardiovascular disease, so the whole idea that alcohol raises the wrong form of HDL has pretty much been discarded.

Gaziano: There is probably a duration effect as well. Alcohol intake increases HDL_3 acutely, and this is detected in short-term studies. However, the effect on HDL_2 is probably a more chronic one. This suggests that the two components of HDL are raised by different mechanisms.

Assuming that levels of lipoproteins change, as we begin to look at the particles contained within these rather crude subfractions, I don't think we can assume that a change in the level of a plasma marker will give us the predicted clinical effect. This is an oversimplification. There's a lot of work being done now on triglyceride-carrying particles that suggests that fluffy, buoyant triglycerides are different functionally.

Marmot: One might have predicted, given what has been said about increased insulin sensitivity, that alcohol would cause triglyceride to go down and HDL to go up, but alcohol actually raises triglycerides.

Gaziano: We don't know why this is. These two effects don't occur at the same dose: to raise triglycerides you would have to give a bigger dose than is necessary to raise HDL. It's not a single mechanism.

Criqui: It is basically a misconception that triglycerides go up with alcohol consumption in most individuals. They don't, particularly in moderate consumers. We published the Lipid Research Clinic's study data in 1986, in which we found no statistically significant association between alcohol consumption and triglycerides in three different age- and sex-specific groups (Criqui et al 1986). There are some individuals, however, who get a dramatic hypertriglyceridaemia with alcohol consumption. There are at least three areas where the so-called inverse relationship between triglycerides and HDL cholesterol doesn't occur: one is in alcohol consumption, and another is in post-menopausal oestrogen therapy (particularly with oestrogens that raise HDL but also raise triglycerides significantly). That has been looked at very carefully and these are all the fluffy-puffy triglycerides. They do not metabolize to the small VLDL which is thought to be atherogenic. The third area is the resins, which actually raise HDL slightly but raise triglycerides more. These again are thought to be the fluffy-puffy kind. Also the evidence so far is that the triglycerides which are raised by high carbohydrate diets are thought to be fluffy-puffy triglycerides.

Marmot: How solid are the data that the fluffy triglycerides are not associated with the risk of atherosclerosis?

Gaziano: I don't think the data are very solid at all.

Criqui: There are a couple of observations. The first noted that persons with triglycerides of 2000–3000 are not typically at increased risk of cardiovascular disease, whereas those with triglycerides of 300–500 are at risk. Then the observations were made that the particles were not uniform. The only evidence I have seen that directly answers your question of the atherogenicity of the particles by size, is Walsh et al's data from Boston, looking at oestrogen therapy (Walsh et al 1991). They looked at the change in the triglyceride composition with oestrogen therapy. Oestrogen therapy, which raises HDL and triglycerides, does not produce small atherogenic particles. It's limited evidence: it all tends to point in the same direction, but it's certainly not conclusive.

Hendriks: In the post-prandial phase, when alcohol is taken together with food, triglycerides are indeed increased above control. This does not relate to risk factors for coronary heart disease, but it may say a little bit about the metabolism of alcohol and the mechanisms through which alcohol may have a protective effect.

Criqui: But the post-prandial triglycerides, if anything, are a better predictor of cardiovascular risk than fasting triglycerides. In the very limited clinical studies that have been done, alcohol augments the post-prandial triglycerides. Therefore one might argue that alcohol should worsen cardiovascular risk since triglycerides are increased. However, the time course is unknown.

Shaper: Just how big a rise in HDL is necessary for a protective effect? Looking at our own data, the very heavy drinkers (more than six UK units per day) get about an 18% increase in their HDL level over abstainers (Shaper et al 1985). In moderate/light drinkers the rise is much less — only about a 7.5% increase — and in the occasional drinkers it is almost negligible (about 1%). If occasional drinking is protective, as many studies seem to show, how can one attribute that benefit to HDL?

Keil: I agree: in the meta-analysis by Maclure (1993), he claims that 10 g of alcohol per day can be protective, but this cannot cause a great rise in HDL. When we look at our Augsburg data, and take HDL as the mediator of the alcohol–CHD relationship and filter it out by controlling for it, there's actually not a big difference. Mechanisms other than HDL must therefore be involved in the beneficial effects of alcohol, such as the anti-thrombosis effects.

Gaziano: I think that focusing on a single mechanism is probably simplistic. However, the rise in HDL is an incredibly potent predictor of heart disease, and so I would not be surprised if small amounts of HDL were to yield significant relative changes in risk. The rises in HDL with alcohol consumption are comparable to those we see with exercise.

Criqui: To be specific, Dave Gordon's meta-analysis of all the HDL studies shows that the expected change in coronary risk from a 1% change in HDL is about 3% (Gordon et al 1989). So if one takes an HDL of 50 in a middle-aged man, a 1% change is a 0.5 mg. Thus a 1 mg change would be associated with a 6% change of coronary risk, which is a huge change of coronary risk for what is a very small lipid change.

Klatsky: With respect to the amount of alcohol that may be involved in these effects, we all need to keep in mind the probable underestimation of consumption in many surveys. A reported intake of 10 g/day is a minimum amount, on the basis of the very reasonable assumption that a large proportion of people report a consumption that is lower than what they actually take.

Anderson: For how many years do you need to drink to get this protective effect?

Gaziano: There are studies that show an age effect of various risk factors, and there are competing risks and benefits. Cholesterol reduction is a good example here: it becomes quite costly to treat someone aged 25 for a lipid abnormality because their absolute risk of cardiovascular disease is small. The same effects apply to any other mechanism that is acting through lipids. The differences in the shape of the J curve between men and women may well be explained by an overall lower risk of coronary heart disease in women. We would expect to see that, similarly, in a group of younger men. The competing risks and benefits differ according to the baseline cardiovascular risk.

Criqui: If there is benefit from drinking, and heart attacks are rare before age 40, the key question concerns whether there is any benefit from drinking between ages 20 and 40. Arthur Klatsky has published data showing that in the Kaiser-Permanente study there is no benefit for anyone at any level of alcohol consumption before the age 40 (Klatsky et al 1992). Probably half of the benefit or more from alcohol drinking is acute, in my judgement. That half occurs over minutes or hours, so drinking at a younger age obviously can't confer that. But is it possible that the changes in lipid and insulin resistance slow down atherogenesis in early adulthood and thus help to prevent later events? We really don't know. My concern from a policy issue is that those are the high risk years for addiction, and so encouraging alcohol consumption in early adulthood is inappropriate because those starting to drink only at age 40 may well gain the full beneficial effect from lowered lipid levels.

Klatsky: I agree entirely. However, thinking about the two hats that I wear, one as a practising physician advising individual patients and their families, and the other as an epidemiologist giving public health advice, I certainly do emphasize the importance of starting young with control of risk factors for coronary disease, if there is reason to be concerned. I'll bet that most people in this room would agree that if you have a bad family history and any risk factors, that you should start in childhood with a proper diet and good exercise habits and so forth. Of course, the risks of alcohol are greater for young people and the cost:benefit ratio of lowering lipids by aggressive means is clearly not going to be favourable in this group. Yet in an ideal world from the strictly scientific viewpoint I think the question raised is a really important one, and I don't know the answer. It's true that in our Kaiser-Permanente data it is not possible to demonstrate benefit in early adulthood (Klatsky et al 1992) — in fact light-to-moderate drinking appears to be harmful in youth, but that's because people seldom die of coronary disease at that age. However, it may well be that to drink in youth protects those at risk when they get to being my age!

Shaper: That is a bit like Michael Oliver's argument that if you are a heavy smoker you ought to eat more fruit and vegetables (Oliver 1996). In the same way, we're saying now that if you're 20–40 and you're on a diet that conduces to high blood lipids, and a smoker and physically inactive, then you ought to drink readily! I find this a very peculiar public health argument.

Criqui: If you look at the data from the USA, it is clear that the average consumption of alcohol drops with age, with the oldest persons drinking the least.

Rehm: That depends on the culture. For example, in Switzerland it rises until age 50 and then drops (Rehm & Arminger 1996). What you describe is the North American pattern.

Bondy: In Canada the average consumption remains relatively stable within drinkers but the distribution of drinking across the week changes with age: it is more spread out in older people. The indicators of heavy drinking drop off markedly with age. It's the young who drink 5–8 drinks per occasion and who drink their total intake on the weekend.

Gaziano: Oxidation of LDL is a real quagmire. In the studies that we have been involved with, I have become convinced that our ability to predict what a pro-oxidant or antioxidant might do *in vivo* is grossly inaccurate. Many factors that basic scientists tell us should perform favourably as antioxidants, turn out in trials not to have any of the anticipated effect in terms of disease prevention. We are in the very early stages of being able to understand what's going on with lipid peroxidation. For example, vitamin E is a pro-oxidant in some conditions and an antioxidant in other conditions. We must be very careful when we attribute its effects either to its antioxidant or its pro-oxidant effects.

Keaney: A perfect example is probucol, a drug that has been used extensively in evaluating the oxidative modification hypothesis. It doesn't prevent atherosclerosis in people and also fails to work in mice. It only works in rabbits.

Gaziano: We did a study on rabbits with vitamin E, where you get wonderful protection of LDL as you march up to superphysiological doses. *In vivo* LDL becomes more and more resistant to oxidation with higher doses of vitamin E, and yet the protection of the rabbit aorta from atherosclerosis which is apparent at low doses of vitamin E disappears at higher doses. We must question whether protection of LDL from oxidation *ex vivo* will necessarily prevent atherosclerosis *in vivo*.

Shaper: Very often we find mechanisms, and if they exist, then we impute that they work. This may not be true.

Farrell: What is the evidence about the duration of the HDL effect in relation to alcohol consumption? How long would does the effect last and what frequency of alcohol consumption is necessary to produce the beneficial effect?

Gaziano: I don't think we have a very good idea. The short term studies demonstrate that it takes days to weeks to see an acute HDL_3 effect. I don't think we have a good handle on the effect on HDL_2. It appears to take longer to raise HDL_2. It's an area that needs a great deal more attention.

Hillbom: A question of general interest. Do people with hereditary hyperlipidaemia benefit more from moderate alcohol consumption than others?

Criqui: There is a study showing that women at higher risk for coronary disease are the only ones in that particular study to show benefit from alcohol consumption (Fuchs et al 1995). There are also two separate papers from the Copenhagen male study, one showing that the benefit of alcohol is limited to insulin-resistant individuals (Hein et al 1993), the other showing in a separate analysis that the benefit is limited to individuals with LDL cholesterol above a certain threshold point (Hein et al 1996). If you take the insulin resistance as being the low HDL and you take the high LDLs as being the hypercholesterolaemics, at least in the Copenhagen male study, those are the only people who benefit from alcohol ingestion.

References

Allai-Hassani A, Martinez SE, Peralba JM et al 1997 Alcohol dehydrogenase of human and rat blood vessels. Role in ethanol metabolism. FEBS Lett 405:26–30

Bello AT, Bora NS, Lange LG, Bora PS 1994 Cardioprotective effects of alcohol: mediation by human vascular alcohol dehydrogenase. Biochem Biophys Res Commun 203:1858–1864

Boyland E 1989 Water could reduce the hazard of cancer from spirits. Br J Ind Med 46:423–424

Criqui MH, Cowan LD, Heiss G, Haskell WL, Laskarzewski PM, Chaubless LE 1986 Frequency and clustering of nonlipid coronary risk factors in dyslipoproteinemia. The Lipid Research Clinics Program Prevalence Study. Circulation 73:140–150

Fuchs CS, Stampfer MJ, Colditz GA et al 1995 Alcohol consumption and mortality among women. N Engl J Med 332:1245–1250

Gordon DJ, Probstfield JL, Garrison RJ et al 1989 High-density lipoprotein cholesterol and cardiovascular disease. Four prospective American studies. Circulation 79:8–15

Haskell WL, Camargo C, Williams PT et al 1984 The effect of cessation and resumption of moderate alcohol intake on serum high-density-lipoprotein subfractions. A controlled study. N Engl J Med 310:805–810

Hein HO, Sorensen H, Suadicani P, Gyntelberg F 1993 Alcohol consumption, Lewis phenotypes, and risk of ischaemic heart disease. Lancet 341:392–396

Hein HO, Suadicani P, Gyntelberg F 1996 Alcohol consumption, serum low density lipoprotein cholesterol concentration, and risk of ischaemic heart disease: six year follow up in the Copenhagen male study. Br Med J 312:736–741

Hendriks HFJ, Veenstra J, Velthuis-te Wierik EJM, Schaafsma G, Kluft C 1994 Effect of moderate dose of alcohol with evening meal on fibrinolytic factors. Br Med J 308:1003–1006

Klatsky AL, Armstrong MA, Friedman GD 1992 Alcohol and mortality. Ann Intern Med 136:646–654

Lieber CS 1991 Pathways of ethanol metabolism and related pathology. In: Palmer TN (ed) Alcoholism: a molecular pathology. Nato ASI Series, vol 206. Plenum Press, New York, p 1–25

Maclure M 1993 Demonstration of deductive meta-analysis: ethanol intake and risk of myocardial infarction. Epidemiol Rev 15:328–351

Mayer EJ, Newman B, Quesenberry CP Jr, Friedman GD, Selby JV 1993 Alcohol consumption and insulin concentrations. Role of insulin in associations of alcohol intake with high-density lipoprotein cholesterol and triglycerides. Circulation 88:2190–2197

Mira L, Maia L, Barreira L, Manso CF 1995 Evidence for free radical generation due to NADH oxidation by aldehyde oxidase during ethanol metabolism. Arch Biochem Biophys 318: 55–58

Morton S, Mitchell MC 1985 Effects of chronic ethanol feeding on glutathione turnover in the rat. Biochem Pharmacol 34:1559–1563

Oliver MF 1996 Which changes in diet prevent coronary heart disease? A review of clinical trials of dietary fats and antioxidants. Acta Cardiol 51:467–490

Peters TJ, Nikolovski S, Raja GK, Palmer TN, Fournier PA 1996 Ethanol acutely impairs glycogen repletion in skeletal muscle following high intensity short duration exercise in the rat. Addict Biol 1:289–295

Rehm J, Arminger G 1996 Alcohol consumption in Switzerland 1987–1993. Adjusting for differential effects of assessment techniques on the analysis of trends. Addiction 91: 1335–1344

Shaper AG, Pocock SJ, Ashby D, Walker M, Whitehead TP 1985 Biochemical and haematological response to alcohol intake. Ann Clin Biochem 22:50–61

Walsh BW, Schiff I, Rosner B, Greenberg L, Ravnikar V, Sacks FM 1991 Effects of postmenopausal estrogen replacement on the concentrations and metabolism of plasma lipoproteins. N Engl J Med 325:1196–1204

Xu D, Dhillon AS, Palmer TN 1996a Metabolic effects of alcohol on skeletal muscle. Addict Biol 1:143–155

Xu D, Dhillon AS, Davey CG, Fournier PA, Palmer TN 1996b Alcohol and glucose metabolism in skeletal muscles in the rat. Addict Biol 1:71–83

Alcohol and the myocardium

P. J. Richardson, V. B. Patel* and V. R. Preedy*

*Molecular and Metabolic Cardiology Group, Departments of Cardiology and *Clinical Biochemistry, King's College School of Medicine and Dentistry, Bessemer Road, London SE5 9PJ, UK*

Abstract. Structural and functional abnormalities are prominent in alcoholic cardiomyopathy (ACM). Histological features in affected subjects are almost identical to the characteristics of dilated cardiomyopathy. Quantitative morphometry, however, can distinguish between ACM and dilated cardiomyopathy. Biopsies from patients with ACM show increases in the activities of some myocardial enzymes (α-hydroxybutyric dehydrogenase, creatine kinase, lactate dehydrogenase, malic dehydrogenase) which are correlated with the bimodal distribution of alcohol intake and may represent an adaptive response. One-third of patients with ACM have serum antibodies against cardiac acetaldehyde–protein adducts. Animal models of ethanol toxicity have shown that acutely, alcohol and acetaldehyde reduce the synthesis of cardiac contractile proteins *in vivo*. Two-dimensional SDS-PAGE has also shown that in rats chronically fed alcohol, the relative amounts of over 10% of heart muscle proteins are altered. The heat shock proteins (HSP) Hsp60 and Hsp70 are decreased in alcohol-fed rats, as is desmin. Reduction in HSPs may indicate reduced myocardial protection whilst a fall in desmin may indicate structural defects. In conclusion, ACM is a complex process that is due to altered protein synthesis, the formation of acetaldehyde adducts and a reduction of cardiac HSPs and desmin. Both acetaldehyde and alcohol are myocardial perturbants.

1998 Alcohol and cardiovascular diseases. Wiley, Chichester (Novartis Foundation Symposium 216) p 35–50

Excessive alcohol ingestion is clearly damaging and induces a diversity of metabolic abnormalities, including diastolic dysfunction, atrial fibrillation and a variety of histological and biochemical changes (Spodick et al 1972, Wu et al 1976, Richardson et al 1986, Urbano-Márquez et al 1989, Kupari & Koskinen 1990, Kupari et al 1990a,b, Koskinen et al 1990). Left ventricular hypertrophy or cardiomegaly may be present. Alcoholic cardiomyopathy (ACM) may be associated with an alcohol consumption of 80 g ethanol/day and a duration of continuous exposure in excess of 10 years or more or at a cumulative ingestion of 250 kg. There is considerable variation in patient susceptibility and numerous studies have used different definitions of heart muscle disease or cardiac impairment. Thus, Gillet et al (1992) examined a group of patients with dilated cardiomyopathy with lifetime intakes of ethanol of over 500 kg, with consumption rates of 60 g per day over 25 years. In the study by Teragaki et al (1993) mean lifetime cumulative intake of 2030 kg was recorded, a figure calculated from the presented mean intakes of 29 kg/kg body weight and an assumed body weight of 70 kg. In the study of Cerqueira et al (1991) patients had an age range of 24–40 years (average 34 years), and consumed alcohol for 5–29 years (average 16 years) with an immediate consumption rate of a six-pack or a bottle of whisky for 5 days a week over 5 years or more. In these patients, mean ejection fractions at rest and diastolic peak filling rates were similar to age-matched control subjects. Similarly, there were no differences in mean ejection fraction and filling rates at peak exercise. Nevertheless, in 3/25 alcoholic subjects, ejection fractions showed abnormal responses during exercise, i.e. reduced or moderate increase in ejection fraction (Cerqueira et al 1991). These authors concluded that ACM is not common in subjects under 40 years of age though a 'pre-clinical' form of ACM is discernible in some alcohol abusers only after stress or additional pathophysiological stimuli (Bertolet et al 1991). More comprehensive relationships between the development of cardiac abnormalities and the duration and quantity of ethanol intake have been reported by Urbano-Márquez et al (1989).

Histological features

Fibrosis (focal or diffuse), increased lipid deposits and inflammatory infiltration are frequently described histological features in myocardial biopsies from subjects with ACM. Mitochondrial abnormalities include swollen or oval-shaped mitochondria, fragmentation, or disruption of the cristae. The cardiac myofibrillary architecture is also disrupted with changes ranging from small localized areas of increased osmification to dissolution or loss of the filaments and striations (Hibbs et al 1965, Bulloch et al 1972, Urbano-Márquez et al 1989). Many of the histological features of ACM are common to dilated cardiomyopathy and traditionally these are thought to be indistinguishable from one another. However, in dilated cardiomyopathy the degree of myocyte hypertrophy, fibrosis and nuclear alterations appears to be greater than in ACM. Although this implies that dilated cardiomyopathy and ACM can be identified from one another by quantitative histology, it is unlikely that such measurements can be applied routinely. Nevertheless, these differences between the two pathologies may be due to the specific way in which alcohol induces cardiac changes at the biochemical level.

Enzymic alterations in myocardial biopsies and the role of acetaldehyde

Enzymic assays have been carried out on myocardial tissues taken by endomyocardial biopsy from alcohol misusers and have been correlated with alcohol ingestion and left ventricular ejection fractions (Table 1; Richardson et al

TABLE 1   Cardiac enzyme activities in subjects consuming alcohol

Enzyme activities (mU/mg protein)	Abstinent or light ethanol consumption	Heavy ethanol consumption	Difference between abstinent or light and heavy ethanol intakes	Correlations with cumulative ethanol intakes
α-hydroxybutyric dehydrogenase	568 ± 39	828 ± 57	$P < 0.001$	$r = 0.59$, $P < 0.001$
Aspartate aminotransferase	510 ± 63	661 ± 61	$P < 0.10$, NS	$r = 0.19$ NS
Creatine kinase	1674 ± 129	2719 ± 226	$P < 0.001$	$r = 0.56$, $P < 0.01$
Lactate dehydrogenase	730 ± 57	1109 ± 69	$P < 0.01$	$r = 0.68$, $P < 0.001$
Malic dehydrogenase	2089 ± 185	2976 ± 185	$P < 0.01$	$r = 0.53$, $P < 0.01$

Data as mean ± SEM. Light drinkers were defined as those who had a life-time intake of less than 250 kg when daily intake exceeded 40 g per day ($n = 13$ for abstinent and light drinkers). Heavy drinkers exceeded 40 g per day and had an accumulative intake of 250 kg or more ($n = 11$). From Richardson et al (1986).

1986). Elevations in cardiac α-hydroxybutyric dehydrogenase, creatine kinase, lactate dehydrogenase and malic dehydrogenase activities were observed in heavy drinkers (Richardson et al 1986). However, it is not known whether these increased activities are causative mechanisms, or simply reflect an adaptive process. Part of the problem in dissecting out pathogenic mechanisms relates to the fact that alcohol affects virtually every organ system and most biochemical pathways, though many studies use extremely high levels of alcohol *in vitro*. For example, in cultured myocytes, ethanol was used in doses of up to 500 mmol/l to demonstrate its ability to alter mitochondrial morphology, although less severe changes were observed using ethanol at much lower concentrations (Mikami et al 1990). In addition, acetaldehyde, the first oxidation product of ethanol metabolism, is an extremely reactive molecule and may induce myocardial damage. Acetaldehyde binds strongly with proteins to form protein adducts, which may be immunogenic (reviewed in Lieber 1996). Acetaldehyde-induced immunogenicity has been investigated in alcoholics with cumulative ethanol intakes of 250 kg or more, with ejection fractions of less than 45% (Harcombe et al 1995). One-third of subjects with ACM were shown to have antibodies to cardiac acetaldehyde adducts (Harcombe et al 1995). Although this is a significant finding, it also suggests that in a substantial proportion of alcohol misusers with ACM, the disease must be a consequence of processes other than the formation of

TABLE 2   Effect of alcohol on cardiac protein synthesis, circulating cardiac troponin-T and tissue ATP *in vivo* and the modulating effect of inhibiting acetaldehyde dehydrogenase with cyanamide

Pre-treatment (30 min) and treatment (150 min)	Cardiac k_s (%/day)	P	Circulating cardiac troponin-T (μg/l)	P	Cardiac ATP (μmol/g)	P
Saline plus saline (control)	17.5 ± 0.6		0.7 ± 0.1		2.34 ± 0.16	
Cyanamide plus saline	18.1 ± 0.5	NS	0.7 ± 0.1	NS	2.39 ± 0.16	NS
Saline plus ethanol	14.4 ± 0.4	<0.01	2.1 ± 0.3	<0.001	2.35 ± 0.16	NS
Cyanamide plus ethanol	6.6 ± 0.2	<0.001[a]	3.1 ± 0.6	<0.001[b]	2.56 ± 0.17	NS

Adapted from unpublished studies by V. B. Patel. k_s is defined as the fractional rate of protein synthesis. All data are mean ± SEM of 4–9 observations in each group. Ethanol was given at a dose of 75 mmol/kg body weight i.p., whilst cyanamide was given at a dose of 0.5 mmol/kg body weight i.p. P values pertain to differences from saline plus saline controls.
[a]Difference in k_s between saline plus ethanol and cyanamide plus ethanol, $P < 0.001$.
[b]Difference in plasma troponin-T between saline plus ethanol and cyanamide plus ethanol, $P < 0.001$. NS, not significant.

acetaldehyde adducts and/or their antibodies. Free radical-mediated damage may be an alternative mechanism. Certainly, in reperfusion injury, cardiac damage may arise as a consequence of free radical activity (Flaherty 1991). Surges in circulating catecholamine levels, which occur in response to acute ethanol dosage, are thought to induce myocardial damage via the oxidation of catecholamines, producing superoxide free radical (Rupp et al 1994).

Ando et al (1993) have suggested that acetaldehyde may induce myocardial ischaemia and coronary vasospasm. In their studies, ischaemia was evaluated by thallium 201 scintograms and ECG. Although these measurements were not altered by treadmill exercise alone, changes occurred after ethanol ingestion and plasma acetaldehyde levels were determined to be 'abnormally high', with peak levels of about 0.150 mmol/l (Ando et al 1993). Increased circulating cardiac troponin-T (cTnT), a marker of ischaemia, occurs in response to acute ethanol dosage in rats (Table 2; Patel et al 1995). When ethanol-dosed animals are pre-treated with cyanamide (an inhibitor of acetaldehyde dehydrogenase which raises endogenous acetaldehyde), plasma levels of cTnT are further increased, to a level higher than that occurring with ethanol alone (Table 2; Patel et al 1995). The toxicity of acetaldehyde is also emphasized by its ability to inhibit the activities of enzymes, such as those involved in DNA repair (Lieber 1996).

Studies in animal models

The ethanol-dosing studies of Patel et al (1995), mentioned above, raise some important issues in alcohol research. Although there is a clear need to dissect out the pathogenic mechanisms responsible for ACM, practical obstacles arise in carrying out patient-based studies. These difficulties occur because of (1) limitations in obtaining suitably sized samples for biochemical analysis; (2) the presence of co-morbidities in alcoholics, such as liver disease, which will complicate the interpretation of the data; (3) some *control* groups contain individuals who consume alcohol in varying amounts; and (4) abstinent alcohol misusers may consume alcohol despite assurances to their attending physicians (also see Preedy et al 1995). The use of animal studies, in which alcohol is administered in defined amounts without inducing overt nutritional deficiencies, has resolved many of these problems. These studies have shown that a reduction in heart muscle protein synthesis is an initial or precipitating response to acute ethanol toxicity (Preedy & Peters 1990). Fractional rates of protein synthesis (k_s, defined as the percentage of tissue protein synthesised per day) measured by the phenylalanine *flooding dose* technique (now considered to be the gold-standard for measuring rates of protein synthesis *in vivo*), are reduced by 20% at 2.5 h, though greater decreases in protein synthesis occur after 6 and 24 h (Table 3; V. B. Patel, M. E. Reilly, P. J. Richardson & V. R. Preedy, unpublished data). The remarkable feature of these time-course studies is the decline in k_s at 24 h when all circulating ethanol has disappeared. The synthesis of the myofibrillary proteins (i.e. the fraction

TABLE 3   Time course changes in cardiac protein synthesis in response to acute alcohol

	k_s (%/day)	Difference as % from control	Statistical significance (P)
Control (saline)	14.8 ± 0.4		
2.5 h ethanol	12.7 ± 0.7	−14	<0.001
6 h ethanol	12.4 ± 0.2	−16	<0.001
24 h ethanol	8.9 ± 0.3	−40	<0.001
Pair-fed control for 24 h ethanol[a]	12.0 ± 0.5	−19	<0.001

Male Wistar rats approximately 150 g body weight were injected i.p. with 0.15 mol/l saline (NaCl); or ethanol 75 mmol/kg body weight, i.p. In the ethanol-injected group, rats were sacrificed at 2.5, 6 and 24 h after treatment. There was no measurable blood alcohol at 24 h. All data are means ± SEM of 6–8 observations. Differences were assessed with Student's *t*-test using the pooled estimate of variance.
[a]Pair-fed controls were introduced for 24 h ethanol-treated rats to compensate for the reduced food intakes at 24 h ethanol, −25%, P <0.001. Thus, reduced heart muscle protein synthesis rates occur independently of any reduction in food intakes and in the absence of circulating ethanol. From unpublished data of V. B. Patel, M. E. Reilly, P. J. Richardson and V. R. Preedy.

containing proteins necessary for force generation in the contractile response) are also reduced by ethanol, as are proteins of subcellular organelles such as the mitochondria (Siddiq et al 1993a,b,c). All regions of the heart (i.e. atria and ventricles) are susceptible to ethanol-induced perturbations in protein synthesis (Siddiq et al 1993b). Stress situations, such as long-standing hypertension, exacerbate these effects of ethanol on cardiac myofibrillary protein synthesis (Siddiq et al 1997). Moreover, acetaldehyde appears to be a particularly potent myocardial perturbant in that the decrease in protein synthesis at 2.5 h is approximately 80% when ethanol-dosed rats are pre-treated with cyanamide (Siddiq et al 1993c, V. B. Patel, P. J. Richardson & V. R. Preedy, unpublished data; Table 2). In these circumstances, of cyanamide pre-dosing, the total cardiac ATP content remains unaltered compared with saline-injected or even ethanol-injected rats, though there may be alterations in nucleotide turnover or metabolic availability at the subcellular level (Table 2; Patel et al 1996). Certainly, cyanamide increases levels of AMP in ethanol dosed rats suggestive of enhanced nucleotide turnover (Patel et al 1996).

Two-dimensional electrophoresis has been used to study specific protein alterations in a variety of conditions, such as developmental growth, where for example differences in myosin light chain were observed between fetal and adult rat ventricular tissue (Srihari et al 1982). In muscular subaortic stenosis, cardiac protein patterns show decreases in proteins ranging from M_r 35 000–41 000 when compared with normal controls (Liew et al 1980). Chronic alcohol feeding studies in rats that show the loss of myofibrillar proteins at 6 weeks are consistent with histological post-mortem studies showing cardiac myofibrillary disarray and loss in chronic alcoholics (Hibbs et al 1965). However, the myofibrillary proteins extracted by differential solubilization and ultra-centrifugation techniques contain a composite mixture of proteins, though myosin predominates. More recently, we have explored changes in cardiac proteins using analytical two-dimensional electrophoresis (Table 4; Patel et al 1997). After 6 weeks ethanol feeding, 10% of total proteins were altered when identical amounts of proteins were loaded on each gel (i.e. relative amounts): 7% of proteins were significantly decreased whilst 3% were increased. Proteins of the heat shock protein (HSP) superfamily Hsp60 and Hsp70 were reduced. The importance of this relates to the involvement of HSPs in protein translocation and folding, and the conferment of cytosolic or mitochondrial protection (Patel et al 1997). This implies that the ethanol-exposed heart may be more susceptible to cardio-derangements. In these studies, desmin was also decreased, and this may represent structural derangements. It should be also be emphasised, however, that the total amounts of cardiac proteins (i.e. absolute amounts) are reduced after chronic ethanol feeding. Thus, the absolute amounts of two isoforms of myosin light chain 2 (sample spot numbers [SSP] 1214 and 1231) decreased by

TABLE 4 Ventricular protein characterization after chronic alcohol treatment in the rat

SSP number protein	Relative amount (ppmpdu)			Absolute amount (ppmpdu × 10^6 per heart)		
	Control	Alcohol	P-value	Control	Alcohol	P-value
Assigned proteins						
1214 MLC2	1903 ± 406	1832 ± 469	NS	2528 ± 130	1980 ± 114	<0.01
1231 MLC2	5236 ± 999	4048 ± 879	NS	6956 ± 357	4375 ± 253	<0.001
1326 MLCI	822 ± 184	906 ± 284	NS	1092 ± 56	979 ± 57	NS
1501 Vimentin	77 ± 12	99 ± 30	NS	102 ± 5	107 ± 6	NS
1642 Desmin	12303 ± 7212	9996 ± 2960	NS	16346 ± 838	10804 ± 624	<0.001
1643 Desmin	806 ± 66	633 ± 48	<0.025	1071 ± 55	684 ± 39	<0.001
2301 MLCI	1859 ± 408	1950 ± 335	NS	2470 ± 127	2107 ± 122	<0.025
2508 Actin	932 ± 147	936 ± 162	NS	1238 ± 63	1012 ± 58	<0.01
2615 Desmin	632 ± 63	377 ± 36	<0.025	840 ± 43	407 ± 23	<0.001
3715 HSP6O	294 ± 30	277 ± 51	NS	391 ± 20	299 ± 17	<0.01
3750 HSP6O	1603 ± 268	623 ± 141	<0.025	2130 ± 109	673 ± 39	<0.001
4702 HSP7O	279 ± 29	257 ± 42	NS	371 ± 19	278 ± 16	<0.01
4801 HSP7O	487 ± 53	320 ± 46	<0.001	647 ± 33	346 ± 20	<0.001
5733 Albumin	1028 ± 170	687 ± 52	NS	1366 ± 70	743 ± 43	<0.001
8507 Creatine kinase	1402 ± 262	1646 ± 422	NS	1863 ± 96	1779 ± 103	NS

(cont.)

TABLE 4 *(cont.)*

SSP number protein	Relative amount (ppmpdu)			Absolute amount (ppmpdu × 10^6 per heart)		
	Control	*Alcohol*	*P-value*	*Control*	*Alcohol*	*P-value*
Unassigned proteins showing significant increases						
1307 Unknown protein	69 ± 18	153 ± 24	<0.05	92 ± 5	166 ± 10	<0.001
1408 Unknown protein	22 ± 6	92 ± 24	<0.05	29 ± 1	100 ± 6	<0.001
1516 Unknown protein	9 ± 3	37 ± 7	<0.01	11 ± 1	40 ± 2	<0.001
2319 Unknown protein	101 ± 28	328 ± 64	<0.05	134 ± 7	355 ± 20	<0.001
3619 Unknown protein	131 ± 29	176 ± 29	<0.025	174 ± 9	190 ± 11	NS
4624 Unknown protein	139 ± 23	167 ± 29	<0.025	185 ± 9	181 ± 10	NS
5314 Unknown protein	41 ± 16	151 ± 21	<0.01	54 ± 3	163 ± 9	<0.001
5424 Unknown protein	37 ± 8	81 ± 11	<0.01	49 ± 3	88 ± 5	<0.001
6608 Unknown protein	33 ± 9	79 ± 14	<0.01	44 ± 2	86 ± 5	<0.001
7327 Unknown protein	47 ± 11	99 ± 17	<0.05	62 ± 3	107 ± 6	<0.05
7332 Unknown protein	88 ± 11	143 ± 21	<0.05	117 ± 6	154 ± 9	<0.05
Unassigned proteins showing significant decreases						
1620 Unknown protein	1057 ± 135	741 ± 45	<0.05	1405 ± 72	801 ± 46	<0.001
2614 Unknown protein	832 ± 63	547 ± 78	<0.01	1106 ± 57	591 ± 34	<0.001
2627 Unknown protein	155 ± 11	111 ± 12	<0.025	206 ± 11	119 ± 10	<0.001
2707 Unknown protein	201 ± 50	91 ± 14	<0.05	267 ± 14	98 ± 6	<0.001
2824 Unknown protein	46 ± 10	25 ± 6	<0.05	61 ± 3	27 ± 2	<0.001

SSP		Treated		Control	
2913 Unknown protein	297 ± 41	155 ± 29	<0.05	395 ± 20	168 ± 10	<0.001
3509 Unknown protein	170 ± 18	122 ± 14	<0.05	226 ± 12	132 ± 8	<0.001
3602 Unknown protein	704 ± 43	433 ± 50	<0.01	935 ± 48	468 ± 27	<0.001
3732 Unknown protein	516 ± 65	347 ± 31	<0.025	686 ± 35	375 ± 22	<0.001
3819 Unknown protein	230 ± 32	126 ± 16	<0.05	306 ± 16	136 ± 8	<0.001
3824 Unknown protein	188 ± 21	123 ± 24	<0.025	250 ± 13	133 ± 8	<0.001
3829 Unknown protein	175 ± 26	97 ± 22	<0.025	233 ± 12	105 ± 6	<0.001
3833 Unknown protein	150 ± 26	85 ± 19	<0.05	199 ± 10	92 ± 5	<0.001
3841 Unknown protein	155 ± 25	94 ± 15	<0.05	206 ± 11	102 ± 6	<0.001
3843 Unknown protein	125 ± 18	84 ± 16	<0.025	166 ± 9	91 ± 5	<0.001
3853 Unknown protein	276 ± 30	156 ± 21	<0.01	367 ± 19	169 ± 10	<0.001
3870 Unknown protein	155 ± 20	88 ± 16	<0.01	206 ± 11	95 ± 5	<0.001
5110 Unknown protein	1176 ± 203	335 ± 151	<0.025	1562 ± 80	362 ± 21	<0.001
5410 Unknown protein	418 ± 51	126 ± 37	<0.01	555 ± 28	136 ± 8	<0.001
5419 Unknown protein	214 ± 16	151 ± 30	<0.05	284 ± 15	163 ± 9	<0.001
5608 Unknown protein	878 ± 127	452 ± 129	<0.001	1167 ± 60	489 ± 28	<0.001
5617 Unknown protein	811 ± 93	569 ± 82	<0.05	1078 ± 55	615 ± 35	<0.001
6215 Unknown protein	1502 ± 135	1096 ± 132	<0.05	1996 ± 102	1185 ± 68	<0.001
6522 Unknown protein	908 ± 107	645 ± 67	<0.05	1206 ± 62	697 ± 40	<0.001
7319 Unknown protein	2885 ± 338	1306 ± 406	<0.025	3834 ± 197	1412 ± 81	<0.025
7617 Unknown protein	119 ± 6	90 ± 12	<0.025	158 ± 8	98 ± 6	<0.025
8207 Unknown protein	1162[a] ± 96	938 ± 71	<0.05	1545 ± 79	1014 ± 59	<0.05
8524 Unknown protein	776 ± 31	567 ± 49	<0.01	1031 ± 53	613 ± 35	<0.01

ppmpdu, parts per million protein density units; SSP, sample spot number.
Rats were fed on liquid diets containing ethanol as 35% of total calories as ethanol (treated) or a diet in which ethanol was replaced by isocaloric glucose (controls). All data as mean ± SEM (6 pairs of rats). Adapted from Patel et al (1997) and unpublished data of V. B. Patel.

22% ($P < 0.01$) and 37% ($P < 0.001$), respectively (Table 3; Patel et al 1997, V. B. Patel, unpublished observations). Absolute amounts of myosin light; chain 1 (SSP 2301) and actin (SSP 2508) decreased by 18% ($P < 0.025$) and 15% ($P < 0.01$) respectively (Table 4; Patel et al 1997). However, a considerable number of these SSP numbers remain uncharacterized. Thus, the precise qualitative nature of contractile and non-contractile protein in alcohol toxicity awaits further elucidation.

Acknowledgements

The Molecular and Metabolic Cardiology Group thank Professor Timothy J. Peters for encouragement and support. We also thank Drs Mike Dunn and Joe Corbett for 2D electrophoresis studies. Financial support from the British Heart Foundation, The Medical Research Council and The JRC is acknowledged.

References

Ando H, Abe H, Hisanou R 1993 Ethanol-induced myocardial ischemia: close relation between blood acetaldehyde level and myocardial ischemia. Clin Cardiol 16:443–446

Bertolet BD, Freund G, Martin CA, Perchalski DL, Williams CM, Pepine CJ 1991 Unrecognized left ventricular dysfunction in an apparently healthy alcohol abuse population. Drug Alcohol Depend 28:113–119

Bulloch RT, Pearce MB, Murphy ML, Jenkins BJ, Davis JL 1972 Myocardial lesions in idiopathic and alcoholic cardiomyopathy. Study by ventricular septal biopsy. Am J Cardiol 29:15–25

Cerqueira MD, Harp GD, Ritchie JL, Stratton JR, Walker RD 1991 Rarity of preclinical alcoholic cardiomyopathy in chronic alcoholics < 40 years of age. Am J Cardiol 67:183–187

Flaherty JT 1991 Myocardial injury mediated by oxygen free radicals. Am J Med 91 (suppl 3C): 79S–85S

Gillet C, Julliere Y, Pirollet P et al 1992 Alcohol consumption and biological markers for alcoholism in idiopathic dilated cardiomyopathy: a case-controlled study. Alcohol Alcohol 27:353–358

Harcombe AA, Ramsay L, Kenna JG et al 1995 Circulating antibodies to cardiac protein–acetaldehyde adducts in alcoholic heart muscle disease. Clin Sci 88:263–268

Hibbs RG, Ferrans VJ, Black WC, Weilbaecher DG, Walsh JJ, Burch GE 1965 Alcoholic cardiomyopathy. An electron microscopic study. Am Heart J 69:766–779

Koskinen P, Kupari M, Leinonen H 1990 Role of alcohol in recurrences of atrial fibrillation in persons < 65 years of age. Am J Cardiol 66:954–958

Kupari M, Koskinen P 1990 Seasonal variation in occurrence of acute atrial fibrillation and relation to air temperature and sale of alcohol. Am J Cardiol 66:1519–1520

Kupari M, Koskinen P, Hynynen M, Salmenera M, Ventila M 1990a Acute effects of ethanol on left ventricular diastolic function. Br Heart J 64:129–132

Kupari M, Koskinen P, Suokas A, Ventila M 1990b Left ventricular filling impairment in asymptomatic chronic alcoholics. Am J Cardiol 66:1473–1477

Lieber CS 1996 The metabolism of alcohol and its implication to the pathogenesis of disease. In: Preedy VR, Watson RW (eds) Alcohol and the gastrointestinal tract. CRC Press, Boca Raton, FL, p 19–39

Liew CC, Sole MJ, Silver MD, Wigle ED 1980 Electrophoretic profiles of non-histone nuclear proteins of human hearts with muscular subaortic stenosis. Circ Res 46:513–519

Mikami K, Sato S, Watanabe T 1990 Acute effects of ethanol on cultured myocardial cells: an ultrastructural study. Alcohol Alcohol 25:651–660

Patel VB, Sherwood R, Why H, Poyser K, Richardson PJ, Preedy VR 1995 The acute and chronic effects of alcohol toxicity upon rat plasma troponin-T levels. Alcohol Alcohol 30:525 (abstr)

Patel VB, Salisbury JR, Rodrigues LM, Griffiths JR, Richardson PJ, Preedy VR 1996 The acute and chronic effects of alcohol upon cardiac nucleotide status. Addict Biol 1:171–180

Patel VB, Corbett JM, Richardson PJ, Dunn MJ, Preedy VR 1997 Protein profiling in cardiac tissue in response to the chronic effects of alcohol. Electrophoresis 18:2788–2794

Preedy VR, Peters TJ 1990 The acute and chronic effects of ethanol on cardiac muscle protein synthesis in the rat in vivo. Alcohol 7:97–102

Preedy VR, Reilly ME, Why HJF, Bonner AB, Richardson PJ 1995 Protein turnover in alcoholism: should it be considered as a whole body event or tissue specific phenomena? J Am Coll Nutr 14:7–10

Richardson PJ, Wodak AD, Atkinson L, Saunders JB, Jewitt DE 1986 Relation between alcohol intake, myocardial enzyme activity and myocardial function in dilated cardiomyopathy. Br Heart J 56:165–170

Rupp H, Dhalla KS, Dhalla NS 1994 Mechanisms of cardiac cell damage due to catecholamines: significance of drugs regulating central sympathetic outflow. J Cardiovasc Pharmacol 24:S16–S24

Siddiq T, Salisbury JR, Richardson PJ, Preedy VR 1993a Synthesis of ventricular mitochondrial proteins in vivo: effect of acute ethanol toxicity. Alcohol Clin Exp Res 17:894–899

Siddiq T, Richardson PJ, Morton J et al 1993b Rates of protein synthesis in different regions of the normotensive and hypertrophied heart in response to acute alcohol toxicity. Alcohol Alcohol 28:297–310

Siddiq T, Richardson PJ, Mitchell WD, Teare J, Preedy VR 1993c Ethanol-induced inhibition of ventricular protein synthesis in vivo and the possible role of acetaldehyde. Cell Biochem Funct 11:45–54

Siddiq S, Sandhu G, Richardson PJ, Preedy VR 1997 Effects of acute ethanol on ventricular myofibrillary protein synthesis in vivo in normotensive and hypertensive rats. Addict Biol 2:87–93

Spodick DH, Pigott VM, Chirife R 1972 Preclinical cardiac malfunction in chronic alcoholism. Comparison with matched normal controls and with alcoholic cardiomyopathy. N Engl J Med 287:677–680

Srihari T, Tuchscmid CR, Hirzel HO, Schaub MC 1982 Electrophoretic analyses of atrial and ventricular cardiac myosins from foetal and adult rabbits. Comp Biochem Physiol B 72:353–357

Teragaki M, Takeuchi K, Takeda T 1993 Clinical and histologic features of alcohol drinkers with congestive heart failure. Am Heart J 125:808–817

Urbano-Márquez A, Estruch R, Navarro-Lopez F, Grau JM, Mont L, Rubin E 1989 The effects of alcoholism on skeletal and cardiac muscle. N Engl J Med 320:409–415

Wu CF, Sudhakar M, Jaferi G, Ahmed SS, Regan TJ 1976 Preclinical cardiomyopathy in chronic alcoholics: a sex difference. Am Heart J 91:281–286

DISCUSSION

Urbano-Márquez: In our experience the dose of alcohol required to cause cardiomyopathy is higher than in your study. In our studies, the majority of the patients with cardiomyopathy drank more than 20 kg of alcohol per kg of body mass. Furthermore, there are many patients who drink between 15 or 20 kg alcohol/kg body mass and have normal ejection fraction, whereas others drinking just 10 kg/kg have lower ejection fractions than controls although they are higher than 50%. I am sure that this indicates the preliminary stages of cardiomyopathy.

Shaper: If most dilated cardiomyopathies are post-viral in origin — and there is some suggestion of this — could it be that there is an interaction between viral infections and alcoholic cardiomyopathy?

Richardson: We have taken endomyocardial biopsy tissue from our population of patients for examination for enteroviruses such as Coxsackie virus B. We have been surprised by the low pick-up of enterovirus infection in the presence of a history of significant alcohol intake. I rather thought it would be the other way round: that these patients would have had altered immunity and thus less defence against viral infection. Some patients are clearly predisposed to the deleterious effects of alcohol, having had a previous viral infection. All the patients with dilated cardiomyopathy who drink in excess of 60 g alcohol/day may depress their ventricular function.

Gorelick: For how long do these patients have a reversible condition before it becomes permanent? Do any of the histological markers that you measured predict who will have a permanent condition?

Richardson: No. Although we haven't investigated enough patients yet, we did do serial biopsies and then measured the myocardial enzyme activities again. It was possible that the enzyme activity alterations were simply the result of enzyme induction. Underlying all that I said, there is a question mark in my mind as to whether there could be an enzyme alteration which is a primary defect in myocardial metabolism that makes the patients susceptible to alcohol. Seferovic (personal communication) from Yugoslavia has repeated our enzyme activity work with identical findings, but has not yet published this.

Peters: Personally I think there's an adaptive response. One assumes that the mitochondrial changes are pathological, but they might be beneficial. There are some data from the USA that liver biopsies of people showing megamito-chondria have a better prognosis than liver biopsies from patients with cirrhosis without altered mitochondria (Peters 1987). It is often difficult to separate the beneficial compensatory effects from true pathogenic effects.

Anderson: When we talk about sudden coronary death, is this just an arrhythmic effect, or is it also an acute effect on ventricular function?

Richardson: If these patients die suddenly, they're dying because of myocardial instability which is unrelated to coronary artery disease.

Anderson: Is there a dose–response relationship between alcohol ingestion and ventricular function?

Urbano-Márquez: Yes. In our experience there is a linear relationship between the decrease in ejection fraction and increasing intake of alcohol. In the follow-up of a patient we can observe the ventricular function diminishing as they continue to drink alcohol. The more the patient drinks, the more the ejection fraction decreases. However, in those who stop drinking, the ventricular ejection fraction improves.

Puddey: In your definition of ACM, you exclude individuals with coronary artery disease. But can coronary heart disease and alcoholic cardiomyopathy co-exist, since these people are often heavy smokers and have an atherogenic diet?

Richardson: Certainly. The reason we excluded coronary artery disease was to remove this as a factor.

Klatsky: We keep talking about the viral aetiology of idiopathic dilated cardiomyopathy. Yet I have the impression that study of viral titres has a low yield in idiopathic dilated cardiomyopathy.

Richardson: Apart from a study by Cambridge and Goodwin that showed that a high neutralizing antibody titre for Coxsackie virus B was associated with dilated cardiomyopathy (Cambridge et al 1979), viral titres are not applicable in making this diagnosis. The diagnosis is now made on the basis of endomyocardial biopsy tissue subjected to either *in situ* hybridization or PCR for enterovirus. This is very well established; indeed, we have shown a prognostic association with virus in the tissue (Why et al 1994).

Klatsky: So if one takes a group of people with what appears to be idiopathic dilated cardiomyopathy, one can find evidence in a large proportion of them for a viral basis?

Richardson: 30% in most of the studies that are published world-wide (Why et al 1994).

Klatsky: And what would the percentage be where there's a heavy alcohol intake?

Richardson: In our experience, no more than 10%.

Kupari: I'm interested in your chronic animal model. Are you able to produce dilated heart failure in those animals? It would be much easier to label the changes in protein synthesis you describe as causal if you also see heart failure in the animals.

Richardson: One of the problems in this particular area has been the lack of a good animal model of alcoholic cardiomyopathy. Although these changes have been demonstrated, the model that we're looking for isn't produced in the way that we would like.

Kupari: Do you think that alcohol *per se* can produce dilated systolic heart failure, or are other insults necessary, such as toxic effects or interactions with other environmental or genetic factors?

Richardson: I think there is a genetic predisposition, but if you take that away then I'm uncertain how many would develop alcoholic cardiomyopathy even if exposed to the level of alcohol intake seen in our patients.

Urbano-Márquez: It is almost impossible to rule out viral infection from having an influence in alcoholic cardiomyopathy. However, in our biopsies we have never found lymphocytes or anything that resembles myocarditis. Another interesting point is the relationship with the disposition to cardiomyopathy. Some patients with cardiomyopathy drink less than 20 kg alcohol per kg of body mass.

Keil: Perhaps you are studying genetic disposition and not cause. I was a little surprised when you said that there is a *possible* genetic predisposition for cardiomyopathy. In most chronic diseases there is a gene–environment interaction: we know that 'only' about 10% of heavy smokers get lung cancer, so what happens to all the others? They obviously don't have the genetic disposition. I would be surprised if there wasn't a genetic disposition for cardiomyopathy.

Richardson: Our exposure data were carefully assessed and reproduced in six patients to try to make the group that I described to you pretty watertight in terms of the reproducibility of the alcohol histories. The patients that we were interviewing were actually good responders. As we heard this morning, we know there is a tendency always to underestimate the amount of alcohol consumed, but I think these patients' histories were fairly clear.

Gaziano: The case for a causal relationship, even in absence of an animal model, is fairly strong. You have been able to segregate these individuals, you have identified some metabolic characteristics that distinguish these two types of ranges and you see a dose–response relationship. I'm not troubled by the lack of an animal model. What I'm intrigued by is the dose response. Is there a threshold effect beyond which there is a dose response, or are there metabolic derangements that are linear and accumulate over time, and then you end up with a detectable functional abnormality? Is alcohol a low-level myocardial toxin for all of us, or is there a threshold below which there is no damage?

Richardson: The threshold of the effect seemed be at about 60 g alcohol/day. It was only above this level of consumption that there were any detectable changes in ventricular function. The figure of 80 g/day is slightly arbitrary cut-off point. It is impossible to determine an absolute figure. Nevertheless, it was possible to show some effect with regard to the myocardium and hypertension at 60 g/day.

Gaziano: Was the LV dysfunction seen in alcoholic cardiomyopathy comparable to that of dilated cardiomyopathy?

Richardson: Yes. The ejection fractions were 34.5% and 35%, respectively. They were identical in terms of their other demographics.

Gaziano: We've all seen in our clinical practices elevated CK and MB in plasma acutely, and chronic alcoholism has been reported as one of the causes of chronically elevated CK. Aside from the metabolic derangements that are occurring within the cells, does this suggest some low level myocardial necrosis?

Richardson: In the binge drinkers who are admitted to a coronary care unit with chest pain, some get acute CK loss. They look like infarcts but their coronary angiograms are completely normal. So I think you can induce acute myocardial necrosis in response to binge drinking; some of these people have had up to 30 pints of beer at the weekend.

Gaziano: Do the chronic non-binge drinkers have elevated CK?

Richardson: No.

Keaney: There are two different thresholds you are looking at: one is the threshold of alcohol consumption, and the other is the threshold of ejection fraction changes that you are able to detect. If you were able to determine changes in ejection fraction more sensitively, your threshold for alcohol consumption may change.

Richardson: You may see alterations in ejection fraction, dropping from 55–45% with levels of consumption that we might use to define our patients with dilated cardiomyopathy. However, we diagnose dilated cardiomyopathy when the ejection fraction is less than 40. There is an area where there may be effects from alcohol in terms of depression of left ventricular function, but it's not enough to define this as dilated cardiomyopathy.

Shaper: Can one therefore assume that there's no J- or U-shape in the relationship between alcohol intake and myocardial function? In other words, is it correct that there isn't a level of alcohol at which the myocardium is functioning optimally and below which it is not functioning as well?

Urbano-Márquez: The cardiac damage due to alcohol is a continuum. The slope of the line is related to the dose of alcohol. If you drink low doses of alcohol, throughout life you have an ejection fraction of 60–65%. If you increase your intake, five years after the ejection fraction will be 55%, and finally you will reach 45%, and it is admitted that less than 50% ejection fraction is cardiomyopathy. However, this relationship can be influenced by personal sensitivity, genetic factors, etc.

Klatsky: I would like to ask a question having to do with a third kind of threshold, which I think is the most important in a practical sense to doctors dealing with patients. Let's accept that it takes a very high alcohol intake over a long period of time to produce alcoholic cardiomyopathy. There's no public health problem there because nobody should drink that much. There's another threshold having to do with what will produce myocardial depression with the normal myocardium. An increasingly common problem is chronic heart failure due to a range of non-alcoholic causes such as hypertension, diabetes and idiopathic cardiomyopathy. What data can you cite to indicate the threshold of alcohol intake that's OK for people who have already have heart failure for causes having nothing to do with alcohol?

Shaper: The question has been raised as to whether in patients with pre-existing cardiovascular disease, the use of alcohol is contraindicated. What justification is there for this?

Gaziano: That's exactly why we looked at people who have had recent myocardial infarction. We presumed that if you have a damaged myocardium you won't want to expose it to any potential myocardial toxin, even at a low level. We have 5000 physicians who reported a myocardial infarction, but unfortunately we have no information on the degree of their myocardial dysfunction, so we can't segregate out people who have severely depressed ejection fractions. What we see in light-to-moderate drinkers is a profound beneficial effect up to our highest drinking level on total mortality.

Klatsky: My question was actually concerned with people who are in heart failure. In the USA this is the commonest hospital admission diagnosis. There are hundreds of thousands of people with chronic heart failure, and they ask whether it is OK for them to have a drink: what should we tell them?

Puddey: I was interested to hear you describe toxic myocardial necrosis following binge drinking, as a syndrome. How sure can you be that it isn't coronary artery spasm, which has been described in a number of case reports, particularly in orientals (Oda et al 1994)?

Richardson: You can't always be sure of that, of course. The tendency would be that the alcohol would be more likely to vasodilate than constrict the vessels.

References

Cambridge G, MacArthur CG, Waterson AP, Goodwin JF, Oakley CM 1979 Antibodies to Coxsackie B viruses in congestive cardiomyopathy. Br Heart J 41:692–696

Oda H, Suzuki M, Oniki T, Kishi Y, Numano F 1994 Alcohol and coronary spasm. Angiology 45:187–197

Peters TJ 1987 Analytic subcellular studies in alcoholic liver disease. In: Reid E, Cook GMW, Luzio JP (eds) Cell membranes and disease. Plenum, New York, p 25–34

Why GHF, Meany BT, Richardson PJ et al 1994 Clinical and prognostic signs of enteroviral RNA in the myocardium of patients with myocarditis or dilated cardiomyopathy. Circulation 89:2582–2589

Alcohol, free radicals and antioxidants

I. B. Puddey, K. D. Croft, R. Abu-Amsha Caccetta and L. J. Beilin

Department of Medicine, Royal Perth Hospital, University of Western Australia, GPO Box X2213, Perth, Western Australia 6001, Australia

Abstract. Antioxidants in alcoholic beverages, especially polyphenolic compounds in red wine, have been proposed as an important contributory factor to the protective effect of regular alcohol use against atherosclerotic cardiovascular disease. The postulated mechanism involves quenching of free radicals with decreased oxidative damage to low density lipoprotein (LDL) hence reducing its potential atherogenicity. There is definitive *in vitro* evidence that extracts of red wine, white wine, grape juice and beer can inhibit the oxidation of LDL, the degree of inhibition being directly proportional to beverage polyphenolic content and able to be abolished by prior stripping of the polyphenolics from the alcoholic beverage. These *in vitro* antioxidant effects have not been reliably reproduced *in vivo* after acute or short-term administration of alcoholic beverages. In fact, in some studies where white wine or beer have been given over 2–4 week periods, enhanced oxidizability of LDL cholesterol has been reported. Such findings are consistent with the possibility that, depending on the beverage, a predominant pro-oxidant effect of alcohol itself may outweigh any antioxidant effect of beverage polyphenolics. Increased oxidant stress and enhanced lipid peroxidation with alcohol have several biologically plausible explanations and have been reported as possible mechanisms for alcohol-related toxicity and injury in various tissues. Therefore, before the promotion of any particular benefits of ingestion of polyphenolics from alcoholic beverages (especially red wine) for prevention of atherosclerotic cardiovascular disease, the balance of redox effects *in vivo* will need careful further clinical and laboratory evaluation.

1998 Alcohol and cardiovascular diseases. Wiley, Chichester (Novartis Foundation Symposium 216) p 51–67

The most widely embraced current theory for the pathogenesis of atherosclerotic vascular disease proposes as a major initiating factor the oxidation of low density lipoprotein particles (LDL) within the vascular sub-endothelium (Steinberg et al 1989). The subsequent uptake of the oxidized LDL via macrophage scavenger receptors leads to foam cell formation, the genesis of fatty streaks on vascular walls and ultimately atherosclerotic plaques. This current understanding of the development of atherosclerosis has resulted in considerable research into the possibility that certain dietary and lifestyle factors may increase oxidant stress resulting in initiation and acceleration of atherogenesis. Antioxidant compounds that may modulate such oxidant stress have received even greater attention. In particular, the quest for increased pathophysiological understanding of the putative cardiovascular protective effects of alcoholic beverages has led to a sustained focus over recent years on natural antioxidants found in alcoholic beverages—especially those in red wine.

This focus has been predominantly on flavonoids—polyphenolic compounds widely distributed in higher plants and important in contributing to the flavour and colour of many fruits and vegetables as well as the products derived from them, including wine. They are 15-carbon compounds composed of two phenolic rings connected by a three-carbon unit. Variations in the oxygen-containing heterocyclic ring have given rise to thousands of flavonoids in nature, which are further sub-classified as flavonols, flavones, flavanones, catechins and anthocyanidins. Attachment of the second phenolic ring to the 3 instead of the 2 carbon position produces a further class—the isoflavonoids. Some of the major flavonoids found in wines include the flavonols quercetin and myricetin, the anthocyanidins (which are primarily responsible for wine colour), catechin and epicatechin, and gallic acid. The quantity of these flavonoids is significantly higher in red rather than white wines and relates to how much grape seed has been in contact with the must during fermentation (Kovac et al 1995), the degree of cell disruption during grape skin crushing and pressing (Meyer et al 1997), the phenolic composition of the grape itself, and the duration and method of fermentation (Auw et al 1996). Other major phenolic compounds in wines are the simple phenolic acids especially the cinnamic acid derivatives coumaric acid, caffeic acid and protocatechuic acid. Resveratrol, a phytoalexin produced in the grape skin in response to fungal infection, has also been a focus of interest (Belguendouz et al 1997, Frankel et al 1993a) but has extremely variable levels in red wine and has been shown to be less potent an antioxidant than the flavonoid components (Frankel et al 1995).

Early reports of potent free radical scavenging activity of procyanidins isolated from grape seeds (da Silva et al 1991) were followed by the pioneering study of Frankel et al (1993b) who reported that diluted extracts of red wine could significantly inhibit lipid peroxidation of human LDL *in vitro*. This observation has been followed by a plethora of further *in vitro* studies both characterizing the relative antioxidant activities of extracts of red and white wine (Abu-Amsha et al 1996, Teissedre et al 1996, Kanner et al 1994, Frankel et al 1995, Fuhrman et al 1995) and convincingly relating this activity to the beverage polyphenolics. Our own *in vitro* study confirmed that it is the phenolic content of various beverages that determines the extent of inhibition of both serum and LDL oxidation (Abu-Amsha et al 1996). We utilized both a whole serum oxidation system and isolated LDL and showed that the higher the total polyphenolic content of an alcoholic beverage the greater the antioxidative effect measured as a change in lag time (Fig. 1). The effect was most pronounced with dilutions of red wine and high

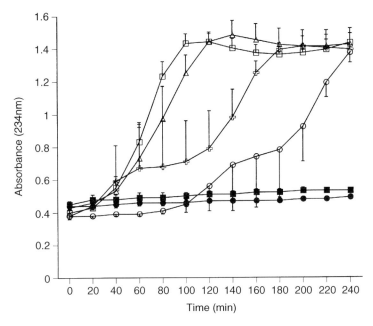

FIG. 1. The mean change ($\pm$ SEM) in conjugated diene absorbance at 234 nm over a 240 min period in LDL after initiation of peroxidation with 8 mM Cu^{2+} at 37 °C. Control oxidation ($\square$) was LDL plus PBS vehicle ($n = 8$), all beverages tested were diluted 1:500; ●, LDL plus red wine ($n = 7$); $\triangle$, LDL plus carboxylic acid mixture ($n = 4$); ○, LDL plus red grape juice ($n = 3$); ■, LDL plus high phenolic content red grape juice, ($n = 3$); ⊕, LDL plus white wine ($n = 4$). (Reproduced with permission from Abu-Amsha et al 1996.)

phenolic content grape juice but substantially less for white wine or lower phenolic content grape juice. Other studies have also reported direct correlations between the total phenolic content of wines and the inhibition of LDL oxidation (Verhagen et al 1996). Others have also found that grape juice alone can similarly inhibit LDL oxidation (Lanningham-Foster et al 1995, Teissedre et al 1996). Reports of the effects of white wine *in vitro* have not been as consistent, with Fuhrman et al (1995) reporting no effect on LDL oxidation and surprisingly observing an increase in plasma oxidation. Isolated dietary phenolic compounds found in wines (Laranjinha et al 1994, Nardini et al 1995) also show a protective effect against LDL oxidation. When we stripped both red wine and grape juice of their phenols, *in vitro* antioxidant activity against LDL oxidation was markedly curtailed (Fig. 2). In our study we also showed that both light and full-strength beers can significantly inhibit LDL oxidation (Fig. 3), suggesting such effects are not unique to the polyphenolics found in wine and grape juice alone. In fact, using a variety of oxidation systems, flavonoids and polyphenolics in a large number of plant

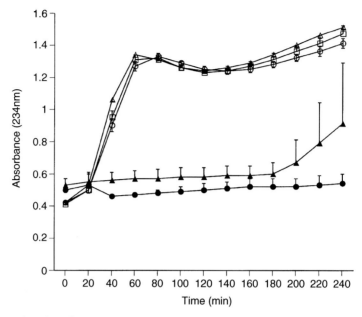

FIG. 2.   The effect of removing more than 90% of phenolics from red wine and grape juice on oxidation of LDL initiated with Cu as described in Fig. 1. The results are of three experiments done in duplicate. Control oxidation (□) was LDL plus PBS; ●, LDL plus 1:500 diluted red wine; ○, LDL plus 1:500 diluted phenolic-stripped red wine; ▲, LDL plus 1:500 diluted high-polyphenolic red grape juice; △, LDL plus 1:500 diluted phenolic-stripped red grape juice. (Reproduced with permission from Abu-Amsha et al 1996.)

products, including tea, liquorice, cola, cocoa and olive oil, have now been reported as showing significant *in vitro* antioxidant effects against oxidative modification of LDL.

In order to differentiate antioxidant effects due to Cu binding or free radical trapping, in our studies we used two different models of LDL oxidation, the Cu-induced oxidation of LDL and oxidation induced by peroxyl radicals generated during the thermal decomposition of AAPH (2,2'-azobis-[2-amidino-propane]hydrochloride). The phenolic compounds were more effective in inhibiting Cu-induced oxidation of LDL compared with AAPH-induced oxidation. This observation was not surprising given that phenolic compounds can actively bind Cu ions as well as trap free radicals (Nardini et al 1995). Since there is some evidence that redox reactive Cu ions may exist in atherosclerotic lesions, the potency of these naturally occurring substances to inhibit Cu-induced oxidation may have pathogenic relevance. Conceivably, similarly to ascorbic acid (Bowry & Stocker 1993), polyphenolics may also act as 'co-antioxidants', sparing

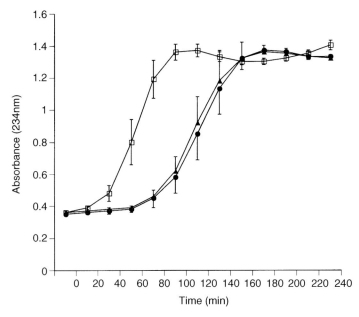

FIG. 3. Mean change ($\pm$ SEM) in conjugated diene absorbance at 234 nm over a 240 min period in LDL after initiation of peroxidation with 8 mM copper at 37 °C ($n = 5$). Control oxidation ($\square$) was LDL plus PBS vehicle. Both beverages tested were diluted 1:500. $\blacktriangle$, LDL plus full-strength beer; $\bullet$, LDL plus light beer. Both beer oxidation curves were significantly different from control: $P < 0.001$.

α-tocopherol from consumption during free radical attack and possibly regenerating α-tocopherol from the α-tocopherol radical.

In order to characterize further the most active antioxidant fractions, we separated acid-hydrolysed red wine by thin layer chromatography followed by GCMS analysis of the fractions (Abu-Amsha et al 1996). This process identified several cinnamic acid derivatives with important LDL antioxidant activity. Caffeic acid was potentially the most potent and significantly inhibited lipid hydroperoxide formation while sparing α-tocopherol consumption during Cu^{2+}-initiated LDL oxidation. We analysed only a single red wine, however, and in other wines catechins and procyanidins have shown the predominant antioxidant activity (Teissedre et al 1996), while Frankel and colleagues, after analysing 20 Californian wines together with their wide variety of polyphenolics, found the highest correlations were between gallic acid content and LDL antioxidant activity (Frankel et al 1995).

Before concluding from the results of these *in vitro* studies that the regular consumption of red wine may have possible health benefits due to antioxidant effects, some caveats need to be issued. Firstly, the chelation of metal ions such as copper and iron by flavonoids in oxidation systems that use catalytic transition metals may theoretically render them pro-oxidant (Cao et al 1997) presumably by reducing Cu^{2+} to Cu^+ and hence allowing the formation of initiating radicals. A similar phenomenon has been demonstrated *in vitro* with caffeic acid, which had significant pro-oxidant activity in the propagation phase of LDL oxidation (Laranjinha et al 1994). This phenomenon may have particular relevance where there is pre-existing tissue injury. In this situation transition metal ions, rather than being largely sequestered, may be released, catalyzing free radical reactions. Such a pro-oxidant effect with caffeic acid has not been seen in the initiation phase of Cu^{2+}-induced LDL oxidation; rather, inhibition has been consistently demonstrated (Nardini et al 1995, Abu-Amsha et al 1996). The second caveat relates to the insufficient attention given to the extent to which wine phenolics may actually be absorbed from the gut. Evidence suggests the flavonoid, quercetin, is absorbed and detectable in both blood and urine and with peak absorption 2–3 h after ingestion (Hollman et al 1995). Catechins have also been shown to be absorbed and are present in the plasma after 1 h and detectable in a 24 h urine sample after a single oral dose (Paganga & Rice-Evans 1997). The determination of the relative bioavailability of the many different red wine phenolics and the demonstration that they exhibit *in vivo* physiological effects needs to be a high priority if future research is to provide unambiguous evidence that they may have favourable effects to prevent atherosclerosis in humans.

Only a limited number of studies have attempted to define the effects of ingestion of wine and other alcoholic beverages on lipid peroxidation *in vivo*. These *in vivo* studies have been notable for their diverse outcomes, a consequence probably of the small numbers of subjects studied and several other methodological short-comings in what have often been quite brief reports. Differences in the polyphenolic profile of the various red wines utilized as well as the absorption and bioavailability of such compounds may be a further explanation. In several, only changes in the antioxidant capacity of serum, but not the oxidizability of LDL or serum, was measured following acute ingestion of red wine (Maxwell et al 1994, Whitehead et al 1995, Day & Stansbie 1995). Furthermore, levels of total or individual polyphenolics were not characterized and it therefore remains unclear whether the augmentation in serum antioxidant capacity reported has actually been due to ingestion of such substances. In this regard, one report noted that port wine acutely increased serum uric acid, a major serum antioxidant (Nyyssonen et al 1997), with a time course that matched the increase in total serum antioxidant capacity (Day & Stansbie 1995). In a recent study (R. Abu-Amsha Caccetta, personal communication) we have assessed 12 subjects after acute ingestion of red wine, de-alcoholized red wine, red wine which has been phenol-stripped, or water as a control. All three wines caused an acute increase in uric acid during the

4 h after ingestion but no acute influence on Cu^{2+}-initiated serum or LDL oxidation was seen. The claim therefore, that ingestion of antioxidant polyphenolics in red wine acutely increases serum antioxidant capacity or acutely reduces the oxidizability of LDL is not yet sustainable.

The results of longer-term feeding studies have also not led to consistent or definitive outcomes. Red wine has been administered for 2–4 week periods using either white wine (Fuhrman et al 1995, de Rijke et al 1995) or vodka (Kondo et al 1994) as control beverages. In the study by Fuhrman et al (1995), 17 men were divided into two groups, one that received white wine and the other red wine for 2 weeks (400 ml/day, both beverages 11% alcohol by volume). Whether allocation of subjects to each study group was random was not stated and no comparison was given of baseline diet or drinking habits to ensure comparability of the two groups. The red wine substantially inhibited LDL oxidation while precisely the opposite effect was seen with white wine. Red wine also resulted in a fourfold increase in LDL-associated polyphenols (as measured by a non-specific spectrophotometric method) but effects of white wine on this endpoint were not reported. Red wine but not white wine increased HDL levels and the implication of this increase in HDL for LDL susceptibility to oxidation (Parthasarathy et al 1990) was not discussed. The results corresponded with those of Kondo et al (1994) who also reported inhibition of LDL oxidation with red wine after it was administered for 2 weeks. However, that study was uncontrolled and the use of a baseline period during which vodka alone was consumed ignored the potential for confounding from effects of alcohol ingestion itself. In this regard, de Rijke et al (1995) found no effect on LDL oxidation of either red or white wine at 550 ml/day for 4 weeks, when both beverages had their alcohol content reduced to 3% alcohol by volume. The possibility of confounding by pro-oxidant effects of alcohol has also been highlighted by our recent study (Croft et al 1996) in which we compared the effects on LDL oxidation of 4 weeks of low versus high alcohol intake in 27 predominantly beer-drinking Australian men. Although we saw no effect of alcohol on LDL oxidation lag time, the change in serum conjugated diene formation when switching from low to high alcohol intake correlated with the self-reported change in alcohol intake (Fig. 4). Furthermore, analysis of the total oxidation curve was consistent with enhanced oxidation during the late propagation phase (Fig. 5). Japanese investigators have also studied the effects of changing alcohol intake on LDL oxidizability (Suzukawa et al 1994), but their two study groups were unbalanced with 12 subjects drinking brandy (0.5 g/kg per day) for 4 weeks compared with only four subjects who remained abstinent for the same period. Although no significant differences in LDL oxidation between the groups was found, LDL β-carotene content fell in those consuming brandy, again consistent with a pro-oxidant effect.

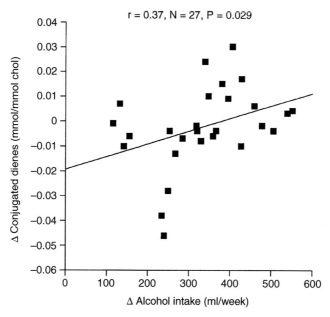

FIG. 4. Scattergam of change in conjugated diene formation when switching from low- to high-alcohol intake versus change in self-reported change in alcohol intake. (Reproduced with permission from Croft et al 1996.)

Apart from potential antioxidant effects of polyphenolic components of alcoholic beverages it has also been proposed that alcohol itself may promote a reductive environment at the level of the blood vessel wall (Bello et al 1994). The $\beta 1\beta 1$-isoenzyme of alcohol dehydrogenase is expressed in the endothelium of human arteries and veins (Bello et al 1994) and is thought to provide a metabolic pathway for defence against cytotoxic aldehydes generated by lipid peroxidation within the vascular wall. Alcohol, at least in low-to-moderate concentrations, may induce this enzyme and hence account for some of the protective influence of alcohol against atherosclerosis. The alternative hypothesis must also be considered, however, that alcohol at higher concentrations could interfere with alcohol dehydrogenase elimination of lipid peroxidation products, thereby contributing to pro-oxidative vascular damage, accelerating atherosclerosis and perhaps contributing to increased vascular tone and hypertension in the long term.

Pro-oxidative effects from the consumption of alcoholic beverages may also be anticipated from the lower levels of plasma selenium and other antioxidants such as α-tocopherol and ascorbic acid reported in alcoholic patients (Lecomte et al 1994). This finding may just reflect poor nutritional status in alcoholics but could equally well be secondary to enhanced antioxidant consumption because of pro-oxidant

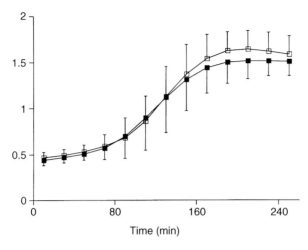

FIG. 5.   Change in absorbance units at 234 nM of LDL after addition of 5 mM of CuCl$_2$ in 27 subjects during low (■)- versus high (□)-alcohol intake periods. (Reproduced with permission from Croft et al 1996.)

stress from excess alcohol intake. In support of the latter possibility, a decrease in both serum and plasma β-carotene levels has been reported with heavy drinking even after adjustment for dietary intake and lipid profiles (Rimm & Colditz 1993). A pro-oxidant effect of excess alcohol use has long been proposed as a major mechanism in the pathogenesis of hepatic cirrhosis (Shaw et al 1983). Such ethanol-induced oxidative stress is also now a recognized phenomenon in extra-hepatic tissues (Nordmann et al 1990) and has been proposed as the basis for alcohol brain pathology, such as stroke (Altura & Gebrewold 1996) and cerebellar degeneration (Nordmann et al 1990), alcohol-related heart muscle disease, alcohol-associated tumour generation and testicular atrophy (Nordmann et al 1990).

Such oxidative stress could be accounted for by free radical generation at several possible steps in the pathways for ethanol metabolism. Ethanol induces microsomal cytochrome P$_{450}$ isozymes (especially 2E1), which in turn reduce NADPH to NADP, generating superoxide radicals and hydrogen peroxide. This mechanism has been proposed as the basis for increased hepatic lipid peroxidation following alcohol (Lieber 1997). Cytochrome P$_{450}$-2E1 induction also results in increased oxidation of ethanol to acetaldehyde. During subsequent acetaldehyde metabolism there is evidence for free radical generation due to NADH oxidation by aldehyde oxidase (Mira et al 1995) or from its metabolism by xanthine oxidase. Acetaldehyde can bind and inactivate both cysteine and glutathione, both potentially important pathways for scavenging free radicals and prevention of lipid peroxidation. It is also proposed that since superoxide radicals can liberate iron from ferritin, the induction of P_{450}-2E1 mobilizes iron from ferritin which in turn catalyzes lipid peroxidation (Song et al 1996). A suggestion that ethanol itself may be metabolized directly to a 1-hydroxyethyl radical (Moore et al 1995) may also be relevant but the toxicological significance of this pathway is uncertain. Ethanol can alter the activities of the antioxidant enzymes Cu/Zn superoxide dismutase and glutathione peroxidase, effects which may be direct but which could also reflect tissue depletion of zinc, copper and selenium.

Although oxidative stress from ethanol metabolism is suggested at least *in vitro* by evidence from a variety of sources, whether such *in vitro* effects translate into increased oxidative stress *in vivo* is less well established. Studies to date are consistent with probable increased pro-oxidant stress in alcoholics with reports of increased diene conjugated linoleic acid which falls during subsequent abstinence from alcohol (Fink et al 1985). Ethane exhalation, another marker of increased lipid peroxidation, however, correlated only weakly with reported daily alcohol intake by alcoholics (Letteron et al 1993). Further evidence is being sought utilizing more sophisticated approaches to the identification of increased *in vivo* lipid peroxidation including the measurement of urinary isoprostane excretion (Delanty et al 1996).

In conclusion, the current evidence for increased oxidative stress following at least heavy alcohol consumption, and the links between such oxidative stress and alcohol-mediated disease, need to be considered in any balanced treatment of the hypothesis that polyphenolic compounds in alcoholic beverages, especially red wine, may have anti-atherosclerotic effects. Future research needs to clarify the overall balance of the redox effects of alcohol and of such polyphenolics in alcoholic beverages using state-of-the-art markers of oxidative stress *in vivo*. It also needs to clarify which specific polyphenolic compounds are absorbed from the gut as well as the extent of any potential *in vivo* physiological effects. In the absence of this information and in the light of those studies so far completed, there is insufficient evidence to justify promotion of the consumption of certain alcoholic beverages on the grounds that they have unique antioxidant properties which will prevent atherosclerotic cardiovascular disease.

References

Abu-Amsha R, Croft KD, Puddey IB, Proudfoot JM, Beilin LJ 1996 Phenolic content of various beverages determines the extent of inhibition of human serum and low-density lipoprotein oxidation *in vitro*—identification and mechanism of action of some cinnamic acid derivatives from red wine. Clin Sci 91:449–458

Altura BM, Gebrewold A 1996 α-tocopherol attenuates alcohol-induced cerebral vascular damage in rats: possible role of oxidants in alcohol brain pathology and stroke. Neurosci Lett 220:207–210

Auw JM, Blanco V, O'Keefe SF, Sims CA 1996 Effect of processing on the phenolics and colour of Cabernet Sauvignon, Chambourcin, and noble wines and juices. Am J Enol Vitic 47:279–286

Belguendouz L, Fremont L, Linard A 1997 Resveratrol inhibits metal ion-dependent and independent peroxidation of porcine low-density lipoproteins. Biochem Pharmacol 53:1347–1355

Bello AT, Bora NS, Lange LG, Bora PS 1994 Cardioprotective effects of alcohol: mediation by human vascular alcohol dehydrogenase. Biochem Biophys Res Commun 203:1858–1864

Bowry VW, Stocker R 1993 Tocopherol-mediated peroxidation. The prooxidant effect of vitamin E on the radical-initiated oxidation of human low-density lipoprotein. J Am Chem Soc 115:6029–6044

Cao G, Sofic E, Prior RL 1997 Antioxidant and prooxidant behavior of flavonoids: structure-activity relationships. Free Radical Biol Med 22:749–760

Croft KD, Puddey IB, Rakic V, Abu-Amsha R, Dimmitt SB, Beilin LJ 1996 Oxidative susceptibility of low-density lipoproteins—influence of regular alcohol use. Alcohol Clin Exp Res 20:980–984

da Silva R, Darmon N, Fernandez Y, Mitjavila S 1991 Oxygen free radical scavenger capacity in aqueous models of different procyanidins from grape seeds. J Agric Food Chem 39:1549–1552

Day A, Stansbie D 1995 Cardioprotective effect of red wine may be mediated by urate. Clin Chem 41:1319–1320

Delanty N, Reilly M, Pratico D, Fitzgerald DJ, Lawson JA, Fitzgerald GA 1996 8-Epi PGF$_{2\alpha}$: specific analysis of an eicosanoid as an index of oxidant stress *in vivo*. Br J Clin Pharmacol 42:15–19

de Rijke YB, Demacker PNM, Assen NA, Sloots LM, Katan MB, Stalenhoef AFH 1995 Red wine consumption and oxidation of low-density lipoproteins. Lancet 345:325–326

Fink R, Marjot DH, Cawood P et al 1985 Increased free-radical activity in alcoholics. Lancet 2:291–294

Frankel EN, Waterhouse AL, Kinsella JE 1993a Inhibition of human LDL oxidation by resveratrol. Lancet 341:1103–1104

Frankel EN, Kanner J, German JB, Parks E, Kinsella JE 1993b Inhibition of oxidation of human low-density lipoprotein by phenolic substances in red wine. Lancet 341:454–457

Frankel EN, Waterhouse AL, Teissedre PL 1995 Principal phenolic phytochemicals in selected California wines and their antioxidant activity in inhibiting oxidation of human low-density lipoproteins. J Agric Food Chem 43:890–894

Fuhrman B, Lavy A, Aviram M 1995 Consumption of red wine with meals reduces the susceptibility of human plasma and low density lipoprotein to lipid peroxidation. Am J Clin Nutr 61:549–554

Hollman PCH, Devries JHM, Vanleeuwen SD, Mengelers MJB, Katan MB 1995 Absorption of dietary quercetin glycosides and quercetin in healthy ileostomy volunteers. Am J Clin Nutr 62:1276–1282

Kanner J, Frankel E, Granit R, German B, Kinsella JE 1994 Natural antioxidants in grapes and wines. J Agric Food Chem 42:64–69

Kondo K, Matsumoto A, Kurata H et al 1994 Inhibition of oxidation of low-density lipoprotein with red wine. Lancet 344:1152

Kovac V, Alonso E, Revilla E 1995 The effect of adding supplementary quantities of seeds during fermentation on the phenolic composition of wines. Am J Enol Vitic 46:363–367

Lanningham-Foster L, Chen C, Chance DS, Loo G 1995 Grape extract inhibits lipid peroxidation of human low density lipoprotein. Biol Pharm Bull 18:1347–1351

Laranjinha JAN, Almeida LM, Madeira VMC 1994 Reactivity of dietary phenolic acids with peroxyl radicals: antioxidant activity upon low density lipoprotein peroxidation. Biochem Pharmacol 48:487–494

Lecomte E, Herbeth B, Pirollet P et al 1994 Effect of alcohol consumption on blood antioxidant nutrients and oxidative stress indicators. Am J Clin Nutr 60:255–261

Letteron P, Duchatelle V, Berson A et al 1993 Increased ethane exhalation, an *in vivo* index of lipid peroxidation, in alcohol-abusers. Gut 34:409–414

Lieber CS 1997 Cytochrome P-450E1: its physiological and pathological role. Physiol Rev 77:517–544

Maxwell S, Cruickshank A, Thorpe G 1994 Red wine and antioxidant activity in serum. Lancet 344:193–194

Meyer AS, Yi OS, Pearson DA, Waterhouse AL, Frankel EN 1997 Inhibition of human low-density lipoprotein oxidation in relation to composition of phenolic antioxidants in grapes (*Vitis vinifera*). J Agric Food Chem 45:1638–1643

Mira L, Maia L, Barreira L, Manso CF 1995 Evidence for free radical generation due to NADH oxidation by aldehyde oxidase during ethanol metabolism. Arch Biochem Biophys 318:55–58

Moore DR, Reinke LA, McCay PB 1995 Metabolism of ethanol to 1-hydroyethyl radicals *in vivo*: detection with intravenous administration of α-(4-pyridyl-1-oxide)-N-t-butylnitrone. Mol Pharmacol 47:1224–1230

Nardini M, D'Aquino M, Tomassi G, Gentili V, Di Felice M, Scaccini C 1995 Inhibition of human low-density lipoprotein oxidation by caffeic acid and other hydroxycinnamic acid derivatives. Free Radical Biol Med 19:541–552

Nordmann R, Ribiere C, Rouach H 1990 Ethanol-induced lipid peroxidation and oxidative stress in extrahepatic tissues. Alcohol Alcohol 25:231–237

Nyyssonen K, Porkkala-Sarataho E, Kaikkonen J, Salonen JT 1997 Ascorbate and urate are the strongest determinants of plasma antioxidative capacity and serum lipid resistance to oxidation in Finnish men. Atherosclerosis 130:223–233

Paganga G, Rice-Evans CA 1997 The identification of flavonoids as glycosides in human plasma. FEBS Lett 401:78–82

Parthasarathy S, Barnett J, Fong LG 1990 High-density lipoprotein inhibits the oxidative modification of low-density lipoprotein. Biochim Biophys Acta 1044:275–283

Rimm E, Colditz G 1993 Smoking, alcohol, and plasma levels of carotenes and vitamin E. Ann N Y Acad Sci 686:323–334

Shaw S, Rubin KP, Lieber CS 1983 Depressed hepatic glutathione and increased diene conjugates in alcoholic liver disease: evidence of lipid peroxidation. Dig Dis Sci 28:585–589

Song BJ, Koop AI, Cederbaum AI, Ingelman-Sundberg M, Nanji A 1996 Ethanol-inducible cytochrome P450 (CYP2E1): biochemistry, molecular biology and clinical relevance: 1996 update. Alcohol Clin Exp Res 20:138A–146A

Steinberg D, Parthasarathy S, Carew TE, Khoo JC, Witzum JL 1989 Beyond cholesterol. Modifications of low-density lipoprotein that increase its atherogenicity. N Engl J Med 320:915–924

Suzukawa M, Ishikawa T, Yoshida H et al 1994 Effects of alcohol consumption on antioxidant content and susceptibility of low-density lipoprotein to oxidative modification. J Am Coll Nutr 13:237–242

Teissedre PL, Frankel EN, Waterhouse AL, Peleg H, German JB 1996 Inhibition of *in vitro* human LDL oxidation by phenolic antioxidants from grapes and wines. J Sci Food Agric 70:55–61

Verhagen JV, Haenen GRMM, Bast A 1996 Nitric oxide radical scavenging by wines. J Agric Food Chem 44:3733–3734

Whitehead TP, Robinson D, Allaway S, Syms J, Hale A 1995 Effect of red wine ingestion on the antioxidant capacity of serum. Clin Chem 41:32–35

DISCUSSION

Grønbæk: Onions, apples and several other fruits and vegetables also contain polyphenols, so why do we focus on wine?

Puddey: That is a good point. Several studies have shown that olive oil (Aviram & Eias 1993) and tea (Ishikawa et al 1997), for instance, have a comparable antioxidant effect to wine. Our group has looked at the skin of mangostin, a tropical fruit, which has potent antioxidant effects (Williams et al 1995). All fruits and vegetables with these polyphenolic compounds and their products must have the potential to cause various degrees of inhibition of serum LDL oxidation.

Shaper: Could you say something about the magnitude of the antioxidant effect? One story doing the rounds is that a single onion has as much polyphenol or flavonoid content as a whole bottle of wine.

Puddey: I can't give you a precise figure, but certainly quercetin is well represented in those food groups. From grape juice and from fruits you can ingest quite high levels of specific polyphenol compounds, each of which inhibits LDL oxidation to varying degrees. Frankel and others have tried to isolate the relative effects of the different polyphenols (Frankel et al 1995, Teissedre et al 1996), but it is still far from clear which are the most potent.

Grønbæk: When you strip red wine of its phenolic compounds, do you also remove other compounds?

Puddey: We're using a PVP (polyvinylpolypyrrolidone) column and, as far as we have been able to ascertain, all we take out are the polyphenolics.

Keaney: Your data are a good demonstration that what happens in the test-tube is not always the same as what goes on *in vivo*, especially with LDL oxidation assays. The important thing to realize is that on the basis of some of the biochemical characteristics of these compounds, you wouldn't expect them to have an effect on isolated LDL, since most of these compounds are water soluble and are removed during the LDL isolation process.

Ascorbic acid and urate are present in plasma at concentrations of 50 μM and up to 300 μM, respectively. The steady-state concentration of these phenolic compounds may well be 5–6 μM. To what extent do you think they can really contribute to any degree of antioxidant protection in your circumstances?

Puddey: This awaits further studies. The literature has been promulgated as showing that these *in vitro* effects translate into *in vivo* effects. I think studies are not clear-cut; they certainly have not been uniform. And, as I tried to show, there are alternative explanations. The increase in uric acid is more likely to be responsible for that initial increase in the antioxidant capacity of serum than any of these polyphenolic compounds.

Shaper: Certainly there is a very linear relationship between alcohol intake and urate levels (Shaper et al 1985).

Puddey: That is a separate issue. Neither our group nor Whitehead's group (Whitehead et al 1995) were able to show, using just alcohol alone, that there was an increase in urate over the 4 h following acute ingestion. However, in the longer-term you are correct that alcohol is associated with higher uric acid levels.

Keil: If I understood you correctly, the potential daily intake of these polyphenols from food is much greater than that from two or three glasses of wine.

Puddey: I don't know about 'much greater', because the actual polyphenol content in red wine is very high. This is probably a function of the grape skins being crushed, how long the must is in contact with the grape skins and the prolonged preparation of the wine over many years. So red wine does provide a quick boost of polyphenols relative to other sources.

A more important question concerns the extent to which the polyphenols are absorbed from all these different sources. And, if they are, do they reach significant concentrations in plasma? Fuhrman et al (1995) looked at isolated LDL and reported, at least with their red wine, a fourfold increase in LDL-associated polyphenols. Water soluble or not, they suggested that there was an increment, but they used a non-specific assay of those polyphenolic compounds: I think we need far more clear-cut and precise measurements of polyphenols in both serum and associated with LDL before we can take it as given that they are absorbed and they do have *in vivo* physiological effects.

Gorelick: How long does the antioxidant effect last *in vitro?* It would seem that the public might be better off eating foods rich in polyphenols to sustain the effect, if that of drinking alcohol is short-lived.

Puddey: In vitro we've only looked at 4 h of oxidation and the curves remain flat for 4 h after a 1:500 dilution, as applied to both LDL and serum. From this we can't discern its significance in terms of the magnitude and duration of any *in vivo* effect.

Rehm: Under the best conditions, what proportion of the overall beneficial effect of alcohol could be apportioned to inhibition of the oxidation process? What would be the approximate differential impact of the different mechanisms we know alcohol is having?

Puddey: At this stage there is insufficient evidence for us to invoke an antioxidant effect from the ingestion of alcoholic beverages in mediating any beneficial effect of alcohol on cardiovascular disease endpoints.

Gaziano: This is even further complicated by the fact that examining plasma LDL *ex vivo* doesn't tell us what's going on in the arterial wall, in the subendothelial space. This is where those who are strong supporters of the notion that oxidative stress may play a role in atherosclerosis tell us that a great deal of oxidation may occur. A further complicating factor is that HDL may act to protect LDL from oxidation. There is probably transfer of substances from LDL to and from HDL, so HDL could have an effect on isolated LDL: it is much more complicated than in an isolated *in vitro* model.

Keaney: Your idea about alcohol causing the pro-oxidant effect in isolated LDL is not without some hazard. The alcohol, of course, would be excluded from your isolation procedure and you would have to then hypothesize that it does something that stably modifies the LDL particle.

Puddey: Given the constraints of time I didn't present you with the data from experiments where we took different concentrations of alcohol, and showed in both the serum and LDL model that there was no impact of just adding alcohol on the oxidation of LDL (Abu-Amsha et al 1996). This doesn't surprise me, given that all of the postulated mechanisms for the pro-oxidant effects of alcohol rely on its metabolism either to the so-called ethyl alcohol radical (if you believe that this occurs *in vivo*) or the other pathways we discussed.

Keaney: You would still have to come up with a mechanism whereby alcohol modifies the LDL particle to explain the increase in oxidation.

Criqui: I just wanted to second the idea that the oxidation hypothesis is still fairly young. The supposed data on the beneficial effects of antioxidants that were taken from population cohort studies have so far been uniformly refuted by the early clinical trials. For example, the epidemiological data that beta carotene helped prevent lung cancer in smokers were so strong that several trials were done, yet all the trials we have to date, despite claims to the contrary, are negative (Gaziano 1996, Jha et al 1995). Something funny is going on at a very elementary level of understanding. Some people suggested that this was because the benefit was derived from multiple separate antioxidants in food, but that argument doesn't hold, because the benefit in some population studies was shown to be due to supplements. The science here is somehow more rudimentary than we think it is.

Peters: So to summarize, there is an epidemiological association, but the intervention studies are negative so far.

Keaney: Yes, although after the epidemiological association studies, there were epidemiologists who went on record as saying people should be taking these compounds.

Criqui: There's a good example of how confusing this area can be. There is a drug called probucol, a powerful antioxidant which is unusual in that it lowers both LDL and HDL cholesterol simultaneously. On the basis of animal work this was thought to be good enough to try in humans, and was sold commercially. The Probucol Quantitative Regression Swedish Trial (PQRST) showed no benefit whatsoever (Walldius et al 1994). Subsequently, a recent study has shown a marked reduction in restenosis with probucol post-angioplasty (Tardif et al 1997) and yet a second arm of the trial was an antioxidant cocktail which showed no benefit: in fact antioxidants appeared to reduce the benefit of probucol in the combined probucol and antioxidant arm, thereby suggesting this antioxidant cocktail somehow produced pro-oxidant effects in the body and partially counteracted the benefit of probucol. It is extremely complicated, and before we start giving people antioxidant drugs we need to know more about what's going on.

Peters: What could the explanation be? Is there a variable we're not considering?

Keaney: In the animal studies the serendipitous event was using rabbits as the first animal model. Rabbits actually metabolize probucol to an active metabolite which may be more responsible for the effect. In mice and humans, probucol doesn't work.

Gaziano: I agree with your assessment of what we know about antioxidant supplements, but I think that we have to uncouple the two questions about whether or not oxidative stress plays a role in atherosclerosis and whether or not we can augment any oxygen defences. We have no idea of whether these substances are really behaving as antioxidants *in vivo*. In observational studies antioxidant supplement intake may be associated with other healthy behaviours. In terms of our understanding of oxidation and antioxidants, we are where the cholesterol hypothesis was 40 years ago.

Renaud: In your introduction you mentioned the effect of polyphenols on α-tocopherol, but you didn't present any data. Have you any results suggesting polyphenols have an effect on α-tocopherol?

Puddey: In our *Clinical Science* paper (Abu-Amsha et al 1996) we did look at the actual content of LDL tocopherol, in the presence and absence of caffeic acid using both the AAPH effect and the Cu^{2+}-induced oxidation models. We showed that the caffeic acid protected the tocopherol from consumption during that early lag phase of LDL decomposition.

References

Abu-Amsha R, Croft KD, Puddey IB, Proudfoot JM, Beilin LJ 1996 Phenolic content of various beverages determines the extent of inhibition of human serum and low density lipoprotein oxidation *in vitro*—identification and mechanism of action of some cinnamic acid derivatives from red wine. Clin Sci 91:449–458

Aviram M, Eias K 1993 Dietary olive oil reduced low-density lipoprotein uptake by macrophages and decreases the susceptibility of the lipoprotein to undergo lipid peroxidation. Ann Nutr Metab 37:75–84

Frankel EN, Waterhouse AL, Teissedre PL 1995 Principal phenolic phytochemicals in selected California wines and their antioxidant activity in inhibiting oxidation of human low-density lipoproteins. J Agric Food Chem 43:890–894

Fuhrman B, Lavy A, Aviram M 1993 Consumption of red wine with meals reduces the susceptibility of human plasma and low-density lipoprotein to lipid peroxidation. Am J Clin Nutr 61:549–554

Gaziano JM 1996 Randomized trials of dietary antioxidants in cardiovascular disease prevention and treatment. J Cardiovasc Risk 3:368–371

Ishikawa T, Suzukawa M, Ito T et al 1997 Effect of tea flavonoid supplementation on the susceptibility of low-density lipoprotein to oxidative modification. Am J Clin Nutr 66:261–266

Jha P, Flather M, Lonn E, Farkouh M, Yusuf S 1995 The antioxidant vitamins and cardiovascular disease. A critical review of epidemiologic and clinical trial data. Ann Intern Med 123:860–872

Shaper AG, Pocock SJ, Ashby D, Walker M, Whitehead TP 1985 Biochemical and haematological response to alcohol intake. Ann Clin Biochem 22:50–61

Tardif JC, Côté G, Lespérance J et al 1997 Probucol and multivitamins in the prevention of restenosis after coronary angioplasty. Multivitamins and Probucol Study Group. N Engl J Med 337:365–372

Teissedre PL, Frankel EN, Waterhouse AL, Peleg H, German JB 1996 Inhibition of *in vitro* human LDL oxidation by phenolic antioxidants from grapes and wines. J Sci Food Agric 70:55–61

Walldius G, Erikson U, Olsson AG et al 1994 The effect of probucol on femoral atherosclerosis: the Probucol Quantitative Regression Swedish Trial (PQRST). Am J Cardiol 74:875–883

Whitehead TP, Robinson D, Allaway S, Syms J, Hale A 1995 Effect of red wine ingestion on the antioxidant capacity of serum. Clin Chem 41:32–35

Williams P, Ongsakul M, Proudfoot J, Croft K, Beilin L 1995 Mangostin inhibits the oxidative modification of human low density lipoprotein. Free Radical Res 23:175–184

Alcohol, cardiac arrhythmias and sudden death

Markku Kupari and Pekka Koskinen

Division of Cardiology (Department of Medicine), Helsinki University Central Hospital, FIN-00290 Helsinki, Finland

Abstract. Studies in experimental animals have shown varying and apparently opposite effects of alcohol on cardiac rhythm and conduction. Given acutely to non-alcoholic animals, ethanol may even have anti-arrhythmic properties whereas chronic administration clearly increases the animals' susceptibility to cardiac arrhythmias. Chronic heavy alcohol use has been incriminated in the genesis of cardiac arrhythmias in humans. The evidence has come from clinical observations, retrospective case-control studies, controlled studies of consecutive admissions for arrhythmias, and prospective epidemiological investigations. Furthermore, electrophysiological studies have shown that acute alcohol administration facilitates the induction of tachyarrhythmias in selected heavy drinkers. The role of alcohol appears particularly conspicuous in idiopathic atrial fibrillation. Occasionally, ventricular tachyarrhythmias have also been provoked by alcohol intake. Several lines of evidence suggest that heavy drinking increases the risk of sudden cardiac death with fatal arrhythmia as the most likely mechanism. According to epidemiological studies this effect appears most prominent in middle-aged men and is only partly explained by confounding traits such as smoking and social class. The basic arrhythmogenic effects of alcohol are still insufficiently delineated. Subclinical heart muscle injury from chronic heavy use may be instrumental in producing patchy delays in conduction. The hyperadrenergic state of drinking and withdrawal may also contribute, as may electrolyte abnormalities, impaired vagal heart rate control, repolarization abnormalities with prolonged QT intervals and worsening of myocardial ischaemia or sleep apnoea. Most of what we know about alcohol and arrhythmias relates to heavy drinking. The effect of social drinking on clinical arrhythmias in non-alcoholic cardiac patients needs to be addressed further.

1998 Alcohol and cardiovascular diseases. Wiley, Chichester (Novartis Foundation Symposium 216) p 68–85

Many clinicians feel that patients admitted with acute and seemingly unexplained atrial fibrillation are heavy alcohol drinkers more often than would be expected. Typically the patient is a middle-aged man who, apart from arrhythmia, has no signs of cardiac disease and who denies anything but social drinking despite laboratory or clinical signs of alcohol abuse. Sinus rhythm is often restored spontaneously and the short-term course appears benign. Pathologists examining victims of sudden unexpected cardiac death also encounter heavy drinkers more often than expected. Frequently, the autopsy shows only fatty degeneration of the liver; no gross abnormalities of the heart or other organs are seen and the coronary arteries are patent. These kind of observations initially raised the idea that alcohol plays a role in the onset of cardiac arrhythmias and in sudden arrhythmic deaths. However, in the era of 'evidence-based medicine' we need more valid data to accept the presence of a true association, let alone causality. In this review we summarize the evidence linking alcohol with cardiac arrhythmias and sudden death. We will focus on human research but begin with a concise presentation of pertinent studies in experimental animals.

Studies in experimental animals

Acute effects of ethanol in non-alcoholic animals

The effects of alcohol on the electrophysiology of the heart have been tested *in vitro* in myocardial preparations as well as *in vivo* in non-alcoholic animals. At concentrations of 100–450 mg/100 ml blood, ethanol acutely shortens the duration of action potential in atrial and ventricular myocardial preparations without influencing the resting membrane potential (Gimeno et al 1962, Williams et al 1980). In anaesthetized dogs, acute alcohol administration inhibits atrioventricular and intraventricular conduction and lengthens the sinus node recovery time (Goodkind et al 1975). Some of the electrophysiological effects of ethanol, such as its influence on the action potential, are similar to those of many antiarrhythmic drugs. Indeed, several studies have suggested that in non-alcoholic animals ethanol suppresses chemically or electrically provoked atrial tachyarrhythmias as well as ischaemic ventricular arrhythmias (Nguyen et al 1987, Gilmour et al 1981, Bernauer 1986). Kostis et al have reported in two papers (Kostis et al 1973, 1977) that atrial and ventricular fibrillation thresholds are increased by acute ethanol administration.

Effects of chronic ethanol administration

In a canine study of the chronic cardiac effects of alcohol (Ettinger et al 1976), long-term ethanol administration (36% of daily calories for 1 year) resulted in prolonged intraventricular but not atrial conduction and morphological changes in the ventricular myocardium. Ventricular fibrillation threshold was unaltered in the basal state but declined by more than 50% after acute ethanol infusion. Neither non-alcoholic control animals receiving ethanol intravenously nor alcoholic animals infused saline showed any changes in ventricular fibrillation threshold. Patterson et al (1987) reported that selective chronic administration of ethanol into one coronary branch of dogs decreased the resting membrane potential as well as the amplitude, upstroke and duration of action potential compared with the control myocardial zone. Myocardial refractoriness was prolonged. Ventricular stimulation caused arrhythmias in 14 of 22 ethanol-treated dogs but in none of six control animals receiving intracoronary saline infusion. Guideri et al (1988) studied rats given alcohol for seven weeks and found that the incidence of malignant ventricular arrhythmias after isoprenaline challenge was highest in 'alcohol withdrawal' group as compared with rats either continuing alcohol ingestion or drinking water.

Altogether the experimental studies suggest that the effects of alcohol on cardiac rhythm and conduction are different in non-alcoholic and alcoholic animals. While alcohol may even have antiarrhythmic and antifibrillatory actions acutely in non-alcoholic animals, chronic drinking increases the propensity to cardiac arrhythmias.

Effects of alcohol on cardiac rhythm and conduction in non-alcoholic patients

The influence of alcohol on intracardiac electrophysiology in non-alcoholic cardiac patients has been assessed in two small studies (Gould et al 1974, 1978). The first work showed that a single moderate dose of alcohol (60 ml of whisky) prolonged conduction in the His-Purkinje system but not in the atrioventricular node or intra-atrially. In the later study, His-Purkinje conduction was not altered after a comparable dose of alcohol but atrioventricular nodal conduction was prolonged and the ventricular refractory period was shortened. Since the data are uncontrolled and are not in agreement, their significance remains very limited.

Kentala et al (1976) studied the influence of alcohol on cardiac rhythm in 10 non-alcoholic postmyocardial infarction patients ingesting ethanol 'as much as they wanted'. Twenty-four hour ambulatory electrocardiographic recordings showed a slightly higher number of ventricular ectopic beats after alcohol than prior to drinking, but no significant arrhythmias were seen. Rossinen et al (1996) did not find any effect of ethanol intake (1.25 g/kg) on the number of ventricular ectopic beats in 20 patients with stable angina pectoris and angiographically documented coronary artery disease even though the patients had more myocardial ischaemia after ethanol. Dolly & Block (1983) studied patients with chronic obstructive pulmonary disease and found that alcohol intake increased the number of cardiac ectopic beats and periods of sleep apnoea; peak blood alcohol concentration was 40 mg/100 ml. Altogether the data on the acute effects of alcohol on cardiac rhythm in non-alcoholic persons are clearly insufficient. Whether social drinking provokes or prevents clinically significant arrhythmias, or has no effects, remains unknown.

Cardiac arrhythmias and electrophysiology in alcoholic patients

Clinical observations and ambulatory electrocardiography

A number of well-documented case histories have suggested that alcoholic persons may suffer from post-drink premature contractions, atrial fibrillation and even ventricular tachycardia in the absence of clinical heart disease (Singer & Lundberg 1972, Greenspon et al 1979). In a widely cited observational study, Ettinger et al (1978) reported 32 admissions for atrial tachyarrhythmias, mainly atrial fibrillation, in 24 chronic heavy drinkers. The patients had no clinically detectable heart disease and the arrhythmias disappeared with abstinence without evident residual. Curiously, many episodes occurred during weekends or year-end holidays which led the investigators to coin the term 'holiday heart syndrome'.

The prevalence of cardiac arrhythmias in larger and less selected alcoholic populations have been studied by ambulatory electrocardiography both during withdrawal and after varying periods of abstinence. In general, these studies have shown little or no differences in the rate of cardiac arrhythmias like atrial fibrillation or unsustained ventricular tachycardia between alcoholics free of heart disease and the general population (Abbasakoor et al 1976, Buckingham et al 1985).

Acute-on-chronic effects of alcohol by intracardiac electrophysiology

The effects of acute alcohol intake on intracardiac electrophysiology in alcoholics have been assessed in small groups of patients presenting with symptoms of clinically significant arrhythmias (Greenspon & Schaal 1983, Engel & Luck 1983). Greenspon & Schaal (1983) studied 14 alcoholics of whom 11 had identifiable cardiac disease and 6 had left ventricular dysfunction. They observed prolongation of His to ventricle conduction but no changes in intra-atrial conduction or atrial or ventricular refractory periods after 90 ml of whisky. Atrial or ventricular tachyarrhythmias were provoked by the extrastimulus technique in eight of the 14 patients post-alcohol but in none before alcohol. Engel & Luck (1983) studied 11 chronic alcoholics free of cardiac disease and showed that atrial tachyarrhythmias could be provoked by intracardiac stimulation in the majority either prior to ($n = 4$) or after ingestion of 60–120 ml of whisky ($n = 3$). They also studied three non-alcoholic individuals with sinus node dysfunction and found that atrial arrhythmias could be provoked in two individuals after alcohol ingestion. The value of these studies is undermined by the fact that the study groups were highly selected. The findings confirm that alcohol intake increases the susceptibility to cardiac arrhythmias in alcoholic individuals in whom drinking has previously provoked arrhythmias or palpitations. However, they do not prove that alcoholics in general have an increased vulnerability to cardiac arrhythmias after acute alcohol intake.

Alcohol consumption in patients admitted to hospital for cardiac arrhythmias

Several investigators have focused on the drinking histories of patients admitted for cardiac arrhythmias in an attempt to show the arrhythmogenic role of alcohol. In addition to selected case series (Ettinger et al 1978), there exist retrospective studies of hospital records (Lowenstein et al 1983, Rich et al 1985) and controlled clinical investigations of consecutive admissions for arrhythmias (Koskinen 1991). All works involve patients with atrial arrhythmias; there are no comparable data on alcohol consumption in patients admitted for ventricular arrhythmias.

Retrospective studies of case records

Lowenstein et al (1983) retrospectively studied the causal factors of new-onset atrial fibrillation in 40 patients identified from hospital records. The arrhythmia was attributed to alcohol when ethanol was found in the patient's blood or breath and no other cause was evident. Alcohol was considered the sole aetiological factor in 23% of all episodes and caused or contributed to 63% of arrhythmias in patients less than 65 years of age. Unfortunately, no control group was included. Rich et al (1985) retrospectively studied the records of 64 patients with idiopathic atrial fibrillation to identify heavy alcohol consumers. Records of 64 age and sex-matched control patients selected at random from among general medical admissions were evaluated in an identical way. In total 63% of patients with idiopathic atrial fibrillation but only 33% of the control patients were classified as heavy alcohol consumers.

Controlled studies of consecutive admissions for arrhythmias

We have studied the role of alcohol in consecutive admissions to the Emergency Room of Helsinki University Central Hospital for new-onset atrial fibrillation ($n = 98$), recurrent atrial fibrillation ($n = 98$) or other supraventricular tachy-arrhythmias ($n = 99$) (Koskinen et al 1987, 1990, Koskinen & Kupari 1991). The patients were examined clinically and by echocardiography and questioned regarding their present and past alcohol consumption. For each arrhythmia case, an age and sex-matched control patient was identified from the other Emergency Room patients. In the two later studies (Koskinen et al 1990, Koskinen & Kupari 1991), another control group was selected at random from the local general population. We found that patients with idiopathic new-onset atrial fibrillation

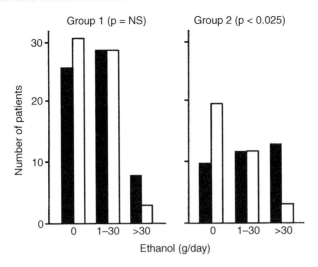

FIG. 1. Average daily alcohol consumption of the patients with new-onset atrial fibrillation (black columns) and of the control patients (white columns). Group 1, disease-related atrial fibrillation. Group 2, idiopathic atrial fibrillation.

had recently drunk more alcohol than their controls whereas patients with disease-related new-onset atrial fibrillation had no excess drinking compared with controls (Fig. 1). Patients with recurrent atrial fibrillation also reported higher alcohol consumption during the week preceding admission than controls derived from the Emergency Room. However, there was no statistically significant difference in self-reported alcohol use between patients with recurrent arrhythmia and the control group derived from the general population. A screening test for alcoholism consisting of four questions (CAGE questionnaire) was administered to all participants. The frequency of individuals responding affirmatively to each of the questions was 12% among patients with recurrent atrial fibrillation and 2% in the population control subjects ($P = 0.06$). Among men, the corresponding frequencies were 16% and none ($P = 0.008$). In logistic regression analysis, the CAGE response and weekly alcohol use were significantly related to the occurrence of recurrent atrial fibrillation in men but not in women. Patients admitted for supraventricular tachyarrhythmias other than atrial fibrillation did not differ from either hospital controls or the population control group regarding alcohol consumption or responses to the CAGE questionnaire.

We also analysed the time of arrhythmia onset in relation to alcohol consumption in the 102 patients who had idiopathic atrial tachyarrhythmias (Kupari & Koskinen 1991). We found that the proportion of problem drinkers by the CAGE questionnaire was statistically significantly higher in weekend

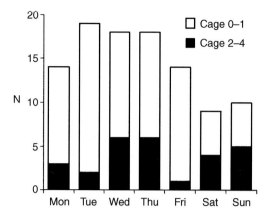

FIG. 2. Relation of the day of onset of idiopathic atrial tachyarrhythmia to the CAGE questionnaire response. The columns show the number (N) of patients and the proportion of individuals with two or more affirmative responses to the CAGE questions each day of the week.

arrhythmias (onset on Saturdays or on Sundays) than in arrhythmias beginning from Mondays through Fridays. However, this was not due to an absolute clustering of problem drinkers' arrhythmias but to a reduced rate of arrhythmias in abstainers and non-problem drinkers during weekends (Fig. 2).

Prospective epidemiological data on alcohol and atrial tachyarrhythmias

In a prospective study of people participating in a health screening examination, Cohen et al (1988) studied the incidence of supraventricular tachyarrhythmias in relation to self-reported alcohol consumption. The combined incidence of atrial fibrillation or flutter and paroxysmal atrial tachycardia was significantly higher among 1322 persons with an intake of six drinks or more per day than in 2344 people consuming less than one drink a day (relative risk, 2.3, $P < 0.05$). The diagnosis of arrhythmias was based on electrocardiograms and medical records available after the initial examination. The follow-up time was not reported.

Alcohol and sudden cardiac death

Necropsy studies

Several necropsy studies have shown that alcohol abusers die suddenly more often than expected and that up to one fourth of sudden cardiac deaths in young and middle-aged adults may be linked to heavy drinking with fatty liver degeneration (Kramer et al 1968, Randall 1980). A number of mechanisms for sudden death in alcoholics free of evident heart disease have been raised including fat embolization and severe withdrawal hypoglycaemia, but ventricular tachyarrhythmia degenerating into fibrillation is believed to be likely cause in most instances.

Prospective epidemiological investigations

Large population studies have supported the presence of a true association between heavy drinking and sudden death. In the 1970s the Social Insurance Institution in Finland conducted a prospective population study comprising 4532 men aged 40–64 years. Suhonen et al (1987) analysed the five year cardiac mortality in relation to the participants' self-reported alcohol consumption. The incidence of sudden coronary death increased statistically significantly with increasing alcohol consumption in men with and without pre-existent coronary artery disease. The predictive value of alcohol consumption was most evident in non-smokers and in the oldest age group. In the British Regional Heart Study, 7735 men aged 40–59 were followed for all cause and cardiovascular mortality for eight years (Wannamethee & Shaper 1992). It was found that men consuming more than six drinks daily ('heavy drinkers') had a significantly higher rate of sudden deaths than men drinking less or not at all; the relative risk was 1.73 (95% CI 1.06–2.86) after adjustment for age, social class and smoking. Further analyses indicated that the association of sudden death incidence with heavy drinking was most apparent in older men (age 50–59) and in men free of coronary heart disease. In men with pre-existent coronary heart disease there was no association between alcohol consumption and the incidence of sudden death. Irrespective of the presence or absence of pre-existent ischaemic heart disease, cardiac deaths were more likely to be sudden in heavy drinkers than in the other drinking groups.

Some epidemiological studies have shown that problem drinking, as defined by registration for alcohol intemperance in society or inability to perform properly at work due to alcohol use, increases the risk of sudden death in particular (Dyer et al 1977, Lithell et al 1987).

Possible mechanisms of alcohol-related cardiac arrhythmias

Table 1 lists some of the mechanisms through which alcohol may contribute to the genesis of cardiac arrhythmias. Subclinical structural changes in the heart muscle are common in alcoholics and may produce patchy delays in conduction promoting re-entry tachyarrhythmias. Alcoholics have prolonged QT intervals without increased QT dispersion (Day et al 1993). This indicates globally prolonged repolarization which may predispose to automatic ventricular arrhythmias. QT interval prolongation predicts mortality in alcoholics with liver disease, particularly in those who continue drinking (Day et al 1993).

TABLE 1 Possible arrhythmogenic mechanisms of alcohol

Subclinical heart muscle injury
Prolongation of ventricular repolarization
Sympathoadrenergic stimulation
Reduced vagal control of heart rate
Electrolyte disturbances
Worsening of sleep apnoea
Worsening of myocardial ischaemia

Alcohol changes the autonomic control of cardiac function in several ways. Circulating catecholamines are elevated both after acute alcohol intake (Perman 1958) and during detoxification (Carlsson & Häggendal 1967). In addition, an accelerated responsiveness to catecholamines may contribute since the density and affinity of lymphocyte β adrenoceptors increases in alcoholic patients during withdrawal (Mäki et al 1990). Augmented adrenergic stimulation of the myocardium can trigger automatic ventricular activity and facilitate the onset of re-entry arrhythmias. Alcohol not only produces adrenergic stimulation but also impairs the parasympathetic cardiac control. Vagally mediated heart rate variability is reduced in chronic alcoholics (Malpas et al 1991), and although the abnormality is often reversible it persists despite prolonged abstinence in some individuals. Furthermore, acute intake of even moderate doses of alcohol impairs vagal modulation of heart rate in healthy persons (Koskinen et al 1994) as well as in non-alcoholic patients with coronary artery disease (Rossinen et al 1997). Reduced vagal influence on the heart may favour cardiac electrical instability, and vagal neuropathy is associated with increased risk of death in chronic alcoholics (Johnson & Robinson 1988). Occasionally, heavy alcohol use may provoke profound vomiting with a sudden strong vagal discharge that can promote atrial arrhythmias.

Electrolyte disturbances like hypopotassaemia and hypomagnesaemia are not uncommon in alcoholics and theoretically favour arrhythmogenesis. The role of alcohol-induced worsening of sleep apnoea also needs to be considered in the onset arrhythmias and in sudden deaths. Since alcohol can rarely act as a coronary vasoconstrictor (Takizawa et al 1984) and may increase the amount of silent ischaemia in patients with coronary artery disease (Rossinen et al 1997), the possibility of ventricular arrhythmias due to ischaemia-triggered activity must be taken into account.

Conclusions

Studies in experimental animals have shown varying acute effects of alcohol on cardiac electrophysiology, some of which may even be antiarrhythmic. Chronic alcohol administration clearly increases the propensity to cardiac arrhythmias in animals. In humans, several lines of evidence suggest that heavy drinking may increase the risk of arrhythmias whether or not heart disease is present. Atrial fibrillation is the most common alcohol-related tachyarrhythmia. Occasionally alcohol may increase the vulnerability to ventricular rhythm disturbances and alcohol-provoked fatal ventricular tachyarrhythmias may explain the increased risk of sudden death in alcoholics. Most of what we currently know about alcohol and arrhythmias relates to heavy drinking. The influence of social use of alcohol on clinically significant arrhythmias in cardiac patients is poorly known and needs to be addressed in the future.

References

Abbasakoor A, Beanlands DS, MacLeod SM 1976 Electrocardiographic changes during ethanol withdrawal. Ann N Y Acad Sci 273:364–370

Bernauer W 1986 The effect of ethanol on arrhythmias and myocardial necrosis in rats with coronary occlusion and reperfusion. Eur J Pharmacol 126:179–187

Buckingham TA, Kennedy HL, Goenjian AK et al 1985 Cardiac arrhythmias in a population admitted to an acute detoxification center. Am Heart J 110:961–965

Carlsson C, Häggendal J 1967 Arterial noradrenaline levels after ethanol withdrawal. Lancet 2:889

Cohen EJ, Klatsky AL, Armstrong MA 1988 Alcohol use and supraventricular arrhythmia. Am J Cardiol 62:971–973

Day CP, James OF, Butler TJ, Campbell RW 1993 QT prolongation and sudden cardiac death in patients with alcoholic liver disease. Lancet 341:1423–1428

Dolly FR, Block AJ 1983 Increased ventricular ectopy and sleep apnoea following ethanol ingestion in COPD patients. Chest 83:469–472

Dyer AR, Stamler J, Paul O et al 1977 Alcohol consumption, cardiovascular risk factors, and mortality in two Chicago epidemiologic studies. Circulation 56:1067–1074

Engel TR, Luck JC 1983 Effect of whisky on atrial vulnerability and "holiday heart". J Am Coll Cardiol 1:816–818

Ettinger PO, Lyons M, Oldewurtel HA, Regan TJ 1976 Cardiac conduction abnormalities produced by chronic alcoholism. Am Heart J 91:66–78

Ettinger PO, Wu CF, De La Cruz C, Weisse AB, Ahmed SS, Regan TJ 1978 Arrhythmias and the "holiday heart": alcohol-associated cardiac rhythm disorders. Am Heart J 95:555–562

Gilmour RF, Ruffy R, Lovelace DE, Mueller TM, Zipes DP 1981 Effect of ethanol on electrogram changes and regional myocardial blood flow during acute myocardial ischemia. Cardiovasc Res 15:47–58

Gimeno AL, Gimeno MF, Webb JL 1962 Effects of ethanol on cellular membrane potentials and contractility of isolated rat atrium. Am J Physiol 203:194–19

Goodkind MJ, Gerber NH, Mellen JR, Kostis JB 1975 Altered intracardiac conduction after acute administration of ethanol in the dog. J Pharmacol Exp Ther 194:633–638

Gould L, Reddy CVR, Patel N, Gomprecht RF 1974 Effects of whisky on heart conduction in cardiac patients. Q J Stud Alcohol 35:26–33

Gould L, Reddy CVR, Becker W, Oh K-C, Kim SG 1978 Electrophysiologic properties of alcohol in man. J Electrocardiol 11:219–226

Greenspon AJ, Schaal SF 1983 The "holiday heart": electrophysiologic studies of alcohol effects in alcoholics. Ann Intern Med 98:135–139

Greenspon A J, Stang JM, Lewis RP, Schaal SF 1979 Provocation of ventricular tachycardia after consumption of alcohol. N Engl J Med 3301:1049–1050

Guideri G, Gutstein WH, Olivetti G, Anversa P 1988 Effects of alcohol on isoproterenol-induced ventricular fibrillation in adult rats. J Cardiovasc Pharmacol 12:479–485

Johnson RH, Robinson B J 1988 Mortality in chronic alcoholics. J Neurol Neurosurg Psychiatry 51:476–480

Kentala E, Luurila O, Salaspuro MP 1976 Effects of alcohol ingestion on cardiac rhythm in patients with ischemic heart disease. Ann Clin Res 8:408–414

Koskinen P 1991 Alcohol consumption and supraventricular tachyarrhythmias: a clinical study of young and middle-aged patients. PhD Thesis, University of Helsinki, Helsinki, Finland

Koskinen P, Kupari M 1991 Alcohol consumption of patients with supraventricular arrhythmias other than atrial fibrillation. Alcohol Alcohol 26:199–206

Koskinen P, Kupari M, Leinonen H, Luomanmäki K 1987 Alcohol and new-onset atrial fibrillation: a case-control study of a current series. Br Heart J 57:468–473

Koskinen P, Kupari M, Leinonen H 1990 Role of alcohol in recurrences of atrial fibrillation in persons <65 years of age. Am J Cardiol 66:954–958

Koskinen P, Virolainen J, Kupari M 1994 Acute alcohol intake decreases short-term heart rate variability in healthy subjects. Clin Sci 87:225–230

Kostis JB, Hortsmann E, Mavrogeorgis E, Radzius A, Goodkind M J 1973 Effect of alcohol on the ventricular fibrillation threshold in dogs. Q J Stud Alcohol 34:1315–1322

Kostis JB, Goodkind M J, Skvaza H, Gerber NH, Kuo PT 1977 Effect of alcohol on the atrial fibrillation threshold in dogs. Angiology 28:583–587

Kramer K, Kuller L, Fisher R 1968 The increasing mortality attributed to cirrhosis and fatty liver in Baltimore (1957–1966). Ann Intern Med 69:273–282

Kupari M, Koskinen P 1991 Time of onset of supraventricular tachyarrhythmias in relation to alcohol consumption. Am J Cardiol 67:718–722

Lithell H, Åberg H, Selinus I, Hedtsrand H 1987 Alcohol intemperance and sudden death. Br Med J 294:1456–1458

Lowenstein A J, Gabow PA, Cramer J, Oliva PB, Ratner K 1983 The role of alcohol in new-onset atrial fibrillation. Arch Intern Med 143:1882–1885

Malpas SC, Whiteside EA, Maling TJB 1991 Heart rate variability and cardiac autonomic function in men with chronic alcohol dependence. Br Heart J 65:84–88

Mäki T, Heikkonen E, Härkönen T, Kontula K, Härkönen M, Ylikahri R 1990 Reduction of lymphocytic beta-adrenoceptor level in chronic alcoholics and rapid reversal after ethanol withdrawal. Eur J Clin Invest 20:313–316

Nguyen TN, Friedman HS, Mkraoui AM 1987 Effects of alcohol on experimental atrial fibrillation. Alcohol Clin Exp Res 11:474–476

Patterson E, Dormer K J, Scherlag B J, Kosanke SD, Schaper J, Lazarra R 1987 Long-term intracoronary ethanol administration. Electrophysiologic and morphologic effects. Alcohol 4:375–384

Perman ES 1958 The effect of ethyl alcohol on the secretion of adrenal medulla in man. Acta Physiol Scand 44:241–247

Randall B 1980 Sudden death and hepatic fatty metamorphosis. A North Carolina study. J AMA 243:1723–1725

Rich EC, Siebold C, Cambion B 1985 Alcohol-related acute atrial fibrillation. A case-control study. Arch Intern Med 145:830–833

Rossinen J, Viitsalo M, Partanen J, Koskinen P, Kupari M, Nieminen MS 1996 Acute heavy alcohol intake increases silent myocardial ischaemia in patients with stable angina pectoris. Heart 75:563–567

Rossinen J, Viitsalo M, Partanen J, Koskinen P, Kupari M, Nieminen MS 1997 Effects of acute alcohol ingestion on heart rate variability in patients with documented coronary artery disease and stable angina pectoris. Am J Cardiol 79:487–491

Singer K, Lundberg WB 1972 Ventricular arrhythmias associated with the ingestion of alcohol. Arch Intern Med 77:247–248

Suhonen O, Aromaa A, Reunanen A, Knekt P 1987 Alcohol consumption and sudden cardiac death in middle-aged Finnish men. Acta Med Scand 221:335–341

Takizawa A, Yasue H, Omote S et al 1984 Variant angina induced by alcohol ingestion. Am Heart J 50:441–447

Wannamethee G, Shaper AG 1992 Alcohol and sudden cardiac death. Br Heart J 68:443–448

Williams ES, Mirro MJ, Bailey JC 1980 Electrophysiological effects of ethanol, acetaldehyde and acetate on cardiac tissues from dog and guinea pig. Circ Res 47:473–478

DISCUSSION

Hillbom: Has anybody looked at whether binge administration of alcohol to experimental animals influences the variability of cardiac arrhythmias?

Kupari: Not that I am aware of.

Anderson: I'm interested in your thoughts about the increase in cardiovascular disease and sudden coronary death in Russia. What is your assessment of this situation? Do you know of any studies looking at arrhythmias and sudden coronary death in Russia or other Baltic states?

Kupari: There was a report published by Vikhert et al (1986) indicating that many sudden deaths in young and middle-aged men in Russia were probably alcohol related. They estimated that about 25% of all sudden deaths were due to alcohol abuse. I think it's highly likely that the recent huge increase in cardiovascular deaths is related to alcohol, but it is important to remember that many other social changes have recently taken place in Russia, such as high unemployment, increasing violence and large-scale societal disintegration. These other factors may also be influencing the cardiovascular system in addition to alcohol. But I agree with you that it's likely that these alcohol-related sudden deaths are responsible for at least a proportion of the recent mortality increase.

Shaper: Does that not conflict with what you told us about Ettinger's work on 'holiday heart' (Ettinger et al 1978)? The arrhythmias were seen in chronic alcoholics or previous heavy drinkers but were not presumably seen in people with a normal heart.

Kupari: Perhaps you must also take into account the fact that the arrhythmias Ettinger reported were mainly atrial tachyarrhythmias. We may be dealing with other mechanisms with ventricular arrhythmias. I don't see a major conflict here.

Shaper: In the data you were showing us, there appeared to be no evidence that acute alcohol ingestion in people with apparently normal hearts provoked arrhythmias: is that correct?

Kupari: Yes, that's correct.

Shaper: So there's an assumption being made about the Russian situation. They must be experiencing acute effects over a background of chronic misuse.

Urbano-Márquez: In your experience, the majority of the patients with sudden death were heavy drinkers. I see many patients that have alcoholic cardio-myopathy but are asymptomatic—in our experience the majority of patients with ventricular arrhythmias were patients with cardiomyopathy, that is to say subclinical cardiomyopathy, not clinical. If you were to study your patients, I suspect that you would be able to detect cardiomyopathy in most of them. Do you agree?

Kupari: Yes. I think that the work by Ettinger and associates on 'holiday heart syndrome' showed that even though these individuals had no signs of clinical heart disease, systolic time intervals and cardiac catheterization revealed evidence of subclinical heart muscle involvement. One might think that these alcohol-related arrhythmias, at least in some instances in these heavy drinkers, could be regarded as an indication of alcoholic heart muscle disease.

Rehm: Are there any human studies on different patterns of drinking, such as binge drinking episodes, and the risk of sudden death?

Kupari: Interestingly, in a recent issue of the *British Medical Journal*, investigators from my country (Kauhanen et al 1997) reported from a prospective study of 1641 men that the risk of cardiac death was substantially increased in men who usually consumed six or more bottles of beer in one session compared with men consuming less than three bottles per session, even after adjustment for total consumption and age. These are the first human data suggesting that binge-type drinking is a risk factor *per se.*

Puddey: There's another potential mechanism that should be considered. If you feed animals ω-3 fatty acids, you raise the threshold for being able to induce ventricular arrhythmia (McLennan et al 1993). Roberts et al (1993) have shown that tissue concentrations and plasma concentrations of linoleic acid are related to an increase in sudden deaths, presumably by ventricular arrhythmia. One of the most potent lifestyle predictors of low linoleic acid in plasma is alcohol (Burke et al 1991). The other major predictor that they have studied is smoking, and there's an additive effect of smoking and alcohol to lead to lower linoleic acid levels and higher saturated fatty acid levels (Simon et al 1996). This may represent a compensatory mechanism for the fluidizing effects of alcohol on membranes. These compositional changes are occurring in nearly every tissue in the body, and the possibility that these compositional changes in fatty acids are particularly relevant to predisposition to arrhythmia probably needs more consideration.

Peters: This is of particular interest in the heart, which is where the fatty acid ethyl esters accumulate in mitochondria. However, I don't think that anybody has investigated the relationship to cardiac dysrhythmias.

You suggested that autonomic neuropathy could be a mechanism. If you look at alcohol misusers who have autonomic neuropathy, are these patients at risk? This is a pretty serious situation. It would be good if we were to be able to predict which people had potentially fatal arrhythmias.

Kupari: It may be an important risk factor. There is at least one small study by Johnson & Robinson (1988) showing that chronic alcoholics who have signs of autonomic neuropathy are at increased risk of sudden cardiac death.

Keil: What is your definition of sudden cardiac death?

Kupari: There is slight variation between different studies. Most define sudden death as a death which occurs within one hour of the onset of symptoms, or which is sudden and unwitnessed.

Klatsky: There is a built-in problem in studying drinking and sudden death, in that the overwhelming majority of all sudden deaths are probably due to coronary disease.

Gaziano: And in the Physicians' health study, we have data showing that among light-to-moderate drinkers, the association of intake with sudden death is U-shaped. I think what is going on here is that a large proportion of people who die suddenly have arrhythmias secondary to thrombosis, rather than a primary arrhythmia.

Klatsky: The data on supraventricular arrhythmias are also a little bit tricky. Hypertension, for example, is an important risk factor for atrial fibrillation in particular. And coronary disease is certainly an important predictor of all types of arrhythmias, not just vagal arrhythmias. Thus there are multiple interactions and it is hard to sort this all out unless one controls for these conditions. One of the reasons that we chose a light-drinking group rather than non-drinkers as a control group in our atrial arrhythmia study, was that we wanted to have at least some degree of control for the presence of coronary disease. Light drinkers might have somewhat similar protection against coronary diseases as heavier drinkers.

Puddey: I guess one of the big problems with any case control study of alcohol-induced disease is the recall bias amongst the people who have the condition. I suspect that could have crept into both your hospital-based and your community-based controls. Have you used biomarkers of alcohol intake to actually give some credence to the self-reports of alcohol intake?

Kupari: In these studies we measured some simple biomarkers of alcohol use, such as liver enzymes (γ-glutamyltranspeptdiase, transaminases) and mean red cell corpuscular volume. We found that patients with atrial arrhythmias had more elevated levels than the control subjects. It is hard to say, however, to what extent these biochemical differences reflect the differences in alcohol consumption.

Marmot: Coming back to the acute mortality story, let's assume for the moment that I'm predisposed to believe that alcohol is making an important contribution to mortality from cardiovascular disease in Russia. Now what I thought I heard in a previous comment was that there's really no good evidence that alcohol is related to acute cardiac deaths. Is that what you said?

Gaziano: No. I think that there is a relationship between alcohol intake and acute death. The key question concerns the mechanism. Cardiovascular disease deaths do turn up, but sorting out the precise mechanism is difficult with a disease that we can't often precisely attribute to arrhythmia. Markku Kupari's definition of sudden death varies from found dead to found dead within one hour.

Marmot: Thinking of Gerry Shaper's question as well, let's take two groups in Russia: one is the young men who presumably have very little atherosclerosis, and so if alcohol were to play a role it would have to be some acute effect, and the second is the middle-aged men, where we know the bulk of the problem is, where you could argue that they have a lot of atherosclerosis and so it could be an acute effect on top of the atherosclerosis. Is there good evidence that alcohol is causing cardiac death to a significant degree in either of those groups?

Kupari: The evidence so far comes from the data that I showed. We must admit that we lack data solid enough to establish a causal link: the evidence is circumstantial for the most part.

Marmot: It's an interesting phenomenon, because I hear people talking all the time about how alcohol is the cause of this major problem in Eastern Europe. It may be true, but it doesn't sound like the evidence supporting that statement is incredibly strong.

Gaziano: I think it is probable in Russia that cardiovascular disease accounts for a substantial portion of the excess death due to alcohol consumption, but we're not talking about light drinking: we're talking about heavy drinking. The average consumption among Russian males is quite heavy, in the order of half a bottle of vodka per day. We know that heavy alcohol consumption increases cardiovascular death. There are probably multiple causes of this, including some catastrophic events that are non-cardiac but get classified as cardiac death. But I don't find it at all improbable that the excess death in Russia is in part due to increased cardiovascular disease. Distinguishing between arrhythmic death, haemorrhagic stroke or some other catastrophic event is difficult.

Anderson: We have looked at sudden cardiovascular deaths in Moscow. Twenty per cent of these individuals had blood alcohol levels of 3.5 g/l or higher. Alcohol must be contributing to the deaths, but the key question concerns the mechanism.

Shaper: The level of drinking in Russia is something which we don't encounter regularly in the UK or the USA. In most US studies the heaviest drinkers consume only 21 drinks a week: we haven't the faintest idea of what heavy drinking is!

Fillmore: As I understand it, the majority of so-called alcohol-related deaths in the former Soviet Union are really due to accidents and violence (Nemstov 1996, Nemstov & Nechayev 1991, Ryan 1995).

Shaper: This is not what they have been classified as in ICD codes. We know there are high levels of violence and accidents, but these are deaths apparently being attributed to CHD.

Marmot: If you look in general at all the Eastern European countries, there is a six year life expectancy gap between East and West. Of those six years, about 3.2 can be attributed to cardiovascular disease, and about 1.2 years is due to external causes (accidents and violence). Just under one year was down to infant mortality. Overwhelmingly, more than half of the East–West difference is because of cardiovascular disease, and the age group concerned is primarily middle-aged.

Rehm: With regard to accidents and injuries, if you consider alcohol-related mortality based on usual epidemiological methodology such as aetiological fractions (English et al 1995), many of the effects of alcohol are not counted because they do not affect the consumers themselves but those around them (Rehm & Fischer 1997). Deaths due to drunk drivers, for example, are not attributed to alcohol in this standard methodology.

Second, there is a structural problem common to most of our cohort studies. All of our big cohorts are selected for coming up with a lot of traceability, i.e. a high response rate after 10–15 years. In order to achieve this, we select populations which are predisposed to still respond in 10–15 years, such as health professionals. Typically, these populations contain very few heavy drinkers: the mean of their highest quintile of alcohol consumption corresponds to the mean of the lowest quintile in some of the high-drinking countries (Rehm & Fichter 1995). Our knowledge of the effects of heavy drinking is therefore based on two or three studies. The Farchi et al (1992) study is one of the few studies where we have alcohol quintiles which are in the realm of what we are now experiencing in Russia.

Keil: In our surveys in the Augsburg region, although we are proud that we had a response rate of 80%, this still means that 20% did not participate. We made a mortality follow-up of the non responders, and found that their relative risk of death is 1.7, which is 70% higher than the responders (Keil et al 1997a,b). So we are looking at a relatively healthy population of 80%, and obviously we don't get the extremes.

Gaziano: The relative risk for total mortality with heavy drinking is so large that it's not a question of whether there's an increased risk of mortality. We don't need additional studies to show that heavy alcohol consumption increases the risk of death from multiple causes, but we do need multiple studies in light-to-moderate range to know exactly what the shape of that curve is.

Rehm: I disagree. I know that for most problems in the USA and western Europe, the concentration on light-to-moderate drinking is relevant, but once we look at heavy drinking and begin to ask whether alcohol can explain the mortality effects in Russia, we lack data. So I would argue that we need further studies on heavy-drinking populations in order to be sure of what we are doing. What we have been discussing has tremendous public health consequences for Russia, and any policy should be based on more data.

Shaper: I'm not sure that's necessary. If you look at the Boffetta & Garfinkel (1990) data, apart from the cardiovascular disease which is flat or dipping, all the other causes of death rise progressively as alcohol intake goes up. You can't make an assumption that somewhere beyond the levels of intake that Boffetta & Garfinkel are recording it's suddenly going to go down: that isn't likely.

Rehm: However, if you look at the data from the large cohort studies of Harvard, they are very scarce in high drinking risk categories for all the cardiac conditions. If you look at the Maclure (1993) meta-analysis cited earlier, the figures are no longer significant after about 9 drinks/day, so we do not know whether there really is an upturn or how this is shaped for cardiovascular diseases. The question of how the upturn is shaped and whether there is an upturn for both males and females is of practical relevance (Rehm et al 1997).

Gaziano: My personal feeling is that better quantitative estimates of the well known risk of heavy drinking are not likely to alter the public health message for the Russian population.

References

Boffetta P, Garfinkel L 1990 Alcohol drinking and mortality among men enrolled in and American Cancer Society Prospective Study. Epidemiology 1:342–348

Burke V, Croft KD, Puddey IB, Cox KL, Beilin LJ, Vandongen R 1991 Effects of alcohol intake on plasma fatty acids assessed independently of diet and smoking habits. Clin Sci 81:785–791

English DR, Holman CDJ, Milne E et al 1995 The quantification of drug-caused morbidity and mortality in Australia. Commonwealth Department of Human Services and Health, Canberra

Ettinger PO, Wu CF, De La Cruz C, Weisse AB, Ahmed SS, Regan TJ 1978 Arrhythmias and the "holiday heart": alcohol-associated cardiac rhythm disorders. Am Heart J 95:555–562

Farchi G, Fidanza F, Mariotti S, Menotti A 1992 Alcohol and mortality in the Italian rural cohorts of the Seven Countries Study. Int J Epidemiol 21:74–81

Johnson RH, Robinson BJ 1988 Mortality in chronic alcoholics. J Neurol Neurosurg Psychiatry 51:476–480

Kauhanen J, Kaplan GA, Goldberg DE, Salonen JT 1997 Beer binging and mortality: results from the Kuopio ischaemic heart disease risk factor study, a prospective population-based study. Br Med J 315:846–851

Keil U, Chambless LE, Döring A, Filipiak B, Steiber J 1997a The relation of alcohol intake to coronary heart disease and all-cause mortality in a beer-drinking population. Epidemiology 8:150–156

Keil U, Chambless LE, Döring A, Filipiak B, Steiber J 1997b Alcohol, coronary heart disease, and mortality (Authors' reply to a letter to the Editor). Epidemiology 8:687–688

Maclure M 1993 Demonstration of deductive meta-analysis: ethanol intake and risk of myocardial infarction. Epidemiol Rev 15:328–351

McLennan PL, Bridle TM, Abeywardena MY, Charnock JS 1993 Comparative efficiency of n-3 and n-6 polyunsaturated fatty acids in modulating ventricular fibrillation threshold in marmoset monkeys. Am J Clin Nutr 58:666–669

Nemstov AV 1996 Overview of national and local alcohol-related problems in the CIS: alcohol situation in Russia. Drugs Education Prev Policy 3:34–36

Nemstov AV, Nechayev AK 1991 Potreblenie alkogolya i nasil'stvennye smerti (Alcohol consumption and violent death). Voprosy Narkologii 1:34–36

Rehm J, Fichter MM 1995 Stichprobenerwägungen bei Verlaufsstudien in der psychiatrischen Epidemiologie. In: Margraf J, Kunath H (eds) Methodische Ansätze in der Public Health Forschung. Roderer, Regensburg, p 180–190

Rehm J, Fischer B 1997 Measuring harm: implications for alcohol epidemiology. In: Plant M, Single E, Stockwell T (eds) Alcohol: minimising the harm. What works. Free Association Books, London, p 248–261

Rehm J, Bondy S, Sempos CT, Vuong CV 1997 Alcohol consumption and CHD morbidity and mortality. Am J Epidemiol 146:495–501

Roberts TL, Wood DA, Riemersma RA, Gallagher PJ, Lampe FC 1993 Linoleic acid and risk of sudden cardiac death. Br Heart J 70:524–529

Ryan M 1995 Alcoholism and rising mortality in the Russian Federation. Br Med J 310:646–648

Simon JA, Fong J, Bernert JT, Browner WS 1996 Relation of smoking and alcohol consumption to serum fatty acids. Am J Epidemiol 144:325–334

Vikhert AM, Tisplenkova VG, Cherpachenko MM 1986 Alcoholic cardiomyopathy and sudden cardiac death. J Am Coll Cardiol 8:3A–11A

Alcohol intake, lipids and risks of myocardial infarction

J. Michael Gaziano* and Julie E. Buring†

*The Massachusetts Veterans Epidemiology and Information Center and the Department of Medicine, Veterans Affairs Medical Center, Brockton/West Roxbury, MA 02132; Division of Preventive Medicine and the Harvard Medical School, Boston, MA 02215-1204; †The Department of Ambulatory Care and Prevention, Harvard Medical School, Boston MA; †The Departments of Epidemiology, Harvard School of Public Health, Boston MA, USA

Abstract. The health effects of alcohol consumption remain complex for several reasons: the risks and benefits accrue over many years, assessment of drinking is generally based on self-report, drinking habits change over time and studies estimate average daily drinking disregarding how or when the beverage was consumed. In addition, alcohol consumption is associated with lifestyle factors which may confound relationship with disease. Despite these methodological difficulties, epidemiological studies are surprisingly consistent, showing that light to moderate intake is associated with a lower risk of total mortality compared with those who drink heavily or do not drink at all. Thus there is a J-shaped association of alcohol intake with risk of total mortality whose basis is likely to be the effect of summing the cause-specific effects at the various drinking levels. Studies using a diversity of methods and populations have consistently reported an inverse relationship between coronary heart disease and light to moderate drinking, with the depth and width of the J-shaped mortality curve depending on the underlying risk of coronary heart disease for that population. The higher risk of death at heavy drinking levels is due to increased risk of cancer, liver diseases, cardiomyopathy and stroke. The precise mechanisms behind these effects of alcohol are only now beginning to be understood. The most plausible mechanism by which alcohol reduces the risk of coronary heart disease is by its effects on blood lipids, particularly increases in high density lipoprotein (HDL) cholesterol: about 50% of the risk reduction attributable to alcohol is explained by changes in total HDL. Further support for the HDL hypothesis comes from the lack of a differential effect of alcohol by beverage type. While the association of alcohol and cardiovascular disease is likely to be causal, any public health recommendations must consider the complexity of alcohol's metabolic, physiological and psychological effects.

1998 Alcohol and cardiovascular diseases. Wiley, Chichester (Novartis Foundation Symposium 216) p 86–110

The consumption of alcohol and its impact on health has been of great interest to researchers for many years, but remains complex for several reasons. First, with the exception of deaths attributable to intoxication, risks and benefits of alcohol are likely to accrue over years or even decades. Second, the assessment of drinking is generally based on self-report and this may lead to some degree of misclassification. Third, drinking habits change over time and, thus, it may be important to update drinking habits periodically during any prospective study. Fourth, most studies tend to estimate average daily intake disregarding issues of how or when the alcoholic beverage was consumed. For example, southern Europeans tend to drink wine with meals, while northern Europeans tend to drink distilled spirits often at times other than mealtimes. The risks and benefits of alcohol consumption certainly seem to be quite different for an individual who consumes seven beers on a Saturday night compared with an individual who consumes half a glass of wine with lunch and dinner every day, despite the obvious similarities in average weekly consumption.

Fifth, consumption of alcoholic beverages tends to be imbedded in cultural practices and associated with a number of lifestyle factors which may confound relationships with disease. For example, age, sex, race, smoking, ethnic background and education are related to alcohol intake and also are predictors of chronic diseases. Further, alcohol is derived from a number of different beverages whose other components may increase or decrease risk of disease aside from, or in addition to, the specific effect of ethanol. Finally, the precise mechanisms by which alcohol raises or lowers risks of various disease are only now beginning to be understood. Despite these inherent methodological difficulties in assessing the risks and benefits of alcohol consumption, data from various epidemiological studies are surprisingly consistent. In this paper, we summarize the strength and consistency of the human observational and experimental data on the relationship between light to moderate alcohol intake and lower risk of coronary heart disease.

Alcohol and total mortality

It is clear that heavy alcohol intake increases the risk of death from all causes (Klatsky et al 1981, Pell & D'Alonzo 1973, Rosengren et al 1988, Thorarinson 1979, Doll & Peto 1994). However, light to moderate intake is associated with lower risk of total mortality compared with those who drink heavily or do not drink at all. This level of alcohol intake is associated with lower risk of cardiovascular disease without increases in liver disease or cancer. Thus, there seems to be a 'J-shaped' association of alcohol intake with risk of total mortality, with the lowest hazard among light to moderate drinkers. While there is some disagreement as to the precise low point of the J-shaped curve, there is general agreement that the relationship is in fact J-shaped. The basis of this J-shaped association is likely to be the effect of summing the cause-specific effects at the various drinking levels. The lower rates of total mortality at light to moderate alcohol consumption levels appears to be due to a reduction in cardiovascular disease without dramatic increases in other causes of death. The lower rates of cardiovascular disease appear to be entirely due to lower rates of coronary heart disease. At higher drinking levels any reduction in risk of death due to coronary heart diseases is overwhelmed by increased risks of death due to liver disease, certain cancers (particularly of the head and neck) and some types of cardiovascular disease, such as cardiomyopathy and haemorrhagic stroke.

Alcohol and coronary heart disease

The association of alcohol consumption with cardiovascular disease has been widely studied using a variety of methodologies (Duetscher et al 1984, Fraser & Upsdell 1981, Hennekens 1983, Hennekens et al 1978, Ross et al 1981, Klatsky et al 1974, Stason et al 1976, Rosenberg et al 1981, Gordon & Kannel 1983, Yano et al 1984, Stampfer et al 1988, Cullen et al 1982, Colditz et al 1985, Dyer et al 1980, Friedman & Kimball 1986, Gordon & Doyle 1985, Rimm et al 1991, Moore & Pearson 1986). Most studies suggest a nadir in total mortality from one to three drinks per day due entirely to lower risk of cardiovascular death. The reduction in cardiovascular disease death at light to moderate levels appears to be largely driven by a reduction in coronary heart disease mortality. At higher drinking levels there appears to be an increase in non-coronary causes of cardiovascular death (cardiomyopathy, sudden death, haemorrhagic stroke) which tend to offset any benefit in terms of coronary heart disease. This then causes the cardiovascular disease curve to turn upward yielding a U-shaped relationship of alcohol consumption with cardiovascular disease death.

With few exceptions, studies using a diversity of methods and populations have consistently reported an inverse association between coronary heart disease and light to moderate alcohol consumption. A dose–response relationship exists in most studies in the range of light drinking and the benefit appears to persist at moderate to heavy drinking levels. In a recent meta-analysis, Maclure (1993) suggests an L-shaped threshold effect for non-fatal coronary heart disease with reduced risks beginning at three drinks per week and no additional benefit for more than one drink per day. This is supported by several autopsy studies which suggest that the burden of atherosclerosis at autopsy among heavy drinkers is lower than controls (e.g. Reubner et al 1961).

Since the reduction in total mortality among those who drink light to moderate amounts of alcohol appears to be due to lower risk of coronary heart disease, the depth and width of the J-shaped mortality curve for a given population depends on the underlying risk of coronary heart disease for that population. Those at lower risk of heart disease, such as young women, derive minimal benefit from light to moderate alcohol intake. On the other hand, those who have had a prior myocardial infarction are at high risk for subsequent coronary heart disease events and thus have a more pronounced reduction in total mortality at light to moderate drinking levels.

The consistency of the epidemiological data suggests more than just a chance association. The available data from cross-cultural, case-control and prospective cohort studies among diverse populations consistently report lower rates of myocardial infarction, angina pectoris and peripheral artery disease among light to moderate drinkers. Some have suggested that the inverse association of alcohol with coronary heart disease is due to the contamination of the non-drinking category with those who have reduced drinking due to preexisting coronary heart disease (Shaper et al 1988). However, this would not explain the apparent dose–response relationship at light drinking levels reported in most studies. In addition, most recent studies exclude recent ex-drinkers from the analysis and the relationship has persisted, so it is unlikely that this potential bias has had a major impact on risk estimates. While the association appears to be strong and consistent, observational data may result in an overestimation or underestimation of the effect due to confounding. The possibility of residual confounding cannot be ruled out, but it is unlikely that residual confounding could fully explain the association. In addition, most of the recent observational studies have controlled for the major predictors of coronary heart disease with little effect on the relationship. Thus, the available epidemiological data strongly suggest that the association of light to moderate alcohol intake with lower risk of coronary heart disease is likely to be causal.

Mechanisms

Establishing causal relationships in human disease where the size of the effect is small-to-moderate can be made much easier if mechanistic explanations for the association are available. A number of mechanistic possibilities have emerged from both experimental and observational epidemiological studies of the past two decades. The most plausible mechanism by which alcohol reduces the risk of coronary heart disease is by its effect on blood lipids.

Other potential mechanisms which may contribute to the cardioprotective effect of light to moderate alcohol consumption include alterations in factors affecting blood clotting. Clot formation is an important step in the development of a myocardial infarction. A number of factors involved in maintaining the delicate balance between clot formation to protect against bleeding and clot dissolution to prevent blood clots from forming in arteries have been implicated as risk factors for myocardial infarction. Alcohol seems to affect several of these factors. One recent study suggests that alcohol consumption increases the levels of a clot-dissolving enzyme, tissue plasminogen activator (tPA) (Ridker et al 1994). Acute ingestion of alcohol can prolong bleeding time and reduce platelet aggregation

(Haut & Cowan 1974, Elmer et al 1984). These data are consistent with the hypothesis that alcohol consumption may reduce the chance of clot formation by enhancing the clot-dissolving system or reducing the stickiness of platelets. While this is a theoretical mechanism by which alcohol may reduce the risk of coronary heart disease mortality, the extent to which this contributes to lower risk beyond that of the lipid effect remains unclear.

Alterations in plasma lipoproteins, particularly increases in high-density lipoprotein (HDL) cholesterol, represent the most plausible mechanism of the apparent protective effect of alcohol consumption on coronary heart disease. HDL cholesterol is produced primarily in the liver and intestines and is released into the blood stream. Commonly referred to as the 'good' cholesterol, HDL binds with cholesterol and brings it back to the liver for elimination or reprocessing, thereby lowering total cholesterol levels in body tissues. In this way, the HDL reduces the cholesterol build-up on the arterial wall, in a sense reversing the atherosclerotic process. In addition, HDL may play a role in rendering the low-density lipoprotein (LDL) less harmful by preventing it from becoming oxidized. Finally, HDL may mediate favourable haemostatic effects.

The evidence from both observational and experimental studies suggests that alcohol raises total HDL, and that approximately 50% of the risk reduction attributable to alcohol consumption is explained by changes in total HDL. Alcohol intake clearly raises HDL cholesterol levels (Castelli et al 1977, Hulley & Gordon 1981, Ernst et al 1980, Langer et al 1992, Suh et al 1992, Glueck et al 1980, Hartung et al 1983, Criqui et al 1987), but until recently it was felt that this may not be the mechanism by which alcohol exerts its protective effect. HDL cholesterol is comprised of two principal types, or subfractions: HDL_2 and HDL_3, each of which have a slightly different function. Early experimental studies of small sample size suggested that moderate alcohol consumption raised HDL_3 but not HDL_2 (Haffner et al 1985, Diehl et al 1988, Haskell et al 1984); however, the protective effect of HDL_2 in reducing risk of myocardial infarction has been well documented, while data on the role of HDL_3 have been less consistent (Goffman et al 1966, Miller et al 1981, Ballantyne et al 1982).

The effect of alcohol on each subfraction of HDL was explored in a large case-control study (Gaziano et al 1993). Total HDL as well as both HDL_2 and HDL_3 levels were strongly associated with alcohol consumption (each P, trend < 0.001). Both subfractions were associated with a reduction in risk of myocardial infarction. The addition of HDL or each of its subfractions to a multivariate model substantially reduced the association of alcohol and myocardial infarction, suggesting that the inverse association is mediated, in large part, by increases in both HDL_2 and HDL_3 subfractions. Thus, the available observational and experimental studies strongly support the hypothesis that the associated risk reduction of coronary heart disease is in large part due to increases in HDL.

Beverage type

Further support for the notion that the beneficial affects of alcoholic beverages is derived from an ethanol-specific effect comes from the lack of differential effect of alcohol by beverage type. Alcohol, regardless of the beverage type in which it is consumed, seems to reduce risks of coronary heart disease.

Recently a great deal of research has focused on the benefits of specific alcoholic beverages. Many have postulated that the antioxidant value of phenolic substances or bioflavonioids in red wine render it more potent in reducing risk of cardiovascular disease. Oxidative damage has been postulated to play an important role in the development of atherosclerosis. Oxidation of LDL cholesterol has been implicated in several steps of atherogenesis, and several antioxidants have been shown to protect LDL against oxidation raising the possibility that they may reduce the risk of atherosclerotic disease. Both *in vitro* and *in vivo* studies have shown that red wine can protect LDL from oxidative damage.

On the basis of these findings, some investigators have postulated that red wine should reduce the risk of atherosclerosis beyond that of other alcoholic beverages. This has been offered as one possible explanation for the lower than expected coronary heart disease mortality rates in France as well as other Mediterranean countries. However, the evidence from available observational data that does not clearly suggest greater benefit for wine compared with beer or distilled spirits. In general, all three have been shown to reduce risks of coronary heart disease. While some studies have suggested greater benefit for wine consumption compared with other beverages (Klatsky & Armstrong 1993), others have reported greatest benefit of beer (Stampfer et al 1988, Yano et al 1984) or liquor (Rimm et al 1991). Those studies which have reported a benefit for wine have not seen a more protective effect for red wine compared with white (Rimm et al 1991). In addition, since wine drinkers tend to be more educated and have higher incomes, it has been speculated that apparent benefits of wine consumption may be due at least in part to confounding. Criqui & Ringel (1994) recently reported that the ethanol content rather than the total volume or type of wine were better predictors of the reduction in risk of coronary heart disease death in a cross-cultural study.

In a recent case-control study the protective effect of each beverage type appeared to be mediated by increases in HDL (Gaziano et al 1998). Alcohol drinkers were defined as those who consumed one half or more drinks on average per day of any alcoholic beverage. Beer, wine and liquor drinkers were defined as those who consumed one half or more drinks per day on average with more than half of their consumption as beer, wine or liquor, respectively. Compared to non-drinkers, after adjustment for age and sex, reductions in risk of myocardial infarction were similar for regular drinkers of any type of alcoholic beverage. Comparable benefits remained apparent even after multivariate adjustment for a wide range of non-lipid coronary risk factors. HDL levels were significantly higher in all four beverage categories as compared to non-drinkers and, as expected, adjustment for total HDL, a major direct effect of alcohol, substantially attenuated the protective effect in all four beverage categories. This strongly suggests that the protective effect of each beverage type is, in large part, mediated by increased HDL. These data indicate that regular consumption of small to moderate amounts of alcoholic beverages, regardless of the type, reduce the risk of myocardial infarction, and further suggest that the benefit is, in large part, from increases in HDL levels.

At this point the majority of data suggest that the major beneficial component of alcoholic beverages is in fact the ethanol itself rather than some other component. Some researchers have speculated that how and when alcoholic beverages are consumed may have more to do with benefits rather than what is consumed. Wine tends to be consumed in modest amounts with meals, which may have metabolic advantages. On the other hand, liquor is often consumed at times other than mealtime. In addition, there may be acute effects of alcohol in risk of coronary heart disease. More analytic data will be required to better answer these questions.

Summary and recommendations

The effects of alcohol consumption on chronic diseases are complex. The basis of the J-shaped mortality curve is likely to be the effect of summing the cause-specific effects at the various drinking levels. The lower rates of total mortality at light to moderate alcohol consumption levels appear to be due to a reduction in cardiovascular disease without dramatic increases in other causes of death. The lower rates of cardiovascular disease appear to be entirely due to lower rates of coronary heart disease. Thus, the depth and width of the J-shaped mortality curve for a given population depends on the underlying risk of coronary heart disease. The higher risk of death at heavy drinking levels is due to increases in risk of death from cancer, liver diseases, and certain cardiovascular causes such as cardiomyopathy and haemorrhagic stroke.

The strength and consistency of the observational and experimental evidence strongly suggests a causal link between light to moderate alcoholic beverage consumption and reduced risks of coronary heart disease. The elucidation of a major mechanistic pathway provides further support for the assertion that the association is causal. The reduction in risk of coronary heart disease appears to be mediated largely by raising HDL cholesterol levels, though additional mechanisms remain possible. Alcohol clearly raises HDL levels, and any factor that raises HDL to the degree that alcohol appears to be able to, would most assuredly lower the risk of coronary heart disease. The precise mechanism by which alcohol raises HDL remains unclear. HDL may have a number of positive effects including reverse cholesterol transport, antioxidant effects and favourable haemostatic effects. Comparisons by beverage type suggest that it is the alcohol itself which is the major factor responsible for the protective association.

While the association of alcohol and coronary heart disease is likely to be causal, any individual or public health recommendations must consider the complexity of alcohol's metabolic, physiological and psychological effects. Maximal benefit in terms of coronary heart disease appears to be at the level of one drink per day. From a public policy standpoint, whether the benefits for coronary heart disease persist at heavy drinking levels or are attenuated is moot, since clear harm in terms of overall mortality outweighs any benefits in the reduction of heart disease. With alcohol, the differences between daily intake of small-to-moderate and large quantities may be the difference between preventing and causing disease.

A discussion of alcohol intake should be a part of routine preventive counselling. One drink per day appears to be safe, in general; however, counselling must be individualized. Other medical problems including diabetes, hypertension, liver disease, tendency toward excess, family history of alcoholism and possibly breast and colon cancer should be taken into account when discussing alcohol consumption. In addition, the dose relationships in men and women appear to be different. Liver toxicities occur at lower levels among women compared with men, which does not appear to be entirely due to the difference in lean body weight. Given the complex nature of alcohol/disease relationships, alcohol consumption should not be viewed as a primary preventive strategy nor should it necessarily be viewed as an unhealthy behaviour.

References

Ballantyne FC, Clarck RS, Simpson HS, Ballantyne D 1982 High density and low density lipoprotein subfractions in survivors of myocardial infarction and in control subjects. Metabolism 31:433–437

Castelli WP, Gordon T, Hjortland MC et al 1977 Alcohol and blood lipids. The cooperative lipoprotein phenotyping study. Lancet 2:153–155

Colditz GA, Branch LG, Lipnick RJ, Rosner B, Hennekens CH 1985 Moderate alcohol and decreased cardiovascular mortality in an elderly cohort. Am Heart J 109:886–889

Criqui MH, Ringel BL 1994 Does diet or alcohol explain the French paradox? Lancet 344:1719–1723

Criqui MH, Cowan LD, Tyroler HA et al 1987 Lipoproteins as mediators for the effects of alcohol consumption and cigarette smoking on cardiovascular mortality: Results from the lipid research clinics follow-up study. Am J Epidemiol 126:629–637

Cullen IK, Stenhouse NS, Wearne KL 1982 Alcohol and mortality in the Busselton study. Internat J Epidemiol 11:67–70

Diehl AK, Fuller JH, Mattock MB, Salter AM, El-Gohari R, Keen H 1988 The relationship of high density lipoprotein subfractions to alcohol consumption, other lifestyle factors, and coronary heart disease. Atherosclerosis 69:145–153

Doll R, Peto R 1994 Mortality in relation to consumption of alcohol: 13 years observation on male British Doctors. Br Med J 309:911–918

Duetscher S, Rockette HE, Krishnswami V 1984 Evaluation of habitual excessive alcohol consumption on myocardial infarction risk in coronary disease patients. Am Heart J 108:988–995

Dyer AR, Stamler J, Paul O et al 1980 Alcohol consumption and 17-year mortality in the Chicago Western Electric Company Study. Prev Med 9:78–90

Elmer O, Goransson G, Zoucas E 1984 Impairment of primary hemostasis and platelet function after alcohol ingestion in man. Haemostatis 14:223–228

Ernst N, Fisher M, Smith W et al 1980 The association of plasma high-density lipoprotein cholesterol with dietary intake and alcohol consumption. The Lipid Research Clinics program prevalence study. Circulation 62(suppl 4):41–52

Fraser GE, Upsdell M 1981 Alcohol and other discriminants between cases of sudden death and myocardial infarction. Am J Epidemiol 114:462–476

Friedman LA, Kimball AW 1986 Coronary heart disease mortality and alcohol consumption in Framingham. Am J Epidemiol 124:481–489

Gaziano JM, Buring JE, Breslow JL et al 1993 Moderate alcohol intake, increased levels of high density lipoprotein and its subfractions, and decreased risk of myocardial infarction. New Engl J Med 329:1829–1834

Gaziano JM, Hennekens CH, Godfried SL et al 1998 Type of alcoholic beverage and risk of myocardial infarction. Am J Cardiol, in press

Glueck CJ, Hogg E, Allen C, Gartside PS 1980 Effects of alcohol ingestion on lipids and lipoprotein in normal men: isocaloric metabolic studies. Am J Clin Nutr 33:2287–2293

Goffman JW, Young W, Tandy R 1966 Ischemic heart disease, atherosclerosis, and longevity. Circulation 34:679–697

Gordon T, Doyle JT 1985 Drinking and coronary heart disease: the Albany Study. Am Heart J 110:331–334

Gordon T, Kannel WB 1983 Drinking habits and cardiovascular disease: The Framingham Study. Am Heart J 105:667–673

Haffner SM, Applebaum-Bowden D, Wahl PW et al 1985 Epidemiological correlates of high density lipoprotein subtractions, apolipoproteins a-I, a-II, and d, and lecithin cholesterol acyltransferase. Effects of smoking, alcohol, and adiposity. Arteriosclerosis 5:169–177

Hartung GH, Foreyt JP, Mitchell RE, Mitchell JG, Reeves RS, Gotto AM 1983 Effect of alcohol intake on high-density lipoprotein cholesterol levels in runners and inactive men. JAMA 249:747–750

Haskell WL, Camargo C, Williams PT et al 1984 The effect of cessation and resumption of moderate alcohol intake on high-density lipoprotein subfractions. N Engl J Med 310:805–810

Haut MJ, Cowan DH 1974 The effect of ethanol on hemostatic properties of human blood platelets. Am J Med 56:22–33

Hennekens CH 1983 Alcohol. In: Kaplan NM, Stamler J (eds) Prevention of coronary heart disease: practical management of the risk factors. WB Saunders, Philadelphia, p 130–138

Hennekens CH, Rosner B, Cole DS 1978 Daily alcohol consumption and fatal coronary heart disease. Am J Epidemiol 107:196–200

Hulley SB, Gordon S 1981 Alcohol and high density lipoprotein cholesterol. Causal inference from diverse study designs. Circulation 64:57–63

Klatsky AL, Armstrong MA 1993 Alcoholic beverage choice and risk of coronary artery disease mortality: do red wine drinkers do best? Am J Cardiol 17:467–469

Klatsky AL, Friedman GD, Seigelaub AB 1974 Alcohol consumption before myocardial infarction. Results from the Kaiser-Permanente epidemiologic study of myocardial infarction. Ann Intern Med 81:294–301

Klatsky AL, Friedman GD, Siegelaub AB 1981 Alcohol and mortality. A ten-year Kaiser-Permanente experience. Ann Intern Med 95:139–145

Langer RO, Criqui MR, Reed DM 1992 Lipoproteins and blood pressure as biological pathways for effect of moderate alcohol consumption on coronary heart disease. Circulation 85:910–915

Maclure M 1993 Demonstration of deductive meta-analysis: Ethanol intake and risk of myocardial infarction. Epidemiologic Reviews 15:1–24

Miller G J, Hammet F, Saltissi S et al 1981 Relation of angiographically defined coronary artery disease to plasma lipoprotein subtractions and apolipoproteins. Br Med J 282:1741–1744

Moore RD, Pearson TA 1986 Moderate alcohol consumption and coronary artery disease: a review. Medicine 65:242–267

Pell S, D'Alzono CA 1973 A five year mortality study of alcoholics. J Occup Med 15:120–125

Reubner BH, Mikai K, Abbey H 1961 The low incidence of myocardial infarction in hepatic cirrhosis. Lancet 1:858–860

Ridker PM, Vaughn DE, Stampfer M J, Glynn R J, Hennekens CH 1994 Association of moderate alcohol consumption and plasma concentrations of endogenous tissue-type plasminogen activator. JAMA 272:929–933

Rimm EB, Giovannucci EL, Willett WC et al 1991 Prospective study of alcohol consumption and risk of coronary disease in men. Lancet 338:464–468

Rosenberg L, Stone D, Shapiro S, Kaufman DW, Miettinem OS, Stolley PD 1981 Alcoholic beverages and myocardial infarction in young women. Am J Publ Health 71:82–85

Rosengren A, Wilhemsen L, Wedel H 1988 Separate and combined effects of smoking and alcohol abuse in middle aged men. Acta Med Scand 223:111–118

Ross RK, Mack TM, Paganini-Hill, Arthur M, Henderson BE 1981 Menopausal estrogen therapy and protection from death from ischemic heart disease. Lancet 1:858–860

Shaper AG, Wannamethee G, Walker M 1988 Alcohol and mortality in British men: explaining the U-shaped curve. Lancet 283:179–186

Stampfer M J, Colditz G A, Willett WC, Speizer FE, Hennekens CH 1988 A prospective study of moderate alcohol consumption and the risk of coronary disease and stroke in women. N Engl J Med 319:267–273

Stason WB, Neff RK, Miettinem OS, Jick H 1976 Alcohol consumption and nonfatal myocardial infarction. Am J Epidemiol 104:603–608

Suh L, Shuten B J, Cutler J A, Kuller LH 1992 Alcohol use and mortality from coronary heart disease: the role of high-density lipoprotein cholesterol. The Multiple Risk Factor Intervention Trial Research Group. Ann Int Med 116:881–117

Thorarinson AA 1979 Mortality among men alcoholics in Iceland 1951–1974. J Stud Alcohol 40:704–718

Yano K, Reed DM, McGee DL 1984 Ten year incidence of coronary heart disease in the Honolulu heart program. Am J Epidemiol 119:653–666

DISCUSSION

Anderson: You showed data indicating that drinking one drink a week gives a significant reduction in risk. I would like to challenge a comment that you made earlier, where you said that perhaps you have got to drink regularly rather than just once a week to get this reduction. It seems that you can get significant reduction in risk at quite infrequent levels of drinking.

Gaziano: It probably depends on the reference group that you use. It is possible that some of what we see in the very light drinkers is artefactual: i.e. that non-drinkers are in some way different from drinkers. If you use very light drinkers as the referent group, the relationship does not really change. Often, what we've done is combine the light drinkers with the referent group or used the light drinkers as the referent group. This may be more appropriate. I don't like to comment too much on the actual quantitative association for one particular data point: it is much more reasonable to look at the trend across the categories, which is a fairly linear trend. This is what we would expect for the observed linear association with HDL.

Anderson: But in public health terms it is very important to know whether one drink a week gives you most of the benefit.

Gaziano: I certainly wouldn't rely on just one data set for the best quantitative estimate. The Maclure meta-analysis suggests that half a drink a day is where you really begin to see a detectable benefit (Maclure 1993). Beyond this level there aren't dramatic changes. The argument about where the nadir of the curve occurs involves two issues that make me sceptical about using any one data set. First, the curves are population-specific. Second, when we are talking about public health we need to look at the total mortality curve, not the MI curve. In the absence of large-scale randomized trial data, the estimates that come from meta-analyses are much better for deriving a public health message.

Anderson: You seem to dismiss the idea that thrombotic factors may play a role. I would welcome your comments on this.

Gaziano: There is certainly a suggestion that they may play a role, and if they do, it is likely to be in the threefold increased risk in haemorrhagic stroke that we see with heavier drinking. As for thrombotic factors explaining the early part of the decline in the MI curve, I think it's biologically plausible, but data which suggest thrombotic factors mediate the protective effect of alcohol are not available. This is in contrast to available data supporting an HDL effect. I don't think thrombotic factors have been fully enough explored in large data sets for us to say definitely whether or not they play a contributing role.

Bondy: I have a question about triglycerides and the fact that there seems to be a threshold effect. Some studies have found lower levels of HDL in very heavy drinkers, but this has been attributed to liver disease. Could the same be true with triglycerides, that what you're actually seeing is some form of liver change?

Gaziano: What we begin to see with respect to triglycerides at two drinks per day does seem to be a threshold effect. There is no linear association with triglycerides. Triglycerides are difficult to measure, because within an individual the fasting triglyceride levels will vary by up to 40%. We don't see any change at all in triglycerides until two drinks per day, but I wouldn't want to postulate that that's due to liver damage, because there's very little evidence of liver damage at these levels of drinking. However, we begin to see the triglyceride effect at about the same point that we begin to see the hypertension effect. This leads me to wonder whether they're metabolically related.

Shaper: Isn't there a strong inverse relationship between HDL and triglycerides?

Gaziano: We often see them inversely related, but this is not always the case. There are certain situations that raise one but don't necessarily lower the other. Here is one case where we have a mechanism that's raising HDL early but it's not having any material effect on triglycerides.

Farchi: What can you say about the temporal relationship between alcohol intake and HDL increase? We see that a drink once a week is associated with a lower risk of myocardial infarction. So is it sufficient to take one drink a week to obtain higher HDL levels or is it necessary to drink regularly the whole week?

Gaziano: Again, we didn't see much of an effect with just one drink a week: it wasn't until we got to one drink a day that we saw a big effect. From what we know from the metabolic studies, the time course of change is probably in the order of days to weeks, at least for HDL_3. There's a suggestion that it might be longer for HDL_2 and there may be more than one mechanism at play. I think that how you drink your alcohol makes a difference, and that's what we would anticipate. Gerry Shaper has HDL data that suggest that binge drinkers don't get as high a rise in their HDL as people who drink regularly during the week (Shaper et al 1985).

Shaper: We can't talk about binge drinkers; we can only talk about heavy weekend drinkers. Heavy weekend drinkers and light daily drinkers have roughly similar HDL levels; in fact, the latter group have slightly higher levels. The effects of prolonged drinking versus intermittent drinking are seen more clearly for blood pressure effects, which can be more easily monitored. Quite persistent drinking is required to keep your blood pressure up. If you measure a group of men between Monday and Friday, as occurs in most surveys, the mean blood pressure drops steadily from Monday to Friday (Wannamethee & Shaper 1991). Hypertension clinics therefore need to be held on Fridays to diminish the effects of alcohol on the prevalence of hypertension.

Puddey: We have recently looked at the effects of alcohol on HDL in an intervention study (Rakic et al 1998). We took 55 men over a four week period and characterized them according to pattern of alcohol intake. Fourteen of them were drinking 80% of their entire intake between Thursday night and Sunday night; the other 41 spread their alcohol intake through the week. We randomized the two groups into a two-way crossover paradigm and compared them while they were on low alcohol and normal beer. We saw a 0.12 mmol/l fall in HDL when they switched to low alcohol intake and the magnitude of the fall was no different in the weekend drinkers compared with the daily drinkers. The weekend drinkers were drinking about 300 g alcohol/week, while the daily drinkers were drinking about 350 g/week. But the weekend drinkers had a much higher daily dose of alcohol. We have therefore been unable to show a difference between pattern of alcohol intake and its effect on HDL or apolipoproteins in an intervention study.

Rehm: Two points. First, I think all measures of linear trends on those relationships between alcohol and myocardial infarction or CHD are somewhat deceptive, because what you see is always a very sharp drop, and then a plateau. Moreover, there are some studies indicating that for females there's an upturn which goes beyond one, meaning that females who drink more than four drinks a day have increased risk of coronary heart disease incidence and mortality. Males rest on the plateau even with quite high levels of drinking. So from the public health perspective it is important to discern when this sharp drop in risk occurs.

Second, can that upturn be explained by a factor such as triglycerides? Is there a sex differential for triglycerides?

Gaziano: We have been looking at the shape of the curve for different risk sets. What we see, whether we look at low risk men or women, or high risk men or women, is that the shape of the MI curve is virtually identical. How that contributes to the total mortality curve depends on the rate of myocardial infarction which will define the shape of the total mortality curve. This is what tells us where the mortality curve begins to turn up. But we see an incredible consistency. The level drops and then plateaus. My suspicion is that we have a protective effect that we think would provide us with a linear decline, but then we may have competing effects as we go up into the heavier-drinking range such that the continued rise in HDL is offset by an increase in possibly hypertension or triglycerides. The shape of the MI curve is consistent through all groups, but how it combines with the other risks to give the overall mortality curve is quite different for each population. I also agree fully with the notion that from a public health standpoint, the main benefit is this reduction in CHD risk, which doesn't seem to increase with heavier drinking.

Shaper: Unfortunately, what people derive from the shape of your curve is that one derives benefit right up to about three or four drinks a day. In fact, a large number of studies have found the greatest benefit at about 3–5 drinks a day. You are pointing out that this benefit has also occurred at lower levels of intake. The trouble is that the pattern of that relationship does not fit with the pattern of HDL increase that one sees as alcohol increases, which is in an almost linear fashion.

Criqui: Gerry Shaper earlier asked a question about inverse correlation between triglycerides and HDL. In free-living individuals there's a strong inverse correlation between the level of HDL cholesterol and the level of triglycerides in the blood. For a variety of behaviours, such as exercise, weight loss and cigarette smoking, the two lipid fractions change in reciprocal fashion, so that if you exercise and lose weight, the HDL cholesterol goes up and the triglyceride goes down.

There are at least four areas where they don't move in synchrony. Each of these I think is illustrative. One is the high carbohydrate diet in which HDL usually stays the same or drops a little, and triglycerides go way up in the early stages. These are thought to be the fluffy-puffy less-atherogenic triglycerides, but the data are somewhat skimpy. The second area, where the data are strong, is post-menopausal oestrogen therapy in which HDL increases substantially and triglyceride also increases statistically significantly. These triglycerides are again of the fluffy-puffy kind (Walsh et al 1991). The third area is with bile acid binding resins, in which HDL goes up a little as do the triglycerides, and yet there is clear protection from coronary disease. The fourth area is alcohol, which, as Mike Gaziano pointed out, causes substantial increase in HDL cholesterol, and in most individuals the triglycerides don't change. In the heavier drinkers there's a subset that appears to experience a sharp elevation in triglycerides. I was very interested in Mike Gaziano's data, because he said that perhaps this increase in triglyceride is somewhat attenuating the benefit occurring with HDL at these high levels of alcohol consumption. This is possible, but it is also possible that there are uncontrolled factors such as blood pressure. But the general principle in looking at triglycerides and HDL is that almost all the population studies show that the risk occurs to individuals who have a simultaneous depression of HDL and increase of triglycerides. In free-living populations where the HDL and the triglycerides are low, as in most third world countries, there is not an increase of coronary disease. In the limited number of individuals, such as women on post-menopausal oestrogen therapy, where both triglycerides and HDLs are high, there is no increase in the risk of cardiovascular disease.

I have a question for Mike: when you talk about thrombotic factors, did you actually put fibrinogen and measures of platelet aggregation in your models?

Gaziano: We didn't.

Klatsky: I have a question that has to do with the relative importance of HDL and anti-thrombotic factors as contributors to the inverse relation of coronary disease. There are studies which suggest that the amount of alcohol taken within the previous 24 h is inversely related to risk of coronary death. Does this not suggest a short-term mechanism? HDL cholesterol is much less likely to act in the short-term than antithrombotic factors.

Gaziano: I have seen contradictory data on the acute effects of alcohol, particularly for heavier or binge drinking. Some data suggest that there may be increases in the rate of MIs in countries where there is heavy weekend drinking, while other data suggest that the previous 24 h of drinking may reduce the risk of MI. It is possible that there's an acute effect that we have not been able to detect. I would suspect that this would operate through some other mechanism.

Klatsky: Do you agree that an acute effect is not likely to be due to HDL?

Gaziano: Yes.

Keil: In our data from southern Germany we see the same L-shaped relationship (starting with alcohol intake of 10 g/day and then the curve is completely flat until an intake of 80 g/day), but the total mortality curve has its lowest point at 30 g/day. My public health recommendation would therefore be that an alcohol intake of 10–20 g/day seems sufficient, but up to 30 g/day doesn't seem to be harmful, at least not for men. I am convinced that besides HDL, antiplatelet aggregation and other antithrombosis factors must play a role in the protective effects of alcohol. I see this parallelism between the protective effect for CHD and for ischaemic stroke: in both events, thrombosis is very important. Besides HDL, I think there must be additional factors, just as with the detrimental effects of smoking where thrombogenesis is an important factor as well as lowered HDL.

Miller: There are several metabolic effects of alcohol on the HDL pathway. These include ApoA1 synthesis via the liver, increased lipoprotein lipase and reduced hepatic lipase activity. There are one or two reports that suggest a more marked increase in the plasma concentration of HDL particles containing ApoA1 and ApoA2 than of particles containing ApoA1 alone (Branchi et al 1997). It may therefore be of benefit to think about HDL particles as Alaupovic thought of them, in terms of ApoA1 and ApoA2. I think the relationship that we're seeing out in the general community, which is reflected in the inverse relationship between HDL and triglyceride, is saying something about lipoprotein lipase: this is why we see an additive effect with alcohol consumption and exercise. When it comes to talking about the sensitivity of the protective response to alcohol levels, it would be useful to know what alcohol dosage does to lipoprotein lipase activity. I don't know of any work in that area, but I wonder just how sensitive lipoprotein lipase is to small intakes of alcohol.

Renaud: We have to remember that aspirin doesn't affect LDL or HDL. None the less, it decreases coronary events by 50% in all studies. Aspirin works by decreasing platelet reactivity, especially aggregation. Alcohol does exactly the same thing by a similar mechanism. This means that in any of these studies there will be a decrease in platelet reactivity. We can't ignore thrombotic effects.

Gaziano: I certainly don't want to dismiss the importance of thrombosis in coronary events. However, non-steroidal agents are also platelet inhibitory, yet they do not have the same effect as aspirin at inhibiting coronary events. Not everything that works in a test-tube to prevent thrombosis prevents myocardial infarctions. Thrombotic or antithrombotic effects remain a possible explanatory variable for certain events, such as haemorrhagic stroke. Different vascular beds are at play here, so we have to remember that we have a two phase process: atherogenesis and plaque rupture followed by thrombosis. We know that preventing both is important. Because of effects in other vascular beds, we don't have to invoke thrombotic mechanisms. We have data from the Physicians' Health Study that alcohol is inversely related to angina, peripheral vascular disease and ischaemic stroke, but not to haemorrhagic stroke. My personal feeling is that we have identified a mechanism for delayed atherogenesis, a chronic effect largely mediated by lipids, that affects peripheral, coronary and cerebral vascular beds, as evidenced by the inverse relationship of all three of those diseases. But we don't have good data that antithrombotic effects are playing a role in explaining lower MI rates among light drinkers. Attractive as the hypothesis might be, the data do not allow us to conclude that they are playing a major role.

Renaud: Are you convinced that atheroslcerosis is lower in people drinking alcohol? In other words, we all learned in pathology that this was the case, but the control autopsies were not done on a random sample of the population. Atherosclerotic lesions of alcoholics were frequently compared to those of patients having died from cardiovascular diseases (Hall et al 1953). By contrast, if autopsy reports from a random sample of the population, let's say road accident victims, were compared to those of alcoholics, you wouldn't find much difference (Viel et al 1966). My point concerns the extent to which we are certain that the protective effect of alcohol on CHD is on atherosclerosis, and not on myocardial infarction (i.e. thrombosis) as observed in the study in Hawaii (Yano et al 1977). I would challenge the hypothesis that the benefits of alcohol are derived through reduced atherosclerosis and not thrombosis.

Fillmore: You mentioned a question you used for evaluating consumption. As I read that question, you were not measuring consumption of alcoholic beverages, but rather frequency of drinking. Is that correct?

Gaziano: Absolutely. This is one of the limitations of many of these studies: we don't have a good characterization of how the subjects consumed the beverage. When we have done small pilot studies in subjects who were healthier than the average, the frequency of binge drinking is low and regular drinking is more common.

Fillmore: I would challenge you that you're not measuring consumption of alcoholic beverages when you are only looking at frequency. There's a lot of work in the alcohol field on measurement and attempts to come to grips with all the problems of measuring patterns of drinking and so on (e.g. Dawson 1998). My impression of a lot of this literature as a sociologist, not as a physician or an epidemiologist, is that the measures of consumption in the mortality literature are typically very poor. In some studies of this genre they are so bad that I couldn't answer the question myself regarding my own consumption. This is worrisome to me.

If you have very different measures of consumption then how can you state that you have cross-study consistency in findings when your major predictor variable is not measuring the same thing?

Gaziano: It is actually quite comforting that people who have measured this parameter in quite a number of different ways find similar associations. If what we were measuring was not a reflection of reality we would find null associations. You are right that there are many problems with the instruments we use. The food frequency questionnaire is not a perfect instrument. We've compared the food frequency questionnaire with a food diary, and for alcohol it turns out to be a reasonable approximation, with correlation coefficients of about 0.6. However, it is comforting that the different methodologies in different study populations have come up with a relatively consistent association, despite the limitations.

Fillmore: How do you explain the fact that the definition of non-drinkers varies radically across the studies? Does this strengthen your point?

Gaziano: I think it's a big problem, and it may explain some of the differences we're seeing in the various studies. Fortunately, in all the studies that our group has been involved in, we've had the luxury of being able to change the definition for the referent group. It really doesn't matter whether we use the never/rare drinkers or the light drinkers as the referent group.

Fillmore: But I'm asking you for consistency across studies, for example when you perform systematic cross-study comparisons such as meta-analysis. When the operational definitions are so different, how can you make comparisons?

Bondy: We all recognize that most of these cohort studies were not designed to study alcohol. They were designed to examine a number of exposure factors, and in some cases alcohol was just an add-on. When you look at the actual measures, they tend to fall into a couple of categories in terms of the underlying construct they really address. Frequency of drinking is how I would describe what is most often covered. This might be why you are seeing consistency across studies. We have also heard a lot over the last couple of days that in looking at frequency of drinking we might have stumbled upon exactly what we should have been measuring. If a person has eight drinks once per week, they're going to sit very low on this frequency scale and we don't think this sort of consumption pattern will be very protective. On the other hand, the drinker who spreads his eight drinks over seven days has a high frequency score and this correlates with the protective effect.

The other common type of measure is a quantity–frequency (QF) scale: most of the food frequency records also have questions about how often you consume, for instance, broccoli, and how much broccoli do you consume at each sitting, and then do the same thing for alcohol.

Fillmore: But are they then converted to volume?

Bondy: Yes, by taking the mid-point of the chosen frequency category, and multiplying that by the usual amount consumed, you get an estimate of the total volume. I'm a little happier with interpreting that as a volume measure than as a single-question frequency scale. However, what still tends to get missed is the contribution to total volume that is attributed to heavier drinking events. People tend to give you a modal intake on drinking occasions, as opposed to their true average number of drinks per occasion. Alcohol consumed during heavy drinking occasions tends to be under-reported in QF scales.

Some of these studies, however, have used beverage-specific quantity scales — asking about the usual frequency and the usual amount for wine, beer and spirits, for example. With the more detailed measure you are getting into instruments which the alcohol sociology literature says aren't so bad. More detailed QF scales are better at measuring volume, and more sensitive to variability in the number of drinks per occasion. For those studies that were fortunate enough to have these more detailed measures, not enough has been done with the data to disaggregate patterns of drinking. These more detailed measures would allow you to compare subjects who drink heavily one day a week with those who drink moderately every day, as well as how this relates to beverage choice.

Fillmore: How are you going to answer my consistency question?

Bondy: Because they're consistently measuring frequency.

Anderson: I would like to make a plea that we should get the measuring instrument right. Of course, the problem is that many of these studies were not set up to study the effect of alcohol. People are embarking on new and hugely costly studies: it seems to me to be totally unacceptable to use the wrong measurement instrument where there is good scientific knowledge about how to get a good one. My plea is therefore for the alcohol field to make sure that what they know gets through to the cardiovascular field or the other epidemiological fields so that people are using good standardized questionnaires.

Peters: You mentioned that in studying people with stroke, when they were unconscious you asked an informant about their alcohol consumption. We know that if you ask an informant about how much someone drinks and you independently ask the person themselves, you get somewhat different results. This is a difficulty in these studies.

Keil: The whole story reminds me of the discussions about smoking. I was asked for a long time whether we were able to assess cigarette smoking accurately. However, we are better off in this area because we have good biological markers, such as cotinine. What measure can you apply at present for assessing alcohol consumption that is better than a seven day nutrition record?

Bondy: It depends on the culture and it depends on how frequently the population under study drinks. If you are studying a population where frequent drinking is common, then the seven day diary has many advantages. The respondent should be able to recall actual recent events quite objectively, as opposed to being faced with the more complex cognitive task of extrapolation — translating their actual behaviour into a statement about usual practices. However, it doesn't work terribly well in the USA and Canada among populations who drink relatively infrequently. In Canadian data where we don't have that many abstainers, at least one third of non-abstainers (people who have had one or more drink in the past 12 months) won't have had a drink in the past week.

We almost always find a seven day diary in the federal general purpose health surveys, and this makes it very difficult to do statistical analyses on the individual level, because so many non-abstainers have had no alcohol in the past week. In the alcohol and drug specific surveys, where you have a variety of measures, you see that many of those people who haven't had a single drink in the previous week drink significant amounts of alcohol. So what needs to be borne in mind is the nature of the population, and what it is about alcohol that we are most interested in studying in terms of the theoretical relationships between the exposure measure and the outcomes we are studying. It may well be that volume is not as important as blood alcohol on peak occasions, for instance.

Farrell: There's a separate problem, which is that when one wishes to quantify the level of consumption, the variation in the type of glasses drunk from may cause major inaccuracy in estimating unit consumption.

Shaper: With due respect to the methodologists, the point that Michael Gaziano was trying to make was that, despite all the problems, most studies ask about frequency and amount which gives a reasonable indication of what people are drinking as a usual event in a week. By and large the studies that you have been telling us about are reasonably consistent in what they're finding.

Peters: I disagree. Recently, we've looked in West London at the alcohol consumption of a group of Indo-Asians. We took medical histories, and they all denied drinking. We then asked one of leaders of the group how much he thought these people were drinking, and it was a significant amount. If drinking is frowned upon for religious or other reasons, you are going to get a totally distorted view.

Shaper: This is an unusual group from which to generalize about the validity of reported intake of alcohol.

Rehm: Consistency of results between different measures for alcohol consumption and consequences varies by the endpoints examined. If the endpoint is a consequence of overall volume of alcohol consumed (e.g. liver cirrhosis) and alcohol consumption was measured by different instruments which all correlated highly with overall volume, consistent results will emerge. Endpoints more related to the pattern of drinking (e.g. traffic accidents, fetal alcohol syndrome) produced varying results, since the causal patterns may be related only indirectly to the measures used in research. This shows that the questionnaire or the specific type of instrument used for alcohol assessment has to be specific for the endpoint, and the biological theory linking alcohol to the endpoint (Rehm et al 1996).

The consistent results found for CHD with different assessment instruments measuring overall volume, or frequency only, can have two explanations: first of all, drinking frequency is important for CHD. Second, by selecting the cohorts —

namely middle-to-upper class males aged 45–64 at baseline — implicitly rather regular drinking patterns were selected (e.g. Willett et al 1985, Rimm et al 1992) where volume correlates highly with frequency. It would be totally disastrous if you were to try the same questionnaires on a young student cohort studying other endpoints related to alcohol such as accidents and injuries. For such studies, we really have to work on our instruments.

Criqui: A point about questionnaires in general. I don't think I've ever done a study where part through we haven't had to tweak the questionnaire. Part of the evolution of epidemiology studies in general is continuing to refine the questionnaire. This is problematic for alcohol, more so than for smoking and cholesterol. The more ethically loaded the question is, the greater the difficulty. If you look at any given population of how much people report in the questionnaire and how much is actually sold, the latter is higher by at least a factor of two. The question is: does this have major implications for results that you obtain? It is possible that that reporting is approximately proportional across categories: i.e. the two per day drinker says one, the four per day drinker says two, and so on. It is also possible that it under-reporting is concentrated in heavy drinkers, where people report honestly up to three drinks a day and then they start attenuating it. If you consider all the biases that can occur in a questionnaire-based study, the majority of them actually tend to support the null hypothesis, that is reduce the possibility of showing an association. Even Dr Shaper's famous point about the sick quitters can cut both ways, because they can quit before baseline, before they enter the study, or after baseline in which case if alcohol is protective it underestimates the benefit.

Quite a large number of epidemiological studies show a consistent relationship between low level alcohol use and reduced risk of death, and also show positive relationships, for instance, between alcohol and accidents, violence, cirrhosis and certain cancers. They are not perfect, but there is a sense of validity. It is difficult to explain all this as an artefact of questionnaires.

Fillmore: It has long been known that populations of abstainers and heavy drinkers share many characteristics in North American and Northern European studies (e.g. Kozlowski & Ferrence 1990). They seem to be in poor health, they both tend to be from dry areas of the country rather than wet areas, and they are both of lower socioeconomic status.

Gaziano: I think we were fortunate that these are all healthy professionals. We didn't see that. We saw a slight increase in risk among abstainers, but we saw the biggest increase risk at the other end of the spectrum. Within this cohort we see a relatively strong association that I think is more likely to be causal than not. When you begin to extrapolate the relative risks to the general population I think you're right, you have to consider that, but we were fortunate that we don't see much of a sick abstainer effect in this cohort of healthy physicians.

Rehm: It really depends on the culture. What has been said is mainly true for American culture. If you look at the Canadian abstainers, they tend to be younger female immigrants with much better than average health status. If you go into the German literature the abstainers are a very different group. In most parts of Italian-speaking Switzerland, more than 60% of females are abstainers, and in no way do these resemble the heavy drinkers. So I am totally against generalizing anything which has been said about abstainers and heavy drinkers because it depends so much on the culture.

Shaper: The point I was trying to make earlier was that because of this cultural variance between populations in the nature and characteristics of the various sub-groups of the non-drinking group, it becomes very difficult in these meta-analyses to combine them, or even to use them at all as a reference group. I agree with what Michael Gaziano was saying, that if you do not use these groups but instead use occasional or very light drinkers, you still observe a benefit for CHD from regular drinking. The shape of the curve will depend on the period of your follow-up, because of the changes in alcohol intake that are taking place over time. If you have a short-term follow-up, most workers will find the curve going up for cardiovascular disease in heavy drinkers.

Keil: We probably all accept that smoking and CHD is causally related and I think we also accept that the CHD risk for smokers is roughly doubled. We find here a protective affect of alcohol on CHD of around 50%, so it's about the same magnitude. We are relying on observational studies in both areas: we have no clinical trial data. In both areas we also have measurement problems. So why is it that one factor — smoking — is universally accepted to have a detrimental effect for CHD, but the protective effect of the other factor — alcohol — causes such controversy? What is the difference in evidence?

Gaziano: I don't think the evidence is quite as clear for alcohol. We know what happens when people stop smoking: their risk of an MI falls back to normal in three to five years. Were we to have the same kind of data on alcohol then I think we would be approaching the same level of certainty. We have multiple mechanisms occurring in alcohol and the shape of the curve is not linear like it is for cigarette smoking. That's why we get into this difficulty of what exactly is going on. It depends on the population and other factors that you put in the model, so it is a bit more complex. And the quantitative estimates I think do vary a bit more than they might for smoking.

Peters: Let me be controversial and suggest that epidemiological studies without biological markers must be interpreted with caution. We've heard about questionnaires, but you wouldn't dream of doing a smoking study without measuring salivary cotinine. There are biological markers for alcohol: should we be using them?

Farrell: The problem is the markers aren't good enough.

Bondy: What health outcomes are you interested in and what is it important to have a marker for? If you want to know how much alcohol a person has in their blood right now, there are some decent markers. But we don't have good markers to tell us how much they drank last week. Show me that the marker is a good estimate of the exposure that you want to study and then I'll be happy.

Peters: There are proxy markers of alcohol toxicity, such as γ-glutamyl-transferase (γGT), mean corpuscular volume and carbohydrate-deficient transferrin (CDT).

Criqui: We have just finished writing a paper looking in an older population, which is where the benefit is liable to be for alcohol, looking at markers of alcohol consumption (Lindenfeld et al 1998). We used the CAGE questionnaire. One of the problems with this is that the questions are phrased for lifetime. We have several people in our population who quit drinking 20 years ago but who are four plus positive because they used to be alcoholics. We also looked at a regular frequency and volume questionnaire, and looked at multiple biochemical markers in 877 men and women. None of the markers were very good. Some red cell parameters and liver enzymes were modestly correlated with drinks per week and CAGE score, but nothing distinguished either abuse or heavy drinking very well. It turns out that HDL cholesterol was as good as anything in distinguishing the level of drinking.

Peters: The CAGE is very convenient, but it is really looking for heavy alcohol misuse. There are better questionnaires. We've done some work on the AUDIT questionnaire: the score from this correlates pretty well with CDT and other markers. If you use the questionnaire that's designed for a continuum from no alcohol to heavy alcohol use, and correlate with these scores, then you are more likely to get a clear result.

Criqui: We used both a regular frequency questionnaire and CAGE. Neither did very well.

Rehm: If we want to use markers quite often we end up using HDL. To some extent this reflects either our ignorance or the poverty of markers available.

Peters: Currently the best marker is probably CDT, which is pretty useful in men but less so in women.

Shaper: More than a decade ago we looked at 25 biochemical and haematological markers in almost 8000 middle-aged men when they came into the study and when we took their alcohol history. On a group basis there is a remarkably good relationship between the biochemical markers and reported alcohol intake (Shaper et al 1985). However, when it comes down to individual drinkers far greater variation will be seen.

Wannamethee: One of the markers that's often used as an indicator of current alcohol consumption is γGT. However, although this is strongly associated with alcohol, it is also strongly affected by other factors such as body mass index. In our own study, when we look at γGT and the risk of coronary heart disease events, we do not get a U-shaped curve but rather a linear positive association. γGT is more strongly associated with many of the major cardiovascular disease risk factors than is alcohol intake (Wannamethee et al 1995).

Peters: γGT is as sensitive as a marker, but CDT is much more specific: it reflects alcohol consumption over the previous two weeks. The early methodological problems have now been ironed out in the latest generation of CDT tests. The previous first and second generation assays did not correct for variations in total transferrin, which is an acute phase protein. This is why, for example, CDT has previously not been very useful in women, because iron deficiency, not uncommon in women, leads to an increase in total transferrin and thus an increase in CDT. However, if you express the CDT as a percentage of the total transferrin, as the new third-generation assays do, it is much more reliable (Keating et al 1998).

Bondy: We should realize that what's wrong with the self-reports we have now is not the respondents but the questions. There is a literature that shows how better measures of self-reports can be obtained with relatively little extra effort, time and money that should be explored first.

Miller: I'm speaking from ignorance, but I've seen literature stating that acetaldehyde reacts with proteins. I have also seen reports that the level of acetaldehyde necessary for this effect are not levels that could be achieved normally *in vivo*. But I wonder whether there have been attempts to develop sensitive tests for small quantities of acetaldehyde-modified proteins with reasonably long half-lives: is this feasible?

Peters: Several people have worked in this area. For example, glycosylated haemoglobin is a good proxy marker for glycaemic control over three months. People thought the same thing might be true for acetaldehyde–haemoglobin complexes. The problem is that the adduct of acetaldehyde and protein is much less stable. People have looked for antibodies raised against protein–acetaldehyde complexes, and although the levels seem to be higher in patients with alcoholic liver disease than people without, some people apparently who have never consumed alcohol do still have antibodies to the adduct!

Shaper: Susan Bondy, you hinted that there are better alcohol questionnaires that are available. What is the nature of these better questionnaires that none of us are using?

Bondy: There is an extensive literature about measuring volume of alcohol. You need to give the respondent something to work with, so you need to give them enough cues to recall so they can recall events. You shouldn't ask them to do a complicated cognitive task: asking them to describe generalities about variable behaviour is difficult. Things like a daily diary are much better in terms of those properties, because they're describing actual behaviour as opposed to a sort of general state of being. It doesn't work terribly well if you don't drink frequently. I would encourage you first to define clearly what it is you want to operationalize.

Peters: I also understand that there is evidence that if you use computers to ask questions the data is more reliable: people are much more less likely to give misleading information.

Bondy: Generally people do not choose to lie to you. If they give false information it is because the question doesn't make sense or isn't interpreted properly. The only exception to that is when they are presently intoxicated, and then they do lie to you.

Peters: Have you any experience of the use of computer-driven questionnaires? They are said to be more reliable, certainly for some of the screening procedures.

Bondy: I can't answer that question specifically, but I wouldn't be surprised if they motivate people and give them time to think.

Hendriks: Is CDT also applicable for moderate alcohol intake measurements? I had the impression that specificity of this parameter is only good at the higher range of alcohol intake.

Peters: Most of these tests are designed to pick up pathological levels of drinking: they're not designed to distinguish between abstainers and those who take, for example one drink a day. They are useful for excluding alcohol misusers.

Puddey: I think you might want to keep an open mind about whether low levels of alcohol intake (I'm talking about 1–5 drinks a day) are correlated with CDT. An abstract presented by Nick Martin's group in Australia (Whitfield et al 1997) suggested that there is a correlation, at least cross-sectionally. We have recently evaluated CDT in an intervention study and have shown tight correlations between CDT and the self-reported change from five down to one drink a day (unpublished results).

References

Branchi A, Rovellini A, Tomella C et al 1997 Association of alcohol consumption with HDL subpopulations defined by apolipoprotein AI and apolipoprotein AII content. Eur J Clin Nutr 51:362–365

Dawson D 1998 Report of the International Workshop on Consumption Measures and Models for use in Policy Development and Evaluation (May 1997). Alcohol Clin Exp Res, in press

Hall EM, Olsen AY, Davies FE 1953 Clinical and pathological review of 782 cases from 16600 necropsies. Am J Pathol 29:993–1027

Keating J, Cheung C, Peters TJ, Przemiosho R, Williams R, Sherwood RA 1998 Carbohydrate-deficient transferrin in alcoholic and non-alcoholic liver disease: a comparison of two assay methods. Addict Biol, in press

Kozlowski T, Ferrence RG 1990 Statistical control in research on alcohol and tobacco: an example from research on alcohol and mortality. Br J Addict 85:271–278

Lindenfeld EA, Barrett-Connor EL, Criqui MH 1998 The pattern of alcohol intake and abuse among older adults. The Rancho Bernardo Study. Submitted

Maclure M 1993 Demonstration of deductive meta-analysis: ethanol intake and risk of myocardial infarction. Epidemiol Rev 15:328–351

Rakic V, Puddey IB, Dimmitt SB, Beilin LJ 1998 A controlled trial of the effects of pattern of alcohol intake on serum lipid levels in regular drinkers. Atherosclerosis 137:243–252

Rehm J, Ashley MJ, Room R et al 1996 On the emerging paradigm of drinking patterns and their social health consequences. Addiction 91:1615–1621

Rimm EB, Giovannucci EL, Stampfer MJ, Colditz GA, Litin LB, Willett WC 1992 Reproducibility and validity of an expanded self-administered semiquantitative food frequency questionnaire among male health professionals. Am J Epidemiol 135:1114–1126

Shaper AG, Pocock SJ, Ashby D, Walker M, Whitehead TP 1985 Biochemical and haematological response to alcohol intake. Ann Clin Biochem 22:50–61

Viel B, Donoso S, Salcedo D et al 1966 Alcoholism and socioeconomic status, hepatic damage and arteriosclerosis. Arch Intern Med 117:84–91

Walsh BW, Schiff I, Rosner B, Greenberg L, Ravnikar V, Sacks FM 1991 Effects of postmenopausal estrogen replacement on the concentrations and metabolism of plasma lipoproteins. N Engl J Med 325:1196–1204

Wannamethee G, Shaper AG 1991 Alcohol intake and variations in blood pressure by day of examination. J Human Hypertens 5:59–67

Wannametheee G, Ebrahim S, Shaper AG 1995 Gamma-glutamyltransferase: determinants and association with mortality from ischaemic heart disease and all causes. Am J Epidemiol 142:699–708

Whitfield JB, Fletcher LM, Murphy TL, Martin NG 1997 Sensitivity of serum carbohydrate-deficient transferrin measurement for detection of hazardous drinking — effects of age, smoking, obesity and lipid profile. Australasian Association of Clinical Biochemists Annual Scientific Meeting, 1997 (abstr)

Willett WC, Sampson L, Stampfer MJ et al 1985 Reproducibility and validity of a semiquantitative food frequency questionnaire. Am J Epidemiol 122:51–65

Yano K, Rhoads GG, Kagan A 1977 Coffee, alcohol and the risk of coronary heart disease among Japanese men living in Hawaii. N Engl J Med 297:405–409

Alcohol, coagulation and fibrinolysis

Henk F. J. Hendriks and Martijn S. van der Gaag

TNO-Nutrition and Food Research Institute, P.O. Box 360, 3700 AJ Zeist, The Netherlands

Abstract. Despite the solid evidence for thrombosis playing a key role in coronary heart disease (CHD) mortality, identifying specific haemostatic risk factors for CHD has been difficult except for fibrinogen. Excessive alcohol consumption clearly affects platelet function. Moderate alcohol consumption may affect several haemostatic factors, including fibrinogen concentration, platelet aggregability and the fibrinolytic factors tissue-type plasminogen activator and plasminogen activator inhibitor. These changes support the hypothesis that moderate alcohol beneficially affects the haemostatic balance in a way that decreases the risk of CHD mortality.

1998 Alcohol and cardiovascular diseases. Wiley, Chichester (Novartis Foundation Symposium 216) p 111–124

The association between alcohol consumption and risk for coronary heart disease (CHD) mortality is U- or L-shaped. Moderate drinking beneficially affects the relative risk for CHD mortality, whereas drinking excessive amounts of alcohol increases the risk for death from other causes (Boffetta & Garfinkel 1990). The inverse association between moderate drinking and CHD mortality is well established. Evidence for a causal relationship comes from over 60 ecological, case-control and cohort studies. Previous reviews have concluded that men and women who drink 1–2 drinks per day have the lowest risk of CHD. In a meta-analysis of cohort studies (Maclure 1993) a summary relative risk of CHD of 0.83 (95% confidence interval 0.77 to 0.89) for moderate drinkers (2–3 drinks per day) compared with teetotallers was calculated. In a recently published review (Rimm et al 1996) covering 10 prospective cohort studies, four found a significant inverse association between CHD risk and moderate wine drinking, four for beer drinking, and four for spirits. The total evidence available so far suggests that all alcoholic drinks are linked with a lower risk, indicating that much of the benefit is from alcohol itself.

Underlying mechanisms

Apart from the epidemiological observation that an association exists between alcohol consumption and CHD risk, a mechanistic support for such an association is essential. The mechanisms underlying the association can be substantiated using many designs measuring biomarkers which need to be causally linked to CHD risk. The processes leading to arteriosclerosis and cardiovascular death include at least two steps:

(1) The deposition of lipids in the vascular wall by the influx of macrophages and modified low density lipoprotein (LDL), and proliferation of smooth muscle cells. A fatty streak or a plaque will develop.
(2) The rupture of a plaque inducing thrombotic events and occlusion of a blood vessel. This may be a life-threatening event if it affects a coronary artery.

Haemostatic factors may play a role in the development of CHD mortality by contributing to each of these steps. Thrombotic factors may contribute to the development of atherosclerotic plaques; fibrin and platelet components are present in plaques, and platelets secrete chemotactic substances and growth factors *in vitro*. Also, at sites of destabilized atherosclerotic plaques, thrombotic factors are involved in occlusion, embolization, or both. The effects of alcohol consumption on factors involved in thrombotic events is the main subject discussed in this presentation.

CHD mortality and thrombosis

The role of thrombotic events in heart infarction has been the subject of some debate, since death from heart infarction has not always corresponded with the occurrence of a coronary thrombus at autopsy. However, later studies have established this relationship by the following observations:

(1) Arteriography within six hours of pain showed a complete occlusion of relevant arteries.
(2) Autoradiographic studies with radiolabelled fibrinogen suggested thrombus formation preceded the infarction.
(3) Angioscopy showed plaque fissures and overlying thrombus in lesions causing unstable angina.
(4) Thrombolytic therapy after acute myocardial infarction showed that occlusions were due to fresh thrombi.
(5) Antiplatelet and anticoagulation therapy (heparin and warfarin) have consistently been shown to reduce coronary and cerebrovascular events.

Haemostatic factors

Haemostatic control is mainly determined by four factors: the endothelium, platelets, coagulation and fibrinolysis. The vascular endothelium is an organ of about 1–2 kg consisting of about 10^{11} cells, with an aggregate surface area exceeding 100 m². The endothelium maintains blood fluidity by inhibiting blood coagulation and platelet aggregation, and promoting fibrinolysis. It also provides a protective barrier that separates blood cells and plasma factors from highly reactive elements in the deeper layers of the vessel wall. When a blood vessel is severed, it constricts and diverts blood from the site of injury. Subsequently, blood is exposed to endothelial structures stimulating haemostatic plug formation by promoting platelet adhesion and aggregation and by activating blood coagulation. The endothelial cell possesses several membrane-oriented molecules that promote the fluidity of blood, including the heparin–antithrombin III system, the thrombin–thrombomodulin–protein C system, and the plasminogen/plasminogen activator system. The second important factor in haemostasis are the platelets. Platelets adhere to areas of disrupted endothelium (providing binding sites for adhesive proteins such as von Willebrand factor through the platelet glycoprotein Ib/IX complex and fibrinogen, as well as fibronectin through integrin receptors), secrete platelet constituents and form large aggregates with clotting factors, forming the clot. The third important factor is coagulation, traditionally subdivided into extrinsic and intrinsic pathways. *In vivo* such a division does not occur because the tissue factor/factor VIIa complex is a potent activator of both pathways of the clotting cascade. Activation of this cascade leads to the activation of thrombin, the enzyme converting fibrinogen into fibrin and cross-linking fibrin. The fourth important factor is fibrinolysis. Fibrinolysis involves the activation of plasminogen into plasmin, the clot-dissolving enzyme. Plasminogen is activated by the tissue-type plasminogen activator (tPA) which itself may be neutralized by its inhibitor the plasminogen activator inhibitor (PAI). The balance between these two proteins determines the fibrinolytic capacity in blood. Overall, these four haemostatic factors yield a complex system of checks and balances, allowing the system to react appropriately according to the local circumstances.

Haemostatic risk factors for CHD

The number of established haemostatic risk factors for CHD are limited. Several methodological issues need to be considered before thrombotic factors can be established as a risk factor. These methodological issues include (Pearson et al 1997):

(1) In observational studies: not only associations, but also independencies and specificity of the association, a temporal sequence, consistency among studies, a strong association and a coherent biological mechanism of action.

(2)   Exclusion of confounding, which occurs when both the disease and the risk factor are related to a common third factor.
(3)   Exclusion of extended confounding, occurring when risk factors act through a haemostatic factor.
(4)   Interaction with other risk factors. A condition, such as an atherosclerotic plaque, may have to be present for a factor to be related.
(5)   Prevalence incidence bias. Haemostatic factors are usually also acute phase proteins changing with any other event in the body. Any increase in risk factors in acute cases may therefore be difficult to interpret.
(6)   Paradoxical reactions. A risk factor may increase when a decrease is expected. In addition, technical aspects need to be considered: are the haemostatic factors measured relevant, was the methodology applied correct and could artefacts be introduced by sampling, storage conditions and storage time?

Several haemostatic CHD risk factors will be discussed in this presentation. These include: fibrinogen, factor VII and VIII, lipoprotein(a), platelet aggregability, PAI-1 and tPA.

Fibrinogen

One of the main established haemostatic risk factors for CHD is fibrinogen. This complex glycoprotein is soluble and can be converted into the insoluble fibrin polymer by cleavage, non-covalent assembly and covalent stabilization by cross-linking. Seven prospective studies have consistently shown a positive association between fibrinogen concentrations and cardiovascular disease. Fibrinogen is likely to be causally related and the positive association has been shown to be dose-dependent. Several factors still need to be evaluated (Pearson et al 1997). Twelve recent studies have been listed reporting the association between alcohol consumption and fibrinogen levels (Table 1). Eight out of the 12 studies have shown an inverse or a partial inverse association and four have shown no inverse association, including one which reported a tendency to an inverse association. Experimental studies are limited.

Factor VII and factor VIII

Factor VII is a vitamin K-dependent plasma clotting factor that, in complex with tissue factor, forms a procoagulant enzyme initiating clot formation. Factor VII can be measured in various ways, including measuring zymogen mass, factor VII activity and factor VII antigen. Factor VIIa represents the *in vivo* activated part, because factor VII is not further activated by the substrates included in the assays. Factor VIIc measurement includes the partial *in vitro* activation of factor

TABLE 1 Association between alcohol consumption and fibrinogen

First author	Study	Study population	Association	Year
Balleisen		2880 men and 1306 women	No	1985
Tarallo		1008 men and women 4–60 y	Inverse for 30–40 y	1992
Krobot	Augsburg MONICA study	4434 men and women	Inverse	1992
Rankinen	FIN-MONICA	260 women 60–69 y	No	1993
Iso	Akita population study	1020 Japanese men and women	Inverse	1993
Iso	ARIC study	>15 000 African American and Caucasian men and women	Inverse	1993
Stefanick	PEPI	875 postmenopausal women	Inverse	1995
De Boever		770 male employees	No	1995
Cushman	Cardiovascular Health Study	5201 men and women over 65 y	Inverse in women only	1996
Sato		995 male employees	Inverse	1996
Ishikawa	Jichi Medical Study	1315 males, 1824 females	Tendency to an inverse	1997
Woodward	Glasgow MONICA study	746 men, 816 women	Inverse in men	1997

VII, the extent of activation depending on the origin of the thromboplastin used (rabbit, human, bovine). It is therefore difficult to compare factor VIIc data between studies.

The strongest risk factor correlations with factor VII (mass or activity) are with serum lipids. Correction for other risk factors maintained the strong association between the triglycerides–factor VII association and therefore this correlation should be taken into account. Although non-conclusive, the factor VII–CHD link is supported by four case-control studies of myocardial infarction survivors and defined coronary stenoses patients having higher factor VII concentrations than controls.

Three recent epidemiological studies investigated the association between factor VII concentration and activity and alcohol consumption (Table 2). The two most recent studies reported an inverse association between both factor VII concentration and factor VII activity, and alcohol consumption.

TABLE 2   Alcohol consumption and factor VII and factor VIII

First author	Study	Study population	Association	Year
Factor VII				
Balleisen		2880 men and 1306 women	No (concentration)	1985
Ishikawa	Jichi Medical Study	1315 males, 1824 females	Inverse (concentration)	1997
Cushman	Cardiovascular Health Study	5201 men and women over 65 y	Inverse (activity)	1996
Factor VIII				
Balleisen		2880 men and 1306 women	No	1985
Cushman	Cardiovascular Health Study	5201 men and women over 65 y	Inverse in women only	1996

Factor VIII is a glycoprotein that participates as a cofactor in the middle phase of the intrinsic pathway of blood coagulation. Only two of the three aforementioned studies have studied the association between factor VIII and alcohol consumption (Table 2), and only in one was a partial inverse association between Factor VIII and alcohol consumption shown. In addition, a limited number of experimental studies have been published on these two factors.

Lipoprotein(a)

Lipoprotein(a) has been proposed as an antifibrinolytic compound. It has some homology with plasminogen and can therefore occupy binding sites for plasminogen on streptokinase, tPA, endothelial cells, platelets and fibrin. However, it does not activate fibrinolysis, and consequently may be anti-fibrinolytic. However, patients with high lipoprotein(a) levels have not been shown to have a decreased fibrinolytic activity. Twelve studies have investigated the association between lipoprotein(a) concentrations and alcohol consumption (Table 3). Six of these were population studies finding no association, and only one described a decrease in lipoprotein(a) concentrations, which occurred in men only. The experimental studies, mainly conducted in alcoholics, observed an increase in lipoprotein(a) after withdrawal from alcohol, whereas only a transient effect of (moderate) alcohol consumption on lipoprotein(a) could be observed in healthy volunteers.

TABLE 3   Alcohol consumption and lipoprotein(a)

First author	Study	Study population	Association	Year
Välimäki	Controlled	10 males	Temporary effect	1991
Huang	Controlled	12 alcoholics	Increase after abstinence	1992
Haffner	San Antonio Heart Study	316 Mexican Americans 242 non-Hispanic Whites	No	1992
Jenner	Framingham Offspring Study	1284 men and 1394 women	No	1993
Välimäki	Controlled	11 female alcoholics	Increase after withdrawal	1993
Selby	Kaiser Permanente Twins study	704 men and women	No	1994
Sharpe	Controlled	20 men and women	Decrease after red wine only	1995
Hong	SATSA	294 twin pairs	No	1995
Nago	Jichi Medical Study	1235 men and 1762 women	Decrease in men only	1995
Rodrioguez		423 men	No	1995
Clevidence	Controlled	34 premenopausal women	No	1995
Delarue	Controlled	24 male alcoholics	Increase after withdrawal	1996

Platelet aggregability

Platelet aggregation is the process by which platelets interact with each other to form a haemostatic plug or thrombus. Fibrinogen plays an essential role in platelet aggregation. Evaluation of platelet function may include platelet counts, platelet shape change, platelet aggregability, bleeding time, platelet adhesion and platelet activation. Platelet aggregability has been studied since the 1960s with a wide variety of techniques and aggregating agents (ADP, thrombin, collagen and epinephrine). Platelet aggregation is potentially influenced by several factors and considerable laboratory-to-laboratory variation exists. In 1985, no established method of *in vitro* aggregability or platelet function could characterize patients with thrombosis (Meade et al 1985). However, several risk factors for CHD have been associated with platelet aggregability. These include age, gender and cigarette smoking. A diurnal cycle for platelet aggregability was reported with a peak from 06:00 a.m. to noon, correlating with a peak occurrence of myocardial infarction (Tofler et al 1987).

A prospective study of spontaneous platelet aggregability, following patients surviving myocardial infarction for five years, showed that those patients with a spontaneous platelet aggregability had a 46.2% chance of cardiac death whereas for those without spontaneous platelet aggregability the chance was only 14.9% (Trip et al 1990).

Platelet abnormalities are well documented in alcoholics. Alcohol in large quantities can disturb haemopoiesis, resulting in moderate or severe aregenerative thrombocytopenia in some individuals. The platelet count typically returns to normal 1–2 weeks after discontinuation of alcohol consumption. Platelet transfusion may be used if the patient is bleeding or is at high risk of bleeding. Folic acid should be given because many patients have coexisting nutritional deficiencies, but this does not hasten the platelet count recovery unless folate deficiency is present. Also, actively drinking alcoholics have a significantly reduced aggregability of platelets induced by various agonists. Impairment of aggregation was observed both in alcoholics with and without thrombocytopenia. These changes usually are accompanied by a prolongation of the bleeding time. Following abstinence, however, aggregation in response to all agonists is significantly increased even above that of normal healthy controls.

Several ecological studies have linked moderate alcohol consumption with reduced risk of CHD through the effect of alcohol on platelet aggregatibility (Renaud et al 1978, 1980, 1981, 1986). These ecological studies are usually difficult to interpret, because of interference of several confounding factors, including genetic and behavioural conditions. However, Renaud also showed in his 1992 Caerphilly Heart Study in Wales (Renaud et al 1992) that the intake of alcohol, in a dose-dependent way, was inversely associated with the response of platelets to aggregation induced by collagen and ADP (as well as to the secondary aggregation induced by ADP), but not to aggregation induced by thrombin. There appeared to be a modulatory effect of the fat content of the diet; those consuming a diet high in saturated fats were most significantly affected by alcohol consumption. Studies from our laboratories performed by Pikaar and Veenstra yielded partially contradictory results. Pikaar observed a decreased platelet aggregability stimulated by collagen after both moderate daily alcohol consumption and after 'binge drinking' (14 drinks during the weekend only) (Pikaar et al 1987). However, in another better-controlled experiment by Veenstra et al (1990), no significant effects on platelet aggregability could be observed after a shorter period of moderate alcohol consumption (4 days). Other studies into the acute effects of alcohol consumption are conflicting. Many of these discrepancies may relate to the variation in the methodology applied and the study design. Another possible explanation may be that consumption of a moderate dose of alcohol has no acute effect on platelet aggregation in habitual moderate drinkers. Daily moderate alcohol consumption, on the other hand, may cause a decreased platelet aggregability after a few weeks. This is in agreement with the epidemiological observations of an inverse relationship between alcohol consumption and platelet aggregation.

A more definitive demonstration of the inhibition of platelet thrombus formation by ethanol was provided (Rand et al 1990) in studies of experimentally induced arterial thrombosis in rabbits. In this model, thrombosis was induced by insertion of a catheter continuously injuring the vessel wall. Acute high doses of alcohol reduced both the number of platelets associated with the thrombi and the dry weight of the thrombus. Association of fibrinogen with the thrombi was also reduced. Platelets from these rabbits were also hyporesponsive in the classical platelet aggregation assays. Interestingly, lower doses of alcohol (48 mM) reduced arterial thrombosis but marginally inhibited platelet responses.

PAI and tPA

PAI-1 is a protease inhibitor with a high affinity for tPA. The complexing of PAI-1 with tPA serves to inactivate tPA and to transport it to the liver. Thus elevated concentrations, at least theoretically, may inhibit the fibrinolytic system. PAI has been associated with several CHD risk factors, and in general PAI is associated with the metabolic syndrome X (obesity, high triglyceride concentrations, low HDL cholesterol, hyperglycaemia, hyperinsulinaemia and a low amount of physical activity). In a three-year prospective study (Hamsten et al 1987) in survivors of myocardial infarction, PAI concentrations were independently predictive of reinfarction, and in the ARIC study a dose–response relationship was observed between PAI-1 concentration and the presence of carotid disease. In general, tPA activity is inversely related to PAI-1 activity, thus the association of tPA with risk factors is generally opposite to those for PAI-1. In the Physicians' Health Study (Ridker et al 1994), a direct positive association between moderate alcohol consumption and plasma levels of tPA antigen concentrations was shown. One of the few experimental studies into PAI and tPA was conducted in our laboratory (Hendriks et al 1994) where eight middle-aged men were followed during the night after consumption of 40 g of alcohol. Immediately after dinner, PAI activity rose and tPA activity was reduced, but was again higher than normal early in the next morning after alcohol but not after water. These results suggested that moderate alcohol consumption may induce the local increase in tPA activity, which may help prevent blood clot formation and stimulate the dissolution of existing clots. Furthermore, tPA activity was increased at a time of day that platelet aggregability is increased and a large proportion of heart attacks normally takes place.

References

Boffetta P, Garfinkel L 1990 Alcohol drinking and mortality among men enrolled in an American Cancer Society prospective study. Epidemiology 1:342–348

Hamsten A, de Faire U, Walldius G et al 1987 Plasminogen activator inhibitor in plasma: risk factor for recurrent myocardial infarction. Lancet i:3–9

Hendriks HFJ, Veenstra J, Velthuis-te Wierik EJM, Schaafsma G, Kluft C 1994 Effect of moderate dose of alcohol with evening meal on fibrinolytic factors. Br Med J 308:1003–1006

Maclure M 1993 Demonstration of deductive meta-analysis: ethanol intake and risk of myocardial infarction. Epidemiol Rev 15:328–351

Meade TW, Vickers MV, Thompson SG, Stirling Y, Haines AP, Miller GJ 1985 Epidemiological characteristics of platelet aggregability. Br Med J 290:428–432

Pearson TA, LaCava J, Weil HFC 1997 Epidemiology of thrombotic-hemostatic factors and their associations with cardiovascular disease. Am J Clin Nutr 65 (suppl 1):1674S–1682S

Pikaar NA, Wedel M, van der Beek EJ et al 1987 Effects of moderate alcohol consumption on platelet aggregation, fibrinolysis, and blood lipids. Metabolism 36:538–543

Rand ML, Groves HM, Packham MA, Mustard JF, Kinlough-Rathbone RL 1990 Acute administration of ethanol to rabbits inhibits thrombus formation induced by indwelling aortic catheters. Lab Invest 63:742–745

Renaud S, Dumont E, Godsey F, Suplisson A, Thevenon C 1978 Platelet functions in relation to dietary fats in farmers from two regions of France. Thromb Haemostasis 40:518–531

Renaud S, Dumont E, Godsey F 1980 Dietary fats and platelet factors in French and Scottish farmers. Nutr Metab 24 (suppl 1):90–104

Renaud S, Morazain R, Godsey F et al 1981 Platelet functions in relation to diet and serum lipids in British farmers. Br Heart J 46:562–570

Renaud S, Godsey F, Dumont E et al 1986 Influence of long-term diet modification on platelet function and composition in Moselle farmers. Am J Clin Nutr 43:136–150

Renaud S, Beswick AD, Fehily AM, Sharp DS, Elwood PC 1992 Alcohol and platelet aggregation: the Caerphilly Protective Heart Disease Study. Am J Clin Nutr 55:1012–1017

Ridker PM, Vaughan DE, Stampfer MJ, Glynn RJ, Hennekens CH 1994 Association of moderate alcohol consumption and plasma concentration of endogenous tissue-type plasminogen activator. JAMA 272:929–933

Rimm EB, Klatsky A, Grobbee D, Stampfer MJ 1996 Review of moderate alcohol consumption and reduced risk of coronary heart disease: is the effect due to beer, wine or spirits? Br Med J 312:731–736

Tofler GH, Brezinski D, Schafer AI et al 1987 Concurrent morning increase in platelet aggregability and the risk of myocardial infarction and sudden cardiac death. N Engl J Med 316:1514–1518

Trip MD, Cats VM, van Capelle FJL, Vreeken J 1990 Platelet hyperreactivity and prognosis in survivors of myocardial infarction. N Engl J Med 22:1549–1554

Veenstra J, Kluft C, Ockhuizen Th, van de Pol H, Wedel M, Schaafsma G 1990 Effects of moderate alcohol consumption on platelet function, tissue-type plasminogen activator and plasminogen activator inhibitor. Thromb Haemostasis 63:345–348

DISCUSSION

Hillbom: Are there any experimental studies showing that alcohol can influence fibrinogen?

Hendriks: Very few. We looked briefly at this 10 years ago and were unable to show a clear effect (Pikaar et al 1987).

Puddey: In the intervention study I mentioned earlier, we also looked at a range of coagulation and fibrinolytic factors (Dimmitt et al 1998). When regular drinkers reduced their alcohol intake from approximately five drinks a day down to one drink a day, there was an 11% increase in fibrinogen. This is one of the first intervention studies to conclusively show that alcohol lowers fibrinogen, and this effect was manifest over a four week intervention period.

Peters: When I was at Northwick Park, Tom Meade used to say that raised fibrinogen was a more important predictor of cardiovascular disease than raised cholesterol.

Miller: A paper by Pellegrini et al (1996) reported a randomized cross-over study of the effects of 30 g/day alcohol as red wine, 30 g/day alcohol in fruit juice, and red wine treated by evaporation to remove its alcohol content. Each was taken for three weeks with the usual diet with a washout of four weeks. Alcohol in red wine or juice lowered fibrinogen significantly, but treated red wine had no effect. Studies are few and far between and dose effects may be important here. The excitement about fibrinogen in coronary heart disease is currently on the increase, because there are studies which suggest that fibrinogen is a stronger predictor than some of the lipid factors we have focused on in the past (Meade et al 1986). The question is now turning to the nature of the mechanisms underlying this association. This leads onto current interest in inflammation, fibrinogen being an acute phase protein. Does anyone have any information on what chronic moderate alcohol consumption does to the other acute phase proteins, such as C-reactive protein, and some of the inflammatory markers, such as interleukin (IL)-6? There is some recent evidence that IL-6 is not a bad predictor of atherosclerosis (Brown et al 1997). This may help us a little in our attempts to unravel the association between CHD and alcohol.

Gaziano: Our group has looked at the relationship between C-reactive protein and a number of other haemostatic factors with the risk of myocardial infarction. Alcohol didn't have a dramatic effect in attenuating the effect of C-reactive protein. Perhaps we ought to go back and take a more careful look at the relationship between alcohol consumption and C-reactive protein.

Keil: Has the effect of alcohol on blood fluidity/viscosity been looked at?

Hendriks: It has not been investigated extensively, but I think it would be worth looking at.

Miller: In the Caerphilly and Speedwell studies (Yarnell et al 1991), a good association was found between blood viscosity and coronary risk, and white blood cell count and coronary risk. The main assay for fibrinogen used in epidemiological studies is the thrombin clotting time, which looks at clottable fibrinogen. However, there's a variable, sometimes quite significant amount of fibrinogen in plasma which is non-clottable. If we're interested in viscosity effects, we need to measure total fibrinogen, not just the clottable component. If anyone is thinking of exploring this area, it may therefore be timely to consider other ways of measuring fibrinogen.

Criqui: With regard to platelets, one issue that is repeatedly raised (and which has major public health implications) is the potential interaction between aspirin and alcohol. There is at least one paper showing a rather dramatic affect of alcohol in prolonging the effects of aspirin on platelet aggregation (Deykin et al 1994). This raises the issue of whether there are synergistic effects of aspirin and alcohol that we need to be aware of, both for prevention of CHD and for potential risk of haemorrhagic stroke or other bleeding tendencies.

One paper reported CHD outcomes in men by level of drinking, where half the group was randomized to aspirin (Camargo et al 1997). They found no interaction between the effects of aspirin and alcohol; however, one would presume from this statement that the effects were additive. Bleeding complications were not reported as an endpoint.

Peters: Do the Oxford group have any data on the relationship between alcohol consumption, aspirin use and cardiovascular disease?

Gaziano: They have good data on the lipids. They are beginning to explore the mechanistic underpinnings of alcohol in one large cohort. I have not seen any data on either coagulation factors or platelets. But the Physicians' Health Study has looked at a number of the haemostatic factors. Paul Ridker has looked at the relationship of lipoprotein(a), tPA antigen, PAI-1 and homocysteine to heart disease, and they are all predictors in one way or another. He has also shown that tPA antigen is associated with alcohol intake, but despite looking he has not been able to see a modifying effect of alcohol's beneficial association by any of these factors. We have seen that for HDL. This is a messy business, and it is certainly plausible that there is a mechanistic contribution by haemostatic factors. However, there are two reasons why we might not be seeing the effect. One is that the magnitude of the effect of haemostatic factors may be relatively small in the light drinking range. The other is that many of these factors are inversely associated with HDL, and HDL may be acting through an antithrombotic mechanism as well as an anti-atherogenic one. When all these effects are included in the model, it becomes difficult to tease out the precise mechanism. When Paul Ridker looked at the diurnal variation in risk of MI, he found that the risk goes up in the morning and down in the evening, but this is abolished completely by aspirin. However, it is not abolished by alcohol. This suggests that aspirin prevents early morning thrombotic events but alcohol does not, and that alcohol is therefore not acting as an antiplatelet agent.

Hendriks: We should be careful that we measure the relevant parameters in these studies. tPA antigen may not be representative of tPA activity *in vivo*.

Gaziano: None the less, it was a potent predictor of risk for CHD.

Renaud: I have a comment on the work on platelets and clotting factors in general. Measurement of platelet activity is extremely problematic, because platelets stick to everything. In addition, when they adhere to the wall of the tube during centrifugation, they liberate phospholipids which shorten most clotting tests (Renaud & Gautheron 1973). The implications are that when one observes a high factor VII or VIII activity, this result may not necessarily be due to the clotting factor *per se* when evaluated in a non-specific clotting test, but rather to the more active phospholipids liberated from the platelets during preparation of the samples. The complexity of working with platelets may be one reason that so few people work in this field, but this doesn't mean that it is not important.

Miller: I wanted to extend the discussion we were having on HDL and VLDL with alcohol over to the effects of lipids on haemostatic factors. John Griffin's group in La Jolla has reported on several occasions recently that HDL influences the coagulation pathway in an anti-thrombotic manner, seeming to operate by potentiating the effect of the protein C/protein S system on the degradation of factor V, thus down-regulating thrombin production (Kojima et al 1997). On the other hand, there is increasing evidence that the VLDLs themselves provide a pro-coagulant surface for assembly of the pro-thrombinase complex, for example. There is abundant epidemiological evidence to link high triglyceride levels with high factor VII coagulant activity. It is possible that in addition to the effect of HDL on reverse cholesterol transport, there are also important effects of HDLs on the thrombotic component, and also on the inflammatory component, of coronary disease. There is some evidence that HDLs are anti-inflammatory in their character (Van Lenten et al 1995). By raising HDLs with alcohol, we may influence a number of pathogenic systems in coronary disease; not simply reverse cholesterol transport.

Klatsky: We have discussed the potential synergistic effects of alcohol and aspirin, but there is another important question that involves fewer people but perhaps would be easier to study. This pertains to the increasingly large number of people who are on chronic warfarin therapy. This number is likely to increase as time goes on since it's now generally accepted that almost everybody with chronic atrial fibrillation should be on warfarin. Most of these people have coronary heart disease or some other disease that increases in prevalence with age. I wonder if the interaction of lighter drinking with chronic warfarin therapy has been studied and, if it has not, what the risks are likely to be of the anticlotting effects of alcohol added to the substantial antithrombotic effects of warfarin.

Gaziano: We have seen clotting factors related to coronary disease, and warfarin affects clotting factors, but warfarin does not prevent coronary thrombosis.

Klatsky: Are you sure?

Gaziano: No, but there are no convincing data.

Criqui: In the post-CABG study published recently in the *New England Journal of Medicine*, there was no effect whatsoever of the warfarin arm in terms of angiographic progression (Anonymous 1997).

Miller: I am hoping that the definitive answer to this will come from the MRC thrombosis prevention trial. The principal results should be published sometime in 1998: Professor Tom Meade is currently analysing the data. This was a randomized placebo control trial of low dose warfarin and aspirin in the primary prevention of coronary disease in men at high risk. It was a factorial design by which the men had either aspirin or warfarin, or both, or double placebo. In addition, subgroup analysis may tell us something about the question of alcohol as a complicating factor and predisposing agent to haemorrhage in people taking low-dose warfarin.

References

Anonymous 1997 The effect of aggressive lowering of low-density lipoprotein cholesterol levels and low-dose anticoagulation on obstructive changes in saphenous-vein coronary-artery bypass grafts. The Post Coronary Artery Bypass Graft Trial Investigators. N Engl J Med 336:153–162

Brown AS, Hong Y, de Belder A et al 1997 Megakaryocyte ploidy and platelet changes in human diabetes and atherosclerosis. Arterioscler Thromb Vasc Biol 17:802–807

Camargo CA Jr, Stampfer MJ, Glynn RJ et al 1997 Moderate alcohol consumption and risk for angina pectoris or myocardial infarction in U.S. male physicians. Ann Intern Med 126:372–375

Deykin D, Janson P, McMahon L 1982 Ethanol potentiation of aspirin-induced prolongation of the bleeding time. N Engl J Med 306:852–854

Dimmitt SB, Rakic V, Puddey IB et al 1998 The effects of alcohol on coagulation and fibrinolytic factors: a controlled trial. Blood Coagul Fibrinolysis 9:39–45

Kojima K, Fernandez JA, Banka CL, Curtiss L, Griffin JH 1997 Anticoagulant protein C pathway upregulation by high density lipoprotein. Thromb Haemostasis (suppl) p 399

Meade TW, Mellows S, Brozovic M et al 1986 Haemostatic function and ischaemic heart disease: principal results of the Northwick Park Heart Study. Lancet ii:533–537

Pellegrini N, Pareti FI, Stanile F, Brusamolino A, Simonetti P 1996 Effects of moderate consumption of red wine on platelet aggregation and haemostatic variables in healthy volunteers. Eur J Clin Nutr 1996 50:209–213

Pikaar NA, Wedel M, van der Beek EJ et al 1987 Effects of moderate alcohol consumption on platelet aggregation, fibrinolysis and blood lipids. Metabolism 36:538–543

Renaud S, Gautheron P 1973 Role of platelet factor 3 in the hypercoagulability induced by pregnancy and oral contraceptives. Thromb Diath Haemorrh 30:299–306

Van Lenten BJ, Hama SY, de Beer FC et al 1995 Anti-inflammatory HDL becomes pro-inflammatory during the acute-phase response. J Clin Invest 96:2758–2767

Yarnell JWG, Baker IA, Sweetnam PM et al 1991 Fibrinogen, viscosity, and white blood cell count are major risk factors for ischemic heart disease. The Caerphilly and Speedwell Collaborative Heart Disease Studies. Circulation 83:836–844

Alcohol, blood pressure and hypertension

Ulrich Keil*, Angela Liese*, Birgit Filipiak†, John D. Swales‡ and
Diederick E. Grobbee¶

*Institute of Epidemiology and Social Medicine, University of Münster, Münster, Germany,
†GSF-Institute for Epidemiology, Neuherberg, Germany, ‡Department of Medicine,
University of Leicester, Leicester, UK, and ¶Julius Center for Patient Oriented Research,
Utrecht University Medical School, Utrecht, The Netherlands

Abstract. In the last 30 years a large number of cross-sectional studies, a smaller number of prospective cohort studies and several intervention studies have addressed the alcohol–blood pressure relationship. Although a number of questions — such as the validity of measurement of alcohol intake, shape of the alcohol–blood pressure relationship, threshold dose for hypertension, and plausible pathophysiological mechanisms — have not yet been answered satisfactorily, it is clear that a causal association exists between chronic intake of ⩾ 30–60 g alcohol per day and blood pressure elevation in men and women. To call the alcohol–blood pressure relationship causal is justified because chance and, to a large degree, bias and confounding, have been ruled out as plausible explanations in most observational studies. More importantly, the intervention studies support the observational studies and show a remarkable consistency in demonstrating a potentially valuable decrease in blood pressure when heavy drinkers abstain or restrict their alcohol intake. From the different studies a rule of thumb can be derived: above 30 g of alcohol intake per day an increment of 10 g of alcohol per day increases on average systolic blood pressure by 1–2 mmHg and diastolic blood pressure by 1 mmHg.

1998 Alcohol and cardiovascular diseases. Wiley, Chichester (Novartis Foundation Symposium 216) p 125–151

Aims and objectives

A relationship between alcohol consumption and blood pressure elevation was first suggested by Lian in 1915, who noted that French service men drinking 2.5 litres of wine or more per day had increased prevalence of hypertension (Lian 1915). Since 1967 attention has shifted to the question of whether an association exists between alcohol consumption and blood pressure in populations not selected on the basis of alcohol intake. A large number of cross-sectional studies, a smaller number of prospective cohort studies, and a few experimental studies have addressed this question. Most studies have reported a positive association between alcohol consumption and blood pressure (Keil et al 1993).

The following questions and issues concerning the alcohol–blood pressure relationship will be addressed in this report:

(1) Is the relationship linear, J-shaped or U-shaped?
(2) Is there a threshold dose for hypertension risk?
(3) What are the difficulties in measuring alcohol consumption in population studies?
(4) What are the major putative confounders of the relationship?
(5) What are the effects of modification of alcohol intake on blood pressure?
(6) What are the physiological mechanisms for the alcohol–blood pressure link?
(7) To what extent does alcohol consumption contribute to the prevalence of hypertension in the population?
(8) How must observational studies be improved to provide a better understanding of the alcohol–blood pressure relationship?

Observational and experimental studies concerning alcohol and blood pressure

Cross-sectional studies

The alcohol–blood pressure association has been investigated worldwide in at least 33 cross-sectional studies, 10 in Europe (Gyntelberg & Meyer 1974, Kozarevic et al 1982, Milon et al 1982, Salonen et al 1983, Cairns et al 1984, Kornhuber et al 1985, Kromhout et al 1985, Keil et al 1989, 1991, Bulpitt et al 1987), 12 in North America (Clark et al 1967, Dyer et al 1977, Klatsky et al 1977, 1986, Harburg et al 1980, Criqui et al 1981, Kagan et al 1981, Fortmann et al 1983, Gordon & Kannel 1983, Coates et al 1985, Gruchow et al 1985, Gordon & Doyle 1986), six in Australia (Mitchell et al 1980, Baghurst & Dwyer 1981, Cooke et al 1982, Arkwright et al 1982, Savdie et al 1984, MacMahon et al 1984), two in New Zealand (Paulin et al 1985, Jackson et al 1985), two in Japan (Ueshima et al 1984, Kondo & Ebihara 1984) and the Intersalt Study comprising 50 centres worldwide (Marmot et al 1994).

All of the European studies found evidence of an association of alcohol and blood pressure that was independent of a number of putative confounding factors such as age, weight (body mass index [BMI] = kg/m^2), physical activity, smoking, coffee consumption, educational attainment, and Type A/B behaviour. Dietary intake was not assessed in most studies.

In the Munich Blood Pressure Study (MBS) (Cairns et al 1984) and in the Lübeck Blood Pressure Study (LBS) (Keil et al 1989), in general the blood pressure of non-drinkers was either greater than or no different from that of people consuming 10–20 g alcohol per day. In the LBS, blood pressure was greater in drinkers than it was in non-drinkers at consumption levels of $\geqslant 40$ g of alcohol per day. In the MBS the respective alcohol consumption level was $\geqslant 60$ g/day for men and $\geqslant 40$ g/day for women.

The MONICA Augsburg Survey 1984/85 (Keil et al 1991) confirmed the MBS results in that blood pressure was clearly greater in drinkers than in non-drinkers at alcohol consumption levels of $\geqslant 60$ g/day in men and $\geqslant 40$ g/day in women. Among the three studies performed in Germany with the same methodology, a clear J-shaped curve for the alcohol–systolic blood pressure relationship was found in LBS men (Keil et al 1989) and in 55–64 year old men and women in Augsburg (Keil et al 1991).

In the three German studies a strong interaction between alcohol consumption and smoking was found in older women; in the MONICA Augsburg Survey this interaction was found in men and women (Keil et al 1989, 1991). Apparently, smoking can act as an effect modifier on the alcohol–blood pressure relationship, i.e. Augsburg men who consume $\geqslant 60$ g of alcohol per day and are smokers have 2–8 mmHg higher systolic and/or diastolic blood pressure values compared with non-smokers. In LBS and MBS women aged 45–69 this alcohol–smoking interaction was seen at alcohol levels $\geqslant 20$ g/day. A study in the Netherlands has confirmed this alcohol–smoking interaction (van Leer et al 1994); however a plausible physiological interpretation of this interaction is not yet available.

With the exception of the Canada Health Study (Coates et al 1985) all of the 12 North American studies have reported a statistically significant positive association of alcohol and blood pressure. In the first Kaiser Permanente Study (Klatsky et al 1977), only a small difference was found in systolic or diastolic blood pressure between non-drinking men and those consuming 10–20 g alcohol per day. In women, systolic and diastolic blood pressures were greater in non-drinkers than in those consuming 10–20 g alcohol per day. Thus, a J-shaped relationship was found in women. The findings of this study suggested that there might be a threshold effect of 30 g alcohol per day for blood pressure elevation in men and women. Many more subsequent North American studies confirmed these findings (Criqui et al 1981).

With the exception of one study (Baghurst & Dwyer 1981), the six Australian and two New Zealand studies found linear, J-shaped and U-shaped associations between alcohol and blood pressure. In the National Heart Foundation of Australia Risk Factor Prevalence Study (MacMahon 1984) and in the Auckland Study (Jackson et al 1985) there was evidence of greater blood pressure values in drinkers than in non-drinkers at consumption levels $\geqslant 30$ g/day. Both Japanese studies (Ueshima et al 1984, Kondo & Ebihara 1984) reported independent linear associations of alcohol with blood pressure. The Intersalt study revealed a significant relationship between drinking $\geqslant 36$ g alcohol/day and blood pressure in both men and women, and in younger and older men. This relationship was independent of, and in addition to, the effect of BMI and urinary excretion of sodium and potassium (Marmot et al 1994).

Prospective cohort studies

There are at least seven prospective cohort studies of the alcohol–blood pressure association (Kromhout et al 1985, Dyer et al 1977, 1981, Gordon & Kannel 1983, Gordon & Doyle 1986, Reed et al 1982, Witteman et al 1989). The results of all but the Honolulu Heart Study (Reed et al 1982) are consistent with those of the cross-sectional studies and indicate a positive alcohol–blood pressure association. The prospective association of alcohol with blood pressure has been investigated over four years in the Framingham Study (Gordon & Kannel 1983). In both men and women an increase in alcohol consumption over four years was associated with a significant increase in blood pressure, whereas a decrease in alcohol consumption was associated with a significant decrease in blood pressure. Results from the Nurses' Health Study (Witteman et al 1989) show that of a cohort of 58 000 US nurses free of diagnosed hypertension, 3275 reported an initial diagnosis of elevated blood pressure during a four year follow-up period. When compared with non-drinkers, women drinking 20–34 g of alcohol per day had an approximate 1.4-fold increased risk of occurrence of hypertension during follow-up. In those drinking 35 g or more the relative risk was 1.9.

Table 1 provides an overview of observational studies on the alcohol blood pressure association. In this table the studies are categorized by the unit of measurement of alcohol intake.

The MONICA Augsburg cohort study provides data on changes in alcohol intake and changes in blood pressure in 1818 men and 1832 women, aged 25–64, over the three year period from 1984/85 to 1987/88 (Keil et al 1988). Table 2 shows changes in alcohol intake categories for men and women over this time. Obviously, the net absolute effects for each gender are more persons changing status from drinker to non-drinker than in the other direction. Table 3 depicts the changes in systolic and diastolic blood pressure by changes in alcohol intake in men. Crude differences and adjusted differences have been calculated. Men who lower their alcohol intake show on average a decrease in systolic and diastolic blood pressure whereas men who increase their alcohol intake exhibit an increase in blood pressure values. This applies to the crude and the adjusted changes (differences). The adjusted differences were obtained by applying analysis of covariance for controlling for age, baseline blood pressure, antihypertensive medication and

TABLE 1 Overview of observational studies on the alcohol–blood pressure association, giving examples of the differences in blood pressure between categories with highest and lowest intake[a]

Study by	M/F	Category with highest alcohol consumption	Systolic blood pressure (mm Hg)	Diastolic blood pressure (mm Hg)
Studies reporting alcohol use by 'unit'[b]				
Gyntelberg & Meyer 1974	M	6–10 units/day	8.1	4.8
Kozarevic et al 1982	M	⩾1 unit/day	7.7	4.3
Coates et al 1985	M age: 20–34 yr	⩾2.14 units/day	1.9	0.4
	M age: 35–49 yr	⩾2.14 units/day	2.9	4.0
	M age: ⩾60 yr	⩾2.14 units/day	−3.4	−0.5
	F age: 20–34 yr	⩾2.14 units/day	1.8	−0.1
	F age: 35–49 yr	⩾2.14 units/day	−2.4	−5.4
	F age: ⩾60 yr	⩾2.14 units/day	−5.7	−2.1
Bulpitt et al 1987	M	>10 units/day	20.0	7.3
	F	>10 units/day	5.5	3.4
Lang et al 1987	M	>5 units/day	8.9	5.3
	F	>5 units/day	14.3	6.1
Weissfeld et al 1988	M age: 18–39 yr	>2 units/day	3.3	3.7
	M age: 40–59 yr	>2 units/day	0.7	1.9
	M age: ⩾60 yr	>2 units/day	2.4	4.5
	F age: 18–39 yr	>2 units/day	8.4	6.9
	F age: 40–59 yr	>2 units/day	6.1	2.8
	F age: ⩾60 yr	>2 units/day	9.7	3.3
Wannamethee & Shaper 1991	M	>6 units/day	6.5	4.0

(cont.)

TABLE 1   (*continued*)

Study by	M/F	Category with highest alcohol consumption	Systolic blood pressure (mm Hg)	Diastolic blood pressure (mm Hg)
Studies reporting alcohol use in millilitres (ml)[b]				
Klatsky et al 1977	M	≥ 72 ml/day	5.4	2.1
	F	≥ 72 ml/day	10.9	4.5
Arkwright et al 1981	M	> 50 ml/day	5.1	n.s.
Milon et al 1982	M age: < 40 yr	≥ 12 ml/day	n.s.	n.s.
	M age: 40–49 yr	≥ 12 ml/day	10.6	n.s.
	M age: > 50 yr	≥ 12 ml/day	11.9	n.s.
Fortmann et al 1983	M age: 20–34 yr	≥ 30 ml/day	2.6	− 1.6
	M age: 35–49 yr	≥ 30 ml/day	3.0	1.2
	M age: 50–74 yr	≥ 30 ml/day	15.4	6.6
	F age: 20–34 yr	≥ 30 ml/day	2.3	0.5
	F age: 35–49 yr	≥ 30 ml/day	− 0.4	− 0.2
	F age: 50–74 yr	≥ 30 ml/day	12.8	6.5
Gordon & Kannel 1983	M	≥ 74.7 ml/day	7.3	n.s.
	F	≥ 74.7 ml/day	8.4	n.s.
Elliott et al 1987	M	> 42.8 ml/day	13.2	5.4
Trevisan et al 1987	M	> 114 ml/day	3.0	1.0
	F	> 114 ml/day	6.7	0.4
Dyer et al 1990	M 'white'	> 30 ml/day	2.4	2.0
	M 'black'	> 30 ml/day	2.8	0.9
	F 'white'	> 30 ml/day	1.5	1.5
	F 'black'	> 30 ml/day	− 0.3	2.4

(*cont.*)

TABLE 1 (*continued*)

Study by	M/F	Category with highest alcohol consumption	Systolic blood pressure (mm Hg)	Diastolic blood pressure (mm Hg)
Klag et al 1990	M 'Japanese'	> 58 ml/day	14.1	8.9
	M 'white'	> 30 ml/day	5.6	3.6
Yamada et al 1991	M	> 58 ml/day	4.9	3.9
Marmot et al 1994	M	> 71 ml/day	4.6	3.0
	F	> 43 ml/day	3.9	3.1
Studies reporting alcohol use in grams (g)				
Myrhed 1974	M+F	> 27.4 g/day	9.6	6.7
Dyer et al 1977	M	'alcoholics'	4.7	n.s.
	M	⩾ 25 g/day	9.7	5.9
Marmot et al 1981	M	> 34 g/day	2.8	2.3
Cooke et al 1983	M	> 30 g/day	7.7	4.7
	F	> 30 g/day	5.0	3.8
Ueshima et al 1984	M 'urban'	> 83 g/day	17.4	10.3
	M 'rural'	> 83 g/day	16.9	8.5
Cairns et al 1984	M	⩾ 60 g/day	2.4	1.2
	F	⩾ 40 g/day	n.s.	2.4
Jackson 1985	M age: > 50 yr	> 34 g/day	4.8	1.7
	F age: > 50 yr	> 34 g/day	10.2	4.5
Paulin et al 1985	M	⩾ 42.8 g/day	9.8	8.9
	F	⩾ 42.8 g/day	− 6.0	1.0
Simon et al 1988	M	> 50 g/day	n.s.	n.s.
Keil et al 1989	M age: 30–69 yr	⩾ 40 g/day	5.5	4.5
	F age: 45–69 yr	⩾ 20 g/day	9.6 (association only in smokers)	5.2

(*cont.*)

TABLE 1 *(continued)*

Study by	M/F	Category with highest alcohol consumption	Systolic blood pressure (mm Hg)	Diastolic blood pressure (mm Hg)
Keil et al 1991	M age: 25–34 yr	$\geqslant$ 80 g/day	5	5
	M age: 35–44 yr	$\geqslant$ 80 g/day	8	5
	M age: 45–54 yr	$\geqslant$ 80 g/day	11	6
	M age: 55–64 yr	$\geqslant$ 80 g/day	3	2
	F age: 25–34 yr	$\geqslant$ 40 g/day	3	3
	F age: 35–44 yr	$\geqslant$ 40 g/day	6	5
	F age: 45–54 yr	$\geqslant$ 40 g/day	6	3
	F age: 55–64 yr	$\geqslant$ 40 g/day	2	1
Studies reporting alcohol use in ounces (oz)[b]				
Harburg et al 1980	M	$\geqslant$ 2.27 oz/day	5.8	3.8
	F	$\geqslant$ 1.98 oz/day	2.0	5.5
Kagan et al 1981	M	$\geqslant$ 1.97 oz/day	6.1	3.4
Gordon et al 1986	M	$\geqslant$ 2.96 oz/day	7.3	5.6
Studies reporting miscellaneous measures of alcohol intake				
Clark et al 1967	M	'yes'	1.9	1.6
Schnall et al 1992	M	'regular alcohol consumption'	3.6	2.8

[a]In general, lowest category pertains to abstainers although sometimes low alcohol users have also been included.
[b]Units: one unit = 10–12 g alcohol; one millilitre (ml) = 0.9 g alcohol; one ounce (oz) = 28 g alcohol
Studies are categorized by the unit of measurement of alcohol intake.

smoking. Table 4 shows the respective changes for women; the findings are similar to those in men. As women drink much less alcohol than men the changes in alcohol intake over the three years are much smaller and so are the respective changes in blood pressure.

Like many other studies (Maclure 1993) the MONICA Augsburg cohort study also shows a protective effect of alcohol on the incidence of myocardial infarction

TABLE 2 Change in alcohol intake (categorical) in men ($n = 1818$) and women ($n = 1832$) aged 25–64 from 1984/85–1987/88 (MONICA Augsburg Cohort Study)

Men			Women		
Change (d) in alcohol intake (g/day)	n	%	Change (d) in alcohol intake (g/day)	n	%
d < −30	231	12.7	d < −10	349	19.0
−30 ≤ d < −10	384	21.1	−10 ≤ d < −2	315	17.2
−10 ≤ d < 10	755	41.5	−2 ≤ d < 2	694	37.9
10 ≤ d < 30	303	16.7	2 ≤ d < 10	229	12.5
d ≥ 30	145	8.0	d ≥ 10	245	13.4

TABLE 3 Change in systolic (SBP) and diastolic (DBP) blood pressure by change in alcohol intake in 25–64 year old men (MONICA Augsburg Cohort Study 1984 to 1988)

Change (d) in alcohol intake (g/day)	n	Crude differences		Adjusted differences[a]	
		SBP (mm Hg)	DBP (mm Hg)	SBP (mm Hg)	DBP (mm Hg)
d < −30	231	−3.9[b]	−2.2[b]	−3.2	−1.4
−30 ≤ d < −10	384	−1.8	−0.9	−1.1	−0.6
−10 ≤ d < 10	755	−1.1	−0.5	−1.5	−0.7
10 ≤ d < 30	303	1.1[b]	1.6[b]	0.6[b]	1.1[b]
d ≥ 30	145	2.4[b]	1.8[b]	2.4[b]	1.5[b]

[a]Adjusted with analysis of covariance for age, baseline blood pressure, antihypertensive medication and smoking. [b]Statistically significant difference ($P < 0.05$) to central alcohol category (−10 to 10 g/day).

(MI) (Keil et al 1997). At the same time we see that the mean systolic blood pressure is 4–6 mm Hg higher in those men who drink 40–79 g/day or ≥80 g/day respectively. These higher mean blood pressure values should have an impact on the respective MI incidence rates; what we see however is an L-shaped curve for the alcohol–MI relationship up to the alcohol intake category ≥80 g/day (see Fig. 1).

Intervention trials on alcohol intake and blood pressure

Acute withdrawal. Blood pressure rises when alcohol is acutely withdrawn from very heavy drinkers. This response is associated with clinical evidence of sympathetic nervous system activation (tachycardia and sweating) and raised

TABLE 4   Change in systolic (SBP) and diastolic (DBP) blood pressure by change in alcohol intake in 25–64 year old women (MONICA Augsburg Cohort Study 1984 to 1988)

Change (d) in alcohol intake		Crude differences		Adjusted differences[a]	
(g/day)	n	SBP (mm Hg)	DBP (mm Hg)	SBP (mm Hg)	DBP (mm Hg)
d < −10	349	−1.8	−1.1	−1.7	−1.0
−10 ≤ d < −2	315	−1.1	−0.3	−1.0	−0.3
−2 ≤ d < 2	694	−0.7	−0.3	−0.5	−0.2
2 ≤ d < 10	229	0.2	−0.4	−0.2	−0.4
d ≥ 10	245	0.6	0.6	0.2	0.2

[a]Adjusted with analysis of covariance for age, baseline blood pressure, antihypertensive medication and smoking.

plasma catecholamines, renin activity, aldosterone and cortisol (Bannan et al 1984, Eisenhofer et al 1985). Withdrawal of alcohol in hypertensives may also give rise to postural hypotension. In some but not all patients who show this effect the catecholamine response to standing is inhibited suggesting impaired cardiovascular reflexes (Eisenhofer et al 1985).

Chronic withdrawal studies. A limited number of investigators have examined the effect of withdrawing alcohol for several days or weeks in moderate to heavy

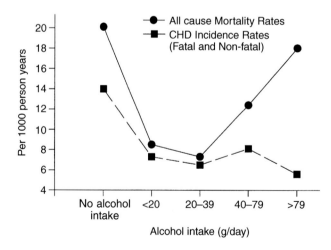

FIG. 1.   Age- and smoking-adjusted coronary heart disease (CHD) incidence rates and all-cause mortality rates in men (per 1000 person years) by alcohol intake categories (from Keil et al 1997)

drinkers. To detect blood pressure lowering effects, such studies have to be carefully designed. To control for potential confounders and possible placebo effects, randomized controlled trials are best suited for approaching this question. Table 5 provides an overview of a number of randomized trials addressing the changes in alcohol intake and their impact on blood pressure of hypertensive and normotensive subjects.

In a randomized trial either a parallel group or crossover design can be adopted. In the latter, subjects are randomly assigned to normal or low alcohol intake but then reallocated to the other group for a second intervention period. Using this design Potter & Beevers (1984) admitted a group of heavy drinking hypertensive patients to hospital and withdrew alcohol from half of the group for three days and maintained the other half on normal alcohol intake. Alcohol was withdrawn from the latter group and given to the former group for the next four days. The period of alcohol withdrawal in both groups was associated with significant lowering of blood pressure. Puddey et al (1985a, 1987) also used a crossover design but employed an intervention period of six weeks. Subjects were also 'blinded' to the level of alcohol intake by being given a low alcohol lager with or without the addition of alcohol. The aims of blinding are to exclude placebo intervention effects and to remove potential observer bias. Both groups were able to demonstrate significant lowering of blood pressure with reduction of alcohol intake in heavy drinkers. This effect was seen both in normotensive and hypertensive subjects. Other reports confirm the blood pressure lowering effect of alcohol withdrawal using both crossover and parallel group designs (Howes & Reid 1986, Parker et al 1990, Maheswaran et al 1992).

The intervention studies show a remarkable consistency in demonstrating a potentially valuable decrease in blood pressure when heavy drinkers abstain or restrict their alcohol intake (Table 5). The decrease in blood pressure induced in these studies is of a similar order of magnitude to that which would be predicted from the population associations if these represented a genuinely causal effect. Taken in conjunction, therefore, the observational and intervention studies create a powerful case for alcohol as an important life-style factor in elevated blood pressure.

From observational and intervention studies a crude rule of thumb can be derived: above 30 g alcohol intake per day an increment of 10 g alcohol per day increases on average systolic blood pressure by 1–2 mmHg and diastolic blood pressure by 1 mmHg.

Interpretation of the findings

Measurement problems

Measurement of alcohol intake is a fundamental issue in all population studies of the alcohol–blood pressure relationship. In these studies alcohol intake is estimated

TABLE 5   Trials of changes in alcohol intake and impact on blood pressure (BP)

Study	Subjects and alcohol intake by day (d) or week (wk)	n	Design	Initial alcohol intake	Final alcohol intake	Duration	Initial BP (mm Hg)	Change in BP (mm Hg)	P-value
Potter & Beevers 1984	H[a] (80 ml/d)	16	Crossover	80 ml/d 0 ml/d	0 ml/d 80 ml/d	3 days 4 days	174/104 156/100	−19/−5 +12/+5	<0.05 <0.01
Puddey et al 1985b	N[b] (366 ml/wk)	46	Crossover	426 ml/wk	85 ml/wk	6 weeks	130/73	−3.7/−1.4	<0.001
Howes & Reid 1986	N[b] (40 ml/d)	10	Crossover	55 ml/d	0 ml/d	7 days	116/60	−3.0/−3.1	<0.05 and <0.01
Puddey et al 1987	H[a] (472 ml/wk)	44	Crossover	452 ml/wk	64 ml/wk	6 weeks	142/84	−5/−3	<0.001
Parker et al 1990	H[a] (480 ml/wk)	59	Parallel group	537 ml/wk	57 ml/wk	4 weeks	138/85	−5.4/−3.2	<0.01
Maheswaran et al 1992	H[a] (480 ml/wk)	41	Parallel group	480 ml/wk	240 ml/wk	8 weeks	149/101	−/5.2	<0.05
								(Systolic blood pressure change n.s.)	

[a]H = hypertensives.
[b]N = normotensives.

on the basis of oral or written information provided by the subject. Self-reports may be obtained by having participants keep daily diaries on their alcohol consumption. Another way is to get the subject to recall consumption over periods ranging from the most recent week to the entire lifetime. One issue is the exact amount of alcohol consumed over a period such as one day, week, month or longer periods. A second issue is the heterogeneity of the group that claims to consume no alcohol at all (Colsher & Wallace 1989).

Assessment of alcohol intake in population studies is conducted retrospectively by a recall method or prospectively by a three or seven day record method. The latter can be incorporated in a seven day nutrition record. When both methods were compared in 45–64 year old men of the MONICA Augsburg survey of 1984/85 it turned out that with regard to the mean daily alcohol intake both methods produced nearly identical results; the Pearson correlation coefficient between the two methods was 0.75 (Schaeffer et al 1991, Döring et al 1993).

The blood alcohol level provides a 'gold standard' for the amount of alcohol consumed recently (Puddey et al 1985b). However, blood alcohol determination becomes impractical when alcohol consumption must be assessed in large numbers of people and over longer periods. Moreover, blood alcohol levels may not be elevated in moderate drinkers several hours after their last drink. A number of biochemical determinations are recommended in order to obtain more insight into alcohol consumption: γGT, SGOT, SGPT, the mean cell volume (MCV) and HDL cholesterol (Chick et al 1981). In general, studies relating biomarkers for alcohol intake to blood pressure levels have obtained results similar to studies relying on reported intake. However, none of these biochemical parameters appears to be sufficiently sensitive or specific to serve as a measure that may replace or substantiate interview or questionnaire data.

The 'no-alcohol-consumption group' is a problem group comprising lifelong abstainers, drinkers who deny their alcohol consumption, those who already suffer from health problems and those who are too sick to drink alcohol (Midanek et al 1990). The effects of such misclassification on the alcohol–blood pressure relationship may be diverse. In this respect, it is important to note that a positive correlation between alcohol consumption and blood pressure was found especially among those with more than an average alcohol intake. The findings for moderate and light alcohol consumption are less clear-cut. Some authors have described a 'threshold phenomenon' whereby the mean blood pressure was only elevated if the alcohol intake exceeded approximately three drinks (30 g alcohol) per day (Klatsky et al 1977, Dyer et al 1977). Others have reported a J-shaped relationship between alcohol and blood pressure whereby moderate alcohol drinkers had a lower blood pressure than total abstainers (Gyntelberg & Meyer 1974, Harburg et al 1980). Inadequate information on low or no alcohol consumption, so that the group of total abstainers becomes 'contaminated' by subjects who do not admit their high alcohol consumption, may explain some of the inconsistency in findings. Such misclassification could cause an inverse relationship at the beginning of the curve although the general view is that this phenomenon, if present, may not completely account for the absence of an association between light to moderate alcohol use and blood pressure.

Another problem is that people might under-report their alcohol intake. Such a general, non-differential, under-reporting will probably result in an overestimate of the association at any specific level of actual alcohol intake, although the overall strength of the association will not be affected. Moreover, if a threshold really exists the estimated threshold level might be higher if there is a systematic under-reporting of alcohol intake by subjects (MacMahon 1987).

Putative confounders

Interpretation of the association between alcohol intake and blood pressure is influenced not only by the quantification and potential misclassification of alcohol intake, but also by various putative confounding factors. This applies in particular to age, sex, and body weight, and in most of the investigations adjustments have been made for these factors. Several other variables have, however, often not been included in the analysis because the relevant information was not available or assessment was too difficult. This applies for example to dietary factors such as electrolyte intake (notably sodium, potassium and magnesium), medication and physical activity. As it has also repeatedly been found that drinkers smoke more cigarettes (Gordon & Kannel 1983), it is not inconceivable that alcohol consumption is related to a lifestyle that could have an effect on blood pressure independent of alcohol intake (Calahan 1981). In addition, a general poor nutritional condition could play a role, especially for heavy drinkers. Perhaps even more difficult to assess is the potentially confounding effect of psychosocial stress. It is generally accepted that alcohol may serve a role in reduction of tension under stressful circumstances (Pohorecky 1991). In view of the potential stress buffering capacity of alcohol at a cognitive level, the blood pressure of subjects who do not drink may be more responsive to stressful conditions and life events. However, the debate about putative confounders can be closed on two grounds:

(1) Analyses in which variables such as age, gender, BMI, smoking, coffee consumption, physical activity, type A/B behaviour, educational attainment were controlled have confirmed the unadjusted associations between alcohol and blood pressure, i.e. have not changed the estimates of the associations (Keil et al 1991).
(2) The randomized trials have confirmed the results from the observational studies. As randomized trials have the advantage of controlling both known

and unknown confounders, the argument that the alcohol-blood pressure association might be due to uncontrolled confounding such as nutrition and/or psychosocial factors or unknown confounders must be refuted.

Mechanisms

Alcohol is widely distributed over body fluids and has important actions upon the physicochemical properties and biological function of cell membranes. Different dose-dependent effects and divergence between acute and chronic actions make the interaction of alcohol and blood pressure a complex one and it is extremely unlikely that a single mechanism accounts for the association between blood pressure and alcohol intake described in population studies. It is likely that chronic alcohol administration directly or indirectly exerts a pressor effect upon the cardiovascular system which is not evident in acute studies where the predominant effect is blood pressure lowering. The pressor effect could be mediated by a neurogenic mechanism, a humoral mechanism, or directly through actions upon the vessels which maintain peripheral resistance. In summary, the acute and chronic physiological effects of alcohol on the cardiovascular system are quite distinct. The pressor effect of chronic ingestion is still poorly understood. At present neural, humoral and direct vascular mechanisms are thought to be possible mediators of the alcohol–blood pressure association. The role of each of these factors, if any, is still unclear (Keil et al 1993).

Implications for prevention and treatment

In most epidemiological studies, blood pressure levels were greater at alcohol consumption levels around $\geqslant 40\,g/day$ than they were at levels of $10–20\,g/day$ (MacMahon 1987, Keil et al 1989). About 25% of studies reported blood pressure elevations at alcohol consumption levels below $30\,g/day$ compared with blood pressure of non-drinkers. About 40% of studies reported blood pressure of non-drinkers to be greater than blood pressure of those consuming $10–20\,g$ alcohol per day. It is doubtful whether these findings actually reflect a blood pressure lowering effect of small amounts of alcohol. Thus, it is still unclear whether the alcohol–blood pressure relationship is linear or curvilinear. One possible explanation for the J-shaped relationship is the finding that 'non-drinkers' are a heterogeneous group. More research is needed to provide a better understanding of the non-drinker group and their potential influence on the shape of the alcohol blood pressure relationship.

If a threshold dose for hypertension risk exists, it is probably around $30–60\,g$ alcohol per day (lower for women than for men).

From the public health perspective it is important to investigate what percentage of hypertension in the community might be caused by alcohol consumption and, more importantly, how much hypertension in the community could be eliminated if intake of e.g. $\geqslant 40$ g of alcohol per day was avoided. Focusing on the population-attributable-risk percentage, it was calculated from LBS data that about 7% of hypertension in men in the community is due to alcohol consumption $\geqslant 40$ g/day (Keil et al 1989). The respective calculations from US and Australian population studies revealed that alcohol consumption could account for as much as 11% of hypertension in men but much less in women because of their much lower alcohol consumption (MacMahon et al 1984, Friedman et al 1982).

In spite of many unanswered questions (e.g. threshold level and shape of the association) concerning the alcohol–blood pressure relationship, it seems clear that a causal association exists between consumption of $\geqslant 30$–60 g alcohol per day and blood pressure elevation in men and women. The statement of a causal relationship is justified because chance and, to a large degree, bias and confounding have been ruled out as plausible explanations of the alcohol–blood pressure association in most observational studies. More importantly, the intervention studies support the observational studies and show a similar quantitative relationship. This indicates that confounding factors are not responsible for the observed relationship. Furthermore, the consistency of the cross-sectional, prospective cohort and intervention studies is high. In addition, a clear time sequence between cause and effect seems present. However, the underlying mechanisms must be clarified further, e.g. the more recent techniques for studying vascular physiology and molecular mechanisms may shed more light on the mechanisms underlying the alcohol–blood pressure relationship.

Chronic alcohol intake $\geqslant 30$–60 g/day can be viewed as the second most important risk factor for hypertension, closely behind the well established risk factor of being overweight.

It is conceivable that a major improvement in the assessment of the exposure variable alcohol will contribute to a more precise delineation of the alcohol–blood pressure association and will transform the frequently found J-shaped curves to a more linear relationship with a more precise estimate of the threshold level in the range of a chronic intake of 30–60 g alcohol per day for hypertension.

References

Arkwright PD, Beilin LJ, Rouse I, Armstrong BK, Vandongen R 1981 Alcohol: effect on blood pressure and predisposition to hypertension. Clin Sci 61:373S–375S

Arkwright PD, Beilin LJ, Rouse I, Armstrong BK, Vandongen R 1982 Effects of alcohol use and other aspects of lifestyle on blood pressure levels and the prevalence of hypertension in a working population. Circulation 66:60–66

Baghurst K, Dwyer T 1981 Alcohol consumption and blood pressure in a group of young Australian males. J Hum Nutr 35:257–264

Bannan LT, Potter JF, Beevers DG, Saunders IB, Walters IRF, Ingram MC 1984 Effect of alcohol withdrawal on blood pressure, plasma renin activity, aldosterone, cortisol and dopamine beta-hydroxylase. Clin Sci 66:659–663

Bulpitt CJ, Shipley MJ, Semmence A 1987 The contribution of a moderate intake of alcohol to the presence of hypertension. J Hypertens 5:85–91

Cairns V, Keil U, Kleinbaum D, Döring A, Stieber J 1984 Alcohol consumption as a risk factor for high blood pressure: Munich Blood Pressure Study. Hypertension 6:124–131

Calahan D 1981 Quantifying alcohol consumption: patterns and problems. Circulation 64:7–14

Chick J, Plant M, Kretiman N 1981 Mean cell-volume and gamma-glutamyltranspeptidase as markers of drinking in working man. Lancet i:1249–1251

Clark VA, Chapman JM, Coulson AH 1967 Effects of various factors on systolic and diastolic blood pressure in the Los Angeles Heart Study. J Chronic Dis 20:571–581

Coates RA, Corey PN, Ashley MJ, Steele CA 1985 Alcohol consumption and blood pressure: analysis of data from the Canada Health Survey. Prev Med 14:1–14

Colsher PL, Wallace RB 1989 Is modest alcohol consumption better than none at all? An epidemiologic assessment. Ann Rev Public Health 10:203–219

Cooke KM, Frost GW, Thornell IR, Stokes GS 1982 Alcohol consumption and blood pressure: survey of the relationship in a health screening clinic. Med J Aust 1:65–69

Cooke KM, Frost GW, Stokes GS 1983 Blood pressure and its relationship to low levels of alcohol consumption. Clin Exp Pharmacol Physiol 10:229–233

Criqui MH, Wallace RB, Mishkel M, Barrett-Conner E, Heiss G 1981 Alcohol consumption and blood pressure: The Lipid Research Clinics Prevalence Study. Hypertension 3:557–565

Döring A, Filipiak B, Stieber J, Keil U 1993 Trends in alcohol intake in a Southern German population from 1984–1985 to 1989–1990: results of the MONICA Project Augsburg. J Stud Alcohol 54:745–749

Dyer AR, Stamler J, Paul O et al 1977 Alcohol consumption, cardiovascular risk factors, and mortality in two Chicago epidemiologic studies. Circulation 56:1067–1074

Dyer AR, Stamler J, Paul O 1981 Alcohol, cardiovascular risk factors and mortality: The Chicago Experience. Circulation (suppl 3) 64:20–27

Dyer AR, Cutter GR, Liu KQ et al 1990 Alcohol intake and blood pressure in young adults: The Cardia Study. J Clin Epidemiol 43:1–13

Eisenhofer G, Whiteside EA, Johnson RH 1985 Plasma catecholamine responses to changes of posture in alcoholics during withdrawal and after continued absence from alcohol. Clin Sci 68:71–78

Elliott P, Fehily AM, Sweetnam PM, Yarnell JWG 1987 Diet, alcohol, body mass and social factors in relation to blood pressure: The Caerphilly Heart Study. J Epidemiol Community Health 41:37–43

Fortmann SP, Haskell WL, Vranizan K, Brown BW, Farquhar JW 1983 The association of blood pressure and dietary alcohol: differences by age, sex and estrogen use. Am J Epidemiol 118:497–507

Friedman GD, Klatsky AL, Siegelaub AB 1982 Alcohol, tobacco and hypertension. Hypertension (suppl 3) 4:143–150

Gordon T, Kannel WB 1983 Drinking and its relation to smoking, blood pressure, blood lipids and uric acid. Arch Intern Med 143:1366–1374

Gordon T, Doyle JT 1986 Alcohol consumption and its relationship to smoking, weight, blood pressure and blood lipids: The Albany Study. Arch Intern Med 146:262–265

Gruchow HW, Sobocinski KA, Barboriak J J 1985 Alcohol, nutrient intake, and hypertension in US adults. JAMA 253:1567–1570

Gyntelberg F, Meyer J 1974 Relationship between blood pressure and physical fitness, smoking and alcohol consumption in Copenhagen males aged 40–59. Acta Med Scand 195:375–380

Harburg E, Ozgoren F, Hawthorne VM, Schork MA 1980 Community norms of alcohol usage and blood pressure. Am J Public Health 70:813–820

Howes LG, Reid JL 1986 Changes in blood pressure and autonomy reflexes following regular moderate alcohol consumption. J Hypertension 4:421–425

Jackson R, Stewart A, Beaglehole R, Scragg R 1985 Alcohol consumption and blood pressure. Am J Epidemiol 122:1034–1044

Kagan A, Yano K, Rhoads GG, McGee DL 1981 Alcohol and cardiovascular disease: The Hawaiian Experience. Circulation (suppl 3) 64:27–31

Keil U, Stieber J, Döring A et al 1988 The cardiovascular risk factor profile in the study area Augsburg. Results from the first MONICA survey 1984/85. Acta Med Scand Suppl 728: 119–128

Keil U, Chambless L, Remmers A 1989 Alcohol and blood pressure: results from the Lübeck Blood Pressure Study. Prev Med 18:1–10

Keil U, Chambless L, Filipiak B, Härtel U 1991 Alcohol and blood pressure and its interaction with smoking and other behavioural variables: results from the MONICA Augsburg Survey 1984/85. J Hypertens 9:491–498

Keil U, Swales JD, Grobbee DE 1993 Alcohol intake and its relation to hypertension. In: Verschuren PM (ed) Health issues related to alcohol consumption. International Life Sciences Institute Europe, Brussels, p 17–42

Keil U, Chambless LE, Döring A, Filipiak B, Stieber J 1997 The relation of alcohol intake to coronary heart disease and all cause mortality in a beer-drinking population. Epidemiology 8:150–156

Klag MJ, Moore RD, Whelton PK, Sakai Y, Comstock GW 1990 Alcohol consumption and blood pressure: a comparison of native Japanese to American men. J Clin Epidemiol 43:1407–1414

Klatsky AL, Friedman GD, Siegeland AB, Gerard MJ 1977 Alcohol consumption and blood pressure. N Engl J Med 296:1194–1200

Klatsky AL, Friedman GD, Armstrong MA 1986 The relationships between alcoholic beverage use and other traits to blood pressure: a new Kaiser Permanente Study. Circulation 73:628–636

Kondo K, Ebihara A 1984 Alcohol consumption and blood pressure in a rural community of Japan. In: Lovenberg W, Yamori Y (eds) Nutritional prevention of cardiovascular disease. Academic Press, Orlando, FL, p 217–224

Kornhuber HH, Lisson G, Suschka-Sauermann L 1985 Alcohol and obesity: a new look at high blood pressure and stroke; an epidemiological study in preventive neurology. Eur Arch Psychiatry Neurol Sci 234:357–362

Kozarevic D, Racic Z, Gordon T, Kaelber CT, MacGee D, Zukel WJ 1982 Drinking habits and other characteristics: the Yugoslavia Cardiovascular Disease Study. Am J Epidemiol 116: 287–301

Kromhout D, Bosschieter EB, de Lezenne Coulander C 1985 Potassium, calcium, alcohol intake and blood pressure: The Zutphen Study. Am J Clin Nutr 41:1299–1304

Lang T, Degoulet P, Aime F, Devries C, Jacquinet-Salord MC, Fouriaud C 1987 Relationship between alcohol consumption and hypertension prevalence and control in a French population. J Chronic Dis 40:713–720

Lian C 1915 L'alcoholisme, cause d'hypertension artérielle. Bull Acad Natl Méd Paris 74: 525–528

Maclure M 1993 Demonstration of deductive meta-analysis: ethanol intake and risk of myocardial infarction. Epidemiol Rev 15:328–351

MacMahon S 1987 Alcohol consumption and hypertension. Hypertension 9:111–121

MacMahon SW, Blacket RB, MacDonald GJ, Hall W 1984 Obesity, alcohol consumption and blood pressure in Australian men and women. The National Heart Foundation of Australia Risk Factor Prevalence Study. J Hypertension 2:85–91

Maheswaran R, Beevers M, Beevers DG 1992 Effectiveness of advice to reduce alcohol consumption in hypertensive patients. Hypertension 19:79–84

Marmot MG, Shipley MJ, Rose G, Thomas BJ 1981 Alcohol and mortality: a U-shaped curve. Lancet ii:580–583

Marmot MG, Elliott P, Shipley MJ et al 1994 Alcohol and blood pressure: the INTERSALT study. Br Med J 308:1263–1267

Midanek LT, Klatsky AL, Armstrong MA 1990 Changes in drinking behaviour: demographic, psychosocial and biochemical factors. Int J Addict 25:599–619

Milon H, Froment A, Gaspard P, Guidollet J, Ripole JP 1982 Alcohol consumption and blood pressure in a French epidemiological study. Eur Heart J 3:59–64

Mitchell PI, Morgan MJ, Boadle DJ et al 1980 Role of alcohol in the etiology of hypertension. Med J Aust 2:198–200

Myrhed M 1974 Alcohol consumption in relation to factors associated with ischemic heart disease. Acta Med Scand Suppl 567:1–93

Parker M, Puddey IB, Beilin LJ, Vandongen R 1990 A 2-way factorial study of alcohol and salt restriction in treated hypertensive men. Hypertension 16:398–406

Paulin JM, Simpson FO, Waal-Manning HJ 1985 Alcohol consumption and blood pressure in a New Zealand community study. N Z Med J 98:425–428

Pohorecky LA 1991 Stress and alcohol interaction: an update on human research. Alcohol Clin Exp Res 15:438–459

Potter JF, Beevers DG 1984 Pressor effect of alcohol in hypertension. Lancet 1:119–122

Puddey IB, Beilin LJ, Vandongen R, Rouse IR, Rogers P 1985a Evidence for a direct effect of alcohol consumption on blood pressure in normotensive men. A randomized controlled trial. Hypertension 7:707–713

Puddey IB, Vandongen R, Beilin LJ, Rouse IL 1985b Alcohol stimulation of renin release in man – its relation to the hemodynamic, electrolyte and sympatho-adrenal responses to drinking. J Clin Endocrinol Metab 61:37–42

Puddey IB, Beilin LJ, Vandongen R 1987 Regular alcohol use raises blood pressure in treated hypertensive subjects — a randomized controlled trial. Lancet 1:647–651

Reed D, McGee D, Yano K 1982 Biological and social correlates of blood pressure among Japanese men in Hawaii. Hypertension 4:406–414

Salonen JT, Tuomilehto J, Tanskanen A 1983 Relation of blood pressure to reported intake of salt, saturated fats and alcohol in a healthy middle aged population. J Epidemiol Community Health 37:32–37

Savdie E, Grosslight GM, Adena MA 1984 Relation of alcohol and cigarette consumption to blood pressure and serum creatinine levels. J Chronic Dis 37:617–623

Schaeffer V, Döring A, Winkler G, Keil U 1991 Erhebung der Alkoholaufnahme: Vergleich verschiedener Methoden. Ernährungs-Umschau 38:490–494

Schnall PL, Schwartz JP, Landsbergis PA, Warren K, Pickering TG 1992 Relation between job strain, alcohol and ambulatory blood pressure. Hypertension 19:488–494

Simon J, Filipovsky J, Rosolova H, Topolcan O, Karlicek V 1988 Cross-sectional study of beer consumption and blood pressure in middle-aged men. J Hum Hypertens 2:1–6

Trevisan M, Krogh V, Farinaro E, Panico S, Mancini M 1987 Alcohol consumption, drinking pattern and blood pressure: analysis of data from the Italian National Research Council Study. Int J Epidemiol 16:520–527

Ueshima H, Shimamoto T, Iida M et al 1984 Alcohol intake and hypertension among urban and rural Japanese populations. J Chronic Dis 37:585–592 van Leer EM, Seidell JC, Kromhout D 1994 Differences in the association between alcohol consumption and blood pressure by age, gender and smoking. Epidemiology 5:576–582

Wannamethee G, Shaper AG 1991 Alcohol intake and variations in blood pressure by day of examination. J Hum Hypertens 5:59–67

Weissfeld JL, Johnson EH, Brock BM, Hawthorne VM 1988 Sex and age interactions in the association between alcohol and blood pressure. Am J Epidemiol 128:559–569

Witteman JCM, Willett WC, Stampfer MJ et al 1989 A prospective study of nutritional factors and hypertension among US women. Circulation 80:1320–1327

Yamada Y, Ishizaki M, Kido T et al 1991 Alcohol, high blood pressure and serum γ-glutamyl transpeptidase level. Hypertension 18:819–826

DISCUSSION

Renaud: Would you conclude that despite increasing blood pressure, alcohol decreases the risk of coronary heart disease?

Keil: That is a key question, and I would like to answer 'yes' to it. Up until an alcohol intake of 80 g/day, the CHD risk curve in our data is L-shaped, despite the fact that blood pressure is increasing beyond an intake of $\geqslant 30$ g/day. We cannot really explain why this blood pressure increase does not have a detrimental effect on CHD.

Peters: Another way of putting this question is to ask about the significance of a 1 mm Hg rise in blood pressure. Each extra 10 g alcohol/day will raise blood pressure by 1 mm Hg: how important is this in terms of morbidity and mortality?

Keil: It is definitely important. In observational studies and clinical trials, a 6 mm difference in diastolic blood pressure accounts for 40% of strokes and 17–25% of CHD. Each extra millimetre of systolic and diastolic blood pressure is important: I don't know where the excess risk due to elevated blood pressure disappears to.

Shaper: While I don't agree with him, Gareth Beevers maintains that the rise in blood pressure associated with alcohol is not pathogenic — it does not increase risk (Lip & Beevers 1995). Our data from the British Regional Heart Study suggest that this is not true (Wannamethee & Shaper 1996). Would you like to comment on this?

Keil: I only have these empirical data showing that there is a rise in blood pressure, yet despite this the CHD risk curve stays L-shaped up until an alcohol intake of 80 g/day.

Shaper: Which would give some support for Gareth Beevers' claim.

Keil: It's a puzzle still.

Criqui: More than 10 years ago, when we first started modelling the effects of alcohol operating through HDL, we also looked at its effects on blood pressure. We were faced with exactly the same question: is the rise in blood pressure that accompanies alcohol consumption pathogenic or is it a transient phenomenon?

We used models looking not only at HDL as a pathway but also at LDL cholesterol and blood pressure. We found that the rise in blood pressure was significantly associated with CHD mortality and cardiovascular disease mortality overall, and that it specifically accompanied alcohol (Criqui 1987, Criqui et al 1987).

Klatsky: We attempted to look at this issue many years ago by studying two fairly large groups (850 hypertensive persons in each) matched for blood pressure and also a number of demographic traits, but differing in alcohol habits: one group took three or more drinks per day and the other were very light or non-drinkers (Klatsky 1995). The alcohol-related mortality seemed to dominate everything: the heavier drinkers had more cirrhosis, accidents and alcohol related cancers, and they also had less CHD. With regard to stroke, however, there was no difference between the two groups. We concluded that in so far as these data were relevant, it appeared that alcohol-associated hypertension had just as much hazard with relationship to stroke as non-alcohol-associated hypertension.

Criqui: In many population studies presenting an alcohol curve the data are adjusted for confounding variables such as age, smoking, BMI and hypertension. It is a tremendous error to adjust the curve for hypertension, because when you do, you are essentially making everybody's blood pressure equal at each level of alcohol consumption, and you therefore don't see the hazard of alcohol-related hypertension.

Puddey: Even if we do accept that alcohol-related hypertension may be benign up to a consumption level of 80 g/day with respect to CHD endpoints, you have still got to take on board the fact if the population attributable risk is in the realm that Ulrich Keil has shown us, one in 10 patients are having a diagnosis of hypertension and being initiated on antihypertensive therapy unnecessarily. More than that, how many people who are already on anti-hypertensive therapy have got inadequate control because of excessive drinking that's leading to a fluctuation of blood pressure? These two questions have to be factored into this equation. Finally, the differential impact of hypertension has always been one of a greater relationship with stroke rather than coronary artery disease, so it should come as no surprise that an agent that's raising HDL but also raising blood pressure is having its major impact on ischaemic and haemorrhagic stroke, not on coronary artery disease.

Keil: Yes, I mentioned that a 6 mm Hg difference in diastolic blood pressure translates into 40% stroke difference and 17–25% CHD difference. Obviously the blood pressure–stroke relationship is stronger than the blood pressure–CHD association.

Gaziano: I don't think that this hypertension is benign. While we call this an L-shaped curve, if we look very carefully at Maclure's data for non-fatal CHD, in the last drinking category it does come back up to 1 (Maclure 1993). I don't find it incongruous that we get a protective effect because, as you pointed out, alcohol doesn't increase blood pressure until an intake level of 30 g/day, and then hypertension begins to march up. By this level, we have already seen much of the benefit from HDL and then we get this competing risk from hypertension that offsets any further benefits from raised HDL levels. We have done modelling that suggests this is what is happening. I hate to have two explanations for a curve, but I would say that in the early part of the curve HDL is playing a big role, but further out there are competing risks and benefits of hypertension and HDL. If we look at stroke, for instance, we see ischaemic protection early on, and then we see the risk offsetting the benefit.

Keil: I think Robert Beaglehole from New Zealand coined the term 'the window of benefit', which describes what is happening up to consumption levels of 30 g/day, where there is no blood pressure increase, but just the protective effect of alcohol.

Shaper: In some of your figures, in the oldest age group (age 55–64 males and females) you showed a J-shaped curve. This is interesting because clearly there is a likelihood for people who have hypertension to be put on medication, which may make them stop drinking. Thus there is a tendency for hypertensives — particularly those with diastolic hypertension, which is the criterion that most general practitioners use in the UK — to congregate in the non-drinking group.

Urbano-Márquez: Is it possible that similar to the situation with salt, there are patients more sensitive to the hypertensive effects of alcohol?

Keil: It is all a matter of interaction between genetic disposition and environmental factors. The figures I have shown are averages. There are quite a number of people with high alcohol intake whose blood pressure is not increasing.

Shaper: One hopes that one of the messages that those reporting on this meeting will take back to the general public is that before we put people on treatment for hypertension we should examine the effect of withdrawing alcohol for at least one week.

Anderson: How confident are we about the effects of alcohol on blood pressure at these low levels of alcohol consumption? I do not think the threshold effect is consistent. I find it difficult to believe that there is not some effect of low levels of consumption in raising blood pressure: could this reflect a measurement problem?

Puddey: One could also ask about how benign alcohol-related hypertension is if it occurs in the setting of decreased platelet adhesiveness, lower fibrinogen levels and maybe even enhanced fibrinolysis. A recent Japanese study has shown quite dramatic synergism between on the one hand, hypertension and consumption of alcohol, and on the other, the incidence of both haemorrhagic and ischaemic stroke (Kiyohara et al 1995).

Keil: I'm surprised that the rather crude measures we are using in epidemiological studies still produce these rather consistent results.

Klatsky: I agree entirely that accuracy of measurement is a crucial factor and I think this is an example where under-reporting of drinking is likely to produce a spurious association, apparently at very low levels of drinking.

But I also want to comment about the smoking interaction, which I find very interesting, especially since we looked at it and did not find an effect. In our first alcohol/blood pressure study we looked at subsets of non-smokers who had never smoked, current non-smokers who were ex-smokers, and current smokers. We found quite similar alcohol/blood pressure relationships in these smoking subsets in men and women in each of three ethnic groups, but we didn't look at age subsets within that. I wonder whether there's an age factor also involved, in that the smokers, if they're middle-aged and beyond, might have generalized atherosclerotic disease which may modulate this response.

I also wanted to comment on another interaction that is not unanimous in all studies but has been surprisingly consistent, and this is the sex disparity. We found (and I believe Mike Criqui found) that there was no J-curve for men: in other words there was either a threshold at heavier drinking levels or a slight increase in blood pressure at lower drinking levels. But there was a rather definite J-curve in lighter-drinking women, in that the women who were lighter drinkers had lower blood pressures than the non-drinkers. We found that in two separate studies done by different statistical methods. I think your data showed that too: can you comment upon that possible interaction?

Keil: The clearest dip (J-shaped curve) we found was in 55–64 year old men with regard to systolic blood pressure. In the younger men we do not see this J-shaped curve. The same applies to women; only in the 55–64 year old females do we see a slight dip in systolic and diastolic blood pressure with the 1–19 g/day alcohol intake group. So obviously our findings are inconsistent with yours. My interpretation here would be that the non-drinkers in this higher age group contain a number of sick people with higher blood pressure who gave up drinking. With regard to the alcohol–smoking interaction, we found this in all age groups in men and women, although the strongest interaction was found in 45–64 year old women (Keil et al 1991).

Hillbom: What are the acute effects of heavy drinking on blood pressure? This could be an important issue when we think about the different mechanisms of haemorrhagic strokes, for example.

Keil: To my knowledge the acute effect of alcohol is a lowering of blood pressure. However, this is a short-term effect.

Grønbæk: I found the data on the changes in alcohol intake and blood pressure interesting. Did you look at the interaction with initial alcohol intake? That is, did the change of alcohol intake have the same effect regardless of the initial alcohol intake? In other words, would you expect the same effect from a change of 50 g/day to 40 g/day, as a change from 10 g/day to zero?

Keil: We have not yet analysed the data in this way, but I would guess that in the alcohol intake range beyond 30 g/day, the changes in alcohol intake have a more clear-cut and larger effect on blood pressure than changes in the lower drinking range.

Rehm: Going back to the point of what low consumption of alcohol means with respect to hypertension, I think we may actually have an exponential curve with a very slow onset. In epidemiology we often model exponential curves as a threshold and then a linear effect. I don't think we have enough data to discern between these two phenomena with just one study.

Did you ever model the effects of hypertension and HDL together on your CHD incidence? If you do this you may well find that the beneficial effect of HDL is actually offset by hypertension. You have the data to do this.

Keil: What you are proposing has been done in a recent paper of ours (Keil et al 1997a). The curve I showed came from this paper. We are presenting the crude data on alcohol and CHD first and then we are adding one variable (confounder, covariate) after the other to the model. We were surprised that when we controlled for HDL, which we regard as a mediator of the alcohol–CHD relationship, the protective effect did not diminish very much. When hypertension was controlled for, the protective effect did not increase.

Criqui: I don't think there's any question that the relationship here is causal. In 1984 a controlled trial in hospitalized patients showed that alcohol challenges caused significant increases in blood pressure (Potter & Beevers 1984). There have been a number of experimental challenge studies since, showing increases of blood pressure with alcohol. Most of them haven't tried to address this issue of very small amounts of alcohol. Arthur Klatsky published a paper some years ago reviewing all the blood pressure alcohol studies, showing that there was some heterogeneity with the lower dose: some studies in fact show no threshold (Klatsky 1995), and other studies show a threshold all the way up to 2–3 drinks a day. In some studies this heterogeneity may reflect misclassification, with people under-reporting their alcohol intake. Alcohol is, at least peripherally, a vasodilator, thus acutely you might expect a slight drop in blood pressure. The question is, why does blood pressure go up when you consume alcohol? We originally suggested in a paper 16 years ago that it was to do with withdrawal (Wallace et al 1981). More recent (within 24 h) consumption is much more important in raising blood pressure than consumption several days previously. If you look at the serum correlates of blood pressure, the increases in plasma arginine vasopressin and renin are much higher during withdrawal phase than they are during the acute ingestion phase. We all know clinically that if we admit somebody to the hospital in acute alcohol withdrawal, hypertension usually disappears completely once the withdrawal is over. We therefore thought that the withdrawal hypothesis was pretty strong. However, some people have done challenge studies in both animals and humans and have shown that there is also a pressor effect and withdrawal may be superimposed on top of this.

Wannamethee: Can I go back to why the shape of the curve may be flattened. How long was your follow-up?

Keil: Eight years.

Wannamethee: One of the things that we do know is that even after five years, many of the heavy drinkers are now abstainers and, among other changes, their blood pressure has regressed. In addition, a lot of the heavy drinkers move into the moderate drinking category, where HDL will still be elevated in terms of a protective effect, but blood pressure will have reduced to non-pathological levels. Thus with short-term studies, one sees more of a U-shaped curve for the effects of drinking on cardiovascular disease. However, as the follow-up time increases the curve flattens out. My suggestion is that the reason you do not see that upturn in heavy drinkers is that some of the heavy drinkers have been reducing their consumption.

Keil: Looking at changes of alcohol intake over time in our cohort clearly reveals that the net effect is a reduction in alcohol consumption over time. In my opinion changes such as these are actually working against the protective effect of alcohol, so it is surprising that we still pick it up so consistently (Keil et al 1997b).

Wannamethee: Yes, but we're not talking about moderate drinkers and light drinkers: we are talking about heavy drinking, where the blood pressure is most elevated. When heavy drinkers cut down their intake, most do not revert to heavy drinking. This is why in a short-term study you might see more of an effect. We saw this very clearly in our own stroke study (Wannamethee & Shaper 1996), where we had a 14 year follow up, and despite all the strong beliefs that heavy drinking predisposes to stroke, the elevation in stroke risk was only about 30%. However, with an eight year follow-up there was a twofold increase in risk.

Klatsky: With respect to the acute effects of alcohol, a number of recent experiments have shown that the acute effects of alcohol (within hours) are to lower blood pressure, so that idea has not been disproved. I think the best data are a series of studies from a Japanese group, where they used ambulatory monitoring instruments that measure the blood pressure automatically every 15 min (Kawano et al 1992, Kojima et al 1993). This is a nice approach, because it studies blood pressure under more-or-less normal living conditions. With substantial alcohol intake — the equivalent of three or four drinks with dinner — blood pressure was quite a bit lower for a number of hours. In some individuals there was a distinct rise above baseline by the next morning, which would support at least the possibility that withdrawal is somewhat involved in this process. Incidentally, they found little difference between flushers and non-flushers. With regard to the withdrawal hypothesis and the intervention studies, starting with the landmark study of Potter & Beevers (1984), they have not shown that this was an acute effect: it takes several days for the blood pressure to rise. In

Potter & Beevers' study, withdrawal did not appear to cause blood pressure rises at those drinking levels.

Criqui: The way that study was done was that they admitted subjects to the hospital and gave them three or four drinks with dinner. The blood pressure measurements were done in the morning when they woke up. They went up a little bit each day and they claimed it was a chronic pressor effect. In my judgement, you need to measure the blood pressure continuously. Blood pressures in the morning could represent withdrawal.

Klatsky: The Japanese data would support the possibility of mild withdrawal, and I suppose that repeated mild withdrawal reactions could add up to chronic hypertension. Then the question becomes does it matter whether it is due to alcohol that's been in the body in the last 8 h, or whether it's due to withdrawal?

Criqui: Unless you have an i.v. line infusing low dose alcohol continuously it is a moot point.

Puddey: We have to agree there is probably a dual mechanism for alcohol-related hypertension, one of which is a withdrawal phenomenon but which is unlikely to be seen with two to three standard drinks a day, which is the range where many of the population studies already show an increase in blood pressure. You are unlikely to have withdrawal the morning after if you have had only 2–3 drinks the previous evening. Having said that, in our time-course studies over six weeks, when regular drinkers have been switched to a low alcohol intake, the predominant fall in blood pressure was within the first two weeks, but we were still seeing further falls after the subjects had been on a lower intake for six weeks (Puddey et al 1985, 1987). This pattern suggests that there is a chronic pressor effect in addition to any acute withdrawal phenomenon. This has been recently reported in alcoholic subjects who have been detoxified for a number of years, where continued blood pressure dysregulation has now been reported (King et al 1994, York & Hirsch 1996).

Keil: The final statement should perhaps be that there is no doubt that the alcohol–blood pressure association is causal. This strong statement is justified because the data from the observational studies and from clinical trials, i.e. experimental studies, correspond very nicely. Regarding this association we are obviously on rather safe ground.

References

Criqui MH 1987 Alcohol and hypertension: new insights from population studies. Eur Heart J 8 (suppl B):19–26

Criqui MH, Cowan LD, Tyroler HA et al 1987 Lipoproteins as mediators for the effects of alcohol consumption and cigarette smoking on cardiovascular mortality: results from the Lipid Research Clinics Follow-up Study. Am J Epidemiol 126:629–637

Kawano Y, Abe H, Kojuma S et al 1992 Acute depressor effect of alcohol in patients with essential hypertension. Hypertension 20:219–226

Keil U, Chambless L, Filipiak B, Härtel U 1991 Alcohol and blood pressure and its interaction with smoking and other behavioural variables: results from the MONICA Augsburg Survey 1984–1985. J Hypertens 9:491–498

Keil U, Chambless LE, Döring A, Filipiak B, Stieber J 1997a The relation of alcohol intake to coronary heart disease and all-cause mortality in a beer-drinking population. Epidemiology 8:150–156

Keil U, Chambless LE, Döring A, Filipiak B, Stieber J 1997b Alcohol, coronary heart disease, and mortality (Authors' reply to a letter to the Editor). Epidemiology 8:687–688

King AC, Parsons OA, Bernardy NC, Lovallo WR 1994 Drinking history is related to persistent blood pressure dysregulation in post-withdrawal alcoholics. Alcohol Clin Exp Res 18:1172–1176

Kiyohara Y, Kato L, Iwamoto H, Nakayama K, Fujishima M 1995 The impact of alcohol and hypertension on stroke incidence in a general Japanese population. The Hisayama Study. Stroke 26:368–372

Klatsky AL 1995 Blood pressure and alcohol intake. In: Laragh JH, Brenner BM (eds) Hypertension: pathophysiology, diagnosis and management, 2nd edn. Raven Press, New York, p 2649–2667

Kojima S, Kawano Y, Abe H et al 1993 Acute effects of alcohol on blood pressure and erythrocyte sodium concentration. J Hypertens 11:185–190

Lip GYH, Beevers DG 1995 Alcohol, hypertension, coronary heart disease and stroke. Clin Exp Pharmacol Physiol 22:189–194

Maclure M 1993 Demonstration of deductive meta-analysis: ethanol intake and risk of myocardial infarction. Epidemiol Rev 15:328–351

Potter JF, Beevers DG 1984 Pressor effect of alcohol in hypertension. Lancet 1:119–122

Puddey IB, Beilin LJ, Vandongen R, Rouse IL, Rogers P 1985 Evidence for a direct effect of alcohol consumption on blood pressure in normotensive men. A randomized controlled trial. Hypertension 7:707–713

Puddey IB, Beilin LJ, Vandongen R 1987 Regular alcohol use raises blood pressure in treated hypertensive subjects. A randomized controlled trial. Lancet 1:647–651

Wallace RB, Lynch CF, Pomrehn PR, Criqui MH, Heiss G 1981 Alcohol and hypertension: epidemiologic and experimental considerations. The Lipid Research Clinics Program. Circulation 64:III 41–III 47

Wannamethee SG, Shaper AG 1996 Patterns of alcohol intake and risk of stroke in middle-aged British men. Stroke 27:1033–1039

York JL, Hirsch JA 1996 Residual pressor effects of chronic alcohol in detoxified alcoholics. Hypertension 28:133–138

General discussion

Alcohol and coagulation

Puddey: I would like to challenge the conclusion that the overall effects of alcohol on coagulation and fibrinolysis are beneficial. This must remain an unproven hypothesis at the present stage. Until we have clearer handles on the activity of both fibrinolysis and coagulation, rather than just measuring changes in these coagulation parameters, we're not going to have a clear understanding of the overall benefits and risks of alcohol.

Hendriks: I have to admit that the evidence for the beneficial effects of haemostatic factors is less strong than for the beneficial effects on high density lipoprotein (HDL) cholesterol. Still, if one looks at how myocardial infarction comes about, one finds that haemostatic processes play an essential role. Furthermore, one should take into account that HDL may explain a large part of the risk, but not all of it.

Urbano-Márquez: What is the literature on alcohol, adhesion molecules and cardiovascular disease?

Criqui: There's a huge literature on adhesion molecules and coronary disease, but I haven't seen anything relating this to alcohol.

Keaney: Part of the problem with those studies is that soluble plasma markers of adhesion molecule activation are controversial. The main question is whether the soluble adhesion molecules which are purportedly shed from endothelial cells actually do represent an accurate marker of endothelial cell activation.

Puddey: Phil Barter in Australia has shown associations at least *in vitro* between HDL and expression of endothelial adhesion factors (Barter 1997). This is another potential link worthy of further explanation.

Renaud: You began this discussion by saying that you don't think that we have enough data to show that alcohol has beneficial effects on clotting. I don't know what you need as a demonstration of this. If you add one drop of alcohol to platelets *in vitro* it blocks aggregation completely and prolongs coagulation. If you give alcohol to animals, the reactivity of platelets is markedly blocked. The same is true in humans, as shown by our group (Renaud & Ruf 1996) and several other investigators (Mikhailidis et al 1983, Meade et al 1985). To my mind, the only problem is the following. When alcohol is given *in vivo*, you get immediately (within 10 min) an effect, which is a lowering of platelet reactivity. Now if you wait several hours, a rebound effect is seen: an increased platelet aggregability. Consequently, depending upon when you take blood after the administration of alcohol to determine platelet reactivity and clotting time, you can obtain opposite results. It is a complicated business. Stroke or sudden death occurring within two days of an intoxication event could well be a consequence of the rebound effect on platelets. In contrast to other alcoholic drinks, red wine doesn't produce this rebound effect. Consequently, this is why certain investigators who have tested platelet reactivity in humans have found it only reduced after wine drinking. Therefore it seems that you can't really say that there are no proven data indicating that alcohol influences platelet parameters and clotting activity.

Puddey: I don't think that's what I said. We've heard that platelets may be less reactive at one stage, there might be might be rebound hyperactivity the next stage, but we have got to think of the full balance of what's happening to coagulation and fibrinolysis. I don't think these data are something we have a complete picture on *in vivo* in humans at the present stage. I don't think we can promote alcohol as an anti-coagulant.

Alcohol and stress

Gorelick: A popular perception amongst the US public is that stress is a risk factor or a mediator of cardiovascular events. As a practising clinician this is a concept that I hear all the time. There may be some truth to this. As of yet we have not heard in this symposium any information relating to psychosocial or physiological measures of stress. I'm wondering whether a subset of the drinking population are 'hot reactors' (i.e. they have a propensity for more marked sympathetic nervous system responses) and that alcohol is mediating its effect through the stress mechanism.

Keil: I didn't show this earlier, but in our paper on 'Alcohol and blood pressure and its interaction with other variables' we also looked at type A and type B behaviour types (Keil et al 1991). We did not see the interaction with type A, which we had expected; nothing came out of it.

Gorelick: Did you measure any physiological markers of stress?

Keil: No.

Shaper: What kind of physiological markers of stress do you suggest should be used?

Gorelick: Catecholamines or cortisol, for instance. It might be interesting to carry out an experiment to administer alcohol, and determine whether there are hot reactors — whether they have more marked elevations in their blood pressure.

Peters: Are there any data on differences between type A and type B personalities in response to acute alcohol ingestion?

Gorelick: We have performed some cold pressor tests in some of our intracranial haemorrhage cases, and found they have markedly elevated blood pressure responses to the stimulus. Sudden high elevations of blood pressure are one of the mechanisms that may underlie haemorrhagic strokes.

Rehm: We have no biological data, but we looked at the potential moderating effect of type A and type B personalities, and of other social variables which have been proposed in the alcohol literature such as social isolation, as moderating effects in the alcohol/mortality and the alcohol/cardiovascular mortality relationship. We were unable to find any significant effects, contrary to what might be expected. Despite the popularity of behavioural indicators, they have no modifying effects in their interaction with alcohol.

Farrell: We have looked within the psychiatric morbidity survey at measures of psychological morbidity scores, and found a correlation with heavy alcohol consumption (Farrell et al 1998). We found increasing scores with heavier drinking. The same applied to tobacco, which would be consistent with the notion that there are other stress factors involved.

Keil: Perhaps the interaction with smoking is an indicator for a stressor effect.

Peters: We have done some work with alcohol misusers and quality of life measures. These indicate that people who misuse alcohol have a much poorer quality of life than even people with head and neck cancer, for instance.

Criqui: The Western Collaborative Group Study in San Francisco about 20 years ago showing a twofold risk for type A versus type B personalities (Rosenman et al 1975). This work has been repeated many times in population studies with very equivocal results. The people who work on stress have distilled a hostility element out which they think still holds predictive value, but the regular type A/ B scale does not seem to hold predictive value. On the other hand, the physiological reactivity measures, such as the cold pressor test, are quite predictive for hypertension or coronary disease, but these are not really dealing with a personality issue so much as a physiological reactivity. This is a separate area, and I don't know anything about alcohol's influence there. It is clear that people who drink heavily are more depressed than those who don't, but which way the causal arrow goes is an important question.

Bondy: I would be very cautious of using measures of perceived stress taken cross-sectionally with a risk factor. For example, smokers who are smoking report that they smoke because of perceived anxiety and stress, and yet they report lower stress levels while they are not smoking and higher stress levels when they return to smoking.

Randomized controlled trials and alcohol

Anderson: I would like to raise the idea of randomized controlled trials with alcohol. I like Ian Puddey's studies in which subjects go from normal to low alcohol beer. Has anyone seriously considered a randomized trial of alcohol against placebo to try to unravel some of these effects on large numbers of people? There are many ethical considerations that would probably rule it out, but at least it would be interesting for us to consider sample sizes, doses and what might be needed to unravel some of these issues.

Shaper: In a clinical trial you would be confronted with trying to persuade moderate and heavy drinkers to become light drinkers, or abstainers to become light or moderate drinkers. The non-drinking group is made up of life-long teetotallers, obviously with a commitment to not drinking, and ex-drinkers who have given up usually for good reasons. Therefore the idea is a non-starter.

Anderson: No, it is not a non-starter. You have to think imaginatively. For example, there is, of course, a whole group of non-drinkers that start drinking at the age of 18 or 21, for instance. It is worth at least exploring these ideas before dismissing them.

Farrell: One problem is the design of the placebo, which would be just about impossible except in a laboratory setting with low levels of consumption.

Puddey: You could easily take moderate to heavy drinkers and randomize them either to continue or to decrease consumption. That would be a reasonable and ethical study to do.

Rehm: It has also been shown that you can experimentally manipulate different dosages of alcohol without the subjects knowing the kind of dosage they have had. This includes designs with placebo. In fact, if you provide a well designed alcohol placebo (cf. Martin & Sayette 1993), 90–95% of the people that are given the placebo will report being intoxicated and having received alcohol. While there is some variability, the good placebo can get people, on average, to report that they have consumed about two drinks in an hour.

The problem with the trials we discuss is that some of the postulated effects occur more in the realm of weeks than days. I cannot see a masking of the alcohol if it goes over from the acute effect of one experiment to a whole week.

Gaziano: I have a comment about the level of data that we need in order to be able to say that an association is causal. Alcohol is in the intermediate category where there's a wealth of consistent observational associations and there's support for causal mechanisms, but we don't have intervention data. Such intervention data would give us two pieces of valuable information. First, they would allow us to be more certain about alcohol relationships with various disease outcomes. Second, they would also allow us to quantitate those estimates much more accurately, and then public policy could flow much more easily from quantitative estimates that were derived from a randomized trial.

Klatsky: Are we talking about prospective randomized clinical trials on these risk factors — which have been done and are feasible — or are we talking about perspective randomized trials on coronary outcomes and mortality? In the latter we would have to modify people's behaviour for decades, not just years — to me that seems almost impossible.

Criqui: Several years ago in Brussels, Dr Renaud, Dr Farchi, Dr Veenstra and I discussed whether or not you could do a clinical trial. We didn't think it was feasible for the following reasons. First, there is no true placebo for alcohol, so the study is not going to be double-blind. Not only is there no placebo, but alcohol has a very specific psychological intoxicating effect which may produce effects beyond a specific disease that will make any outcome difficult to interpret. Second, I don't think the question of what happens when heavy drinkers switch to light/moderate drinking is all that pressing: the key question concerns what happens when you take individuals who are teetotallers and actually assign them to light to moderate drinking. I don't think that's ethical. The population of non-drinkers has very few people who are candidates to be drinkers. The monitoring would be also extremely difficult. The only possibility for a randomized clinical trial is that you use persons who already drink and subclinical measures of disease. Quantitative angiography is a little hazardous, so you can only use that in people who already have coronary disease. In terms of primary prevention of coronary disease, it takes a long time but some of the new subclinical measures such as positron emission tomography scans might give you some information in 3–4 years.

Peters: Our previous Secretary of State for Health has suggested that people who are abstaining at the age of 45 should consider starting moderate drinking of alcoholic beverages.

Rehm: You can use HDL and blood platelet measures as intermediate measures for the endpoints. I think it is of public health relevance to look at the effects of alcohol compared with standardized effects of physical activities which have been done in randomized clinical trials, and there you can see the interaction of alcohol and physical activity in a factorial design. On the other hand, for the platelet you can use something like the effect of alcohol on the platelet and compare it to aspirin and then do a factorial design with aspirin and alcohol together. This would answer some of the questions. I admit that it does not answer any questions about what happens if teetotallers are switched to moderate drinking.

Keaney: The potential problem with that approach is that it pre-supposes mechanisms which we have just been arguing about for the better part of a day.

Dr Klatsky, with reference to your statements that clinical trials of alcohol consumption would require decades of treatment, we must remember that if the effect of alcohol is mediated by HDL, you probably wouldn't have to treat for decades. Our lipid lowering studies tell us that you can detect secondary prevention of cardiovascular events in 4–6 years if you use a high risk population.

Klatsky: In defence of my statement about a clinical trial taking decades, I was of course thinking about primary prevention, which is a public health question that people want answered. I don't think that it would really be feasible to do a trial for secondary prevention studies either. The general public thinks they know not only about light-to-moderate drinking protecting against coronary disease, but that red wine in particular protects against coronary disease. I believe it would be very difficult in the USA to find people willing to randomize themselves in this study if they already knew they had coronary disease. I wouldn't underestimate that problem.

Keaney: I agree. Part of what I do involves clinical studies on vascular effects of antioxidants. We had a very difficult time getting people who weren't already on doses of vitamin C, vitamin E and other supplements.

Keil: We are in an era where nobody believes anything without a clinical trial, but we forget that most decisions in public health are based on observational studies. Think of smoking, asbestos and occupational health, for instance. In most areas clinical trials are not feasible and still we have to make decisions.

Peters: However, using this intuitive approach we have also made wrong decisions, such as treating myocardial infarctions with anticoagulants. Sir Miles Irvine, the surgeon who runs the Health Technology Assessment Programme for the Department of Health, stated that he didn't need a randomized controlled trial to prove that he should ligate a bleeding blood vessel!

Miller: We use clinical trials to address grey areas where there is clinical uncertainty. So we don't need clinical trials, as you said, for ligating bleeding blood vessels. We have never really felt the pressing demand for a clinical trial when it comes to cigarette smoking, and those of us who accept that the data on mild alcohol consumption fit strongly with a protective effect would feel no need to struggle with randomized controlled trials of low dose alcohol. There may be grey areas with regard to subgroups, but my feeling is that we should reserve randomized controlled trials for genuine uncertainties in clinical research. Perhaps what we need is continuing work to tidy up the observational data to satisfy doubters.

References

Barter PJ 1997 Inhibition of endothelial cell adhesion molecule expression by high density lipoproteins. Clin Exp Pharmacol Physiol 24:286–287

Farrell M, Taylor C, Jarvis M et al 1998 Tobacco, alcohol and other drug dependence and psychological morbidity. Br J Psychiatry, in press

Keil U, Chambless L, Filipiak B, Härtel U 1991 Alcohol and blood pressure and its interaction with smoking and other behavioural variables: results from the MONICA Augsburg Survey 1984–1985. J Hypertens 9:491–498

Martin CS, Sayette MA 1993 Experimental design in alcohol administration research: limitations and alternatives in the manipulation of dosage-set. J Stud Alcohol 54:750–761

Meade TW, Vickers MV, Thompson SG, Stirling Y, Haines AP, Miller GJ 1985 Epidemiological characteristics of platelet aggregability. Br Med J Clin Res 290:428–432

Mikhailidis DP, Jeremy JY, Barradas MA, Green N, Dandona P 1983 Effect of ethanol on vascular prostacyclin (prostaglandin I_2) synthesis, platelet aggregation, and platelet thromboxane release. Br Med J Clin Res 287:1495–1498

Renaud S, Ruf JC 1996 Effects of alcohol on platelet functions. Clin Chim Acta 246:77–89

Rosenman RH, Brand RJ, Jenkins D, Friedman M, Straus R, Wurm M 1975 Coronary heart disease in Western Collaborative Group Study. Final follow-up experience of $8\frac{1}{2}$ years. JAMA 1975 233:872–877

Do known cardiovascular risk factors mediate the effect of alcohol on cardiovascular disease?

M. H. Criqui

University of California, San Diego, Department of Family and Preventive Medicine, 9500 Gilman Drive, La Jolla, CA 92093-0607, USA

Abstract. The association between alcohol intake and atherosclerotic cardiovascular disease (CVD) in epidemiological studies is consistent and shows some protection from CVD at consumption levels of one to two drinks per day, but a sharp increase in CVD associated with three or more drinks per day. Analyses of potential mediators of effects of alcohol on CVD show that it increases high density lipoprotein (HDL) cholesterol levels and favourably influences thrombotic factors, especially fibrinogen, and also fibrinolytic factors. Some evidence also suggests moderate alcohol consumption may reduce insulin resistance. However, studies also show an adverse effect of alcohol, particularly at higher doses, on blood pressure (leading to hypertension) and directly on the myocardium (leading to arrhythmias and myocardiopathy). Statistical modelling of the alcohol–CVD relationship is consistent in several studies, with a protective pathway via elevated HDL cholesterol and an adverse pathway through elevated blood pressure. Other possible mediators influenced by alcohol have not yet been examined in this type of analysis. The French Paradox has led to speculation that wine is the only protective alcoholic beverage for CVD, or at least that it has a stronger effect. Multiple non-ethanol components of wine have been studied in the laboratory and have been shown to have antioxidant or anticoagulant effects. Although wine does appear more protective in ecological studies, studies within cohorts show similar effects across alcoholic beverages, suggesting confounding in ecological studies by diet, lifestyle, or other variables. The key component of alcoholic beverages thus appears to be ethanol, consistent with the known potent effects of ethanol on HDL cholesterol and thrombotic factors. The upswing in CVD risk with three or more drinks per day is sharp and emphasizes that benefit from alcohol is limited to moderate consumption only. This upswing also cautions against any public health recommendation to drink alcohol, since many persons will not or cannot limit their intake to moderate levels.

1998 Alcohol and cardiovascular diseases. Wiley, Chichester (Novartis Foundation Symposium 216) p 159–172

Numerous observational studies have consistently reported that light to moderate consumption of alcohol, defined as $\leqslant 2$ drinks per day, is associated with a reduction in coronary heart disease (CHD) (Criqui 1994). These studies have included case-control, cohort, and ecological designs. However, the biological effects of alcohol responsible for this reduction in risk is unclear. Several short-term clinical trials have shown that alcohol affects a number of cardiovascular disease (CVD) risk factors, including high density lipoprotein (HDL) cholesterol, platelets and other coagulation parameters, and blood pressure (Haut & Cowan 1974, Mikhaildis et al 1983, Valimaki et al 1988, Veenstra 1990, Randin et al 1995). Such associations have also been consistently reported in observational studies (Criqui 1987, Criqui et al 1987, Renaud et al 1992). In addition, recent observational studies have suggested alcohol may favorably affect insulin resistance (Razay et al 1992, Kiechl et al 1996), and one cohort study reported the benefits of alcohol consumption for CHD were limited to subjects with the Lewis blood type antigen (a^-b^-), which is associated with the insulin resistance syndrome (Hein et al 1993). In addition to affecting these CVD risk factors, alcohol, at least at higher doses, can directly adversely affect the myocardium, leading to arrhythmias (Ettinger et al 1978) and cardiomyopathy (Urbano-Márquez et al 1989).

Multivariate modelling of alcohol effects

Several years ago we hypothesized that epidemiological cohort studies might be able to help us understand the pathways by which alcohol exerts effects on CHD. Cohort studies of CHD incidence had typically measured subjects' alcohol consumption at baseline, as well as several CVD risk factors which are potential mediators of an alcohol effect. These potential mediators included HDL cholesterol, low-density lipoprotein (LDL) cholesterol and blood pressure. We employed multivariate models with CHD or CVD as the outcome variable, and alcohol consumption as the independent variable. We adjusted these models for what we considered to be true confounding variables; that is risk factor variables that were associated both with alcohol intake and CHD or CVD, but that were not directly biologically affected by alcohol consumption. Examples of such variables are age and cigarette smoking. However, as noted above, a number of other CVD risk factors are directly altered by alcohol consumption. Adjusting for such variables in multivariate analysis could lead to over- or under-estimation of the effect of alcohol on CHD/CVD, since alcohol's effect through such 'pathway' variables would be statistically eliminated. We reasoned, however, that by adding such pathway variables to multivariate models in sequential fashion, we could determine the degree to which alcohol affected CHD/CVD risk through such variables by measuring the change in the strength of alcohol's estimated effect after their addition.

TABLE 1   Relative risks and *P* values of alcohol for cardiovascular disease (CVD) mortality, before and after addition of HDL cholesterol and LDL cholesterol to the Cox model, in men from the Lipid Research Clinics Follow-up Study (4105 men, 130 CVD deaths)

	Model 1 (without lipoproteins)		Model 2 (plus HDL cholesterol)		Model 3 (plus HDL and LDL cholesterol)	
	Relative risk	P	Relative risk	P	Relative risk	P
Alcohol	0.80	0.06	0.91	0.40	0.91	0.38
HDL cholesterol			0.79	<0.01	0.77	<0.01
LDL cholesterol					1.29	<0.01

Relative risks are for 20 ml alcohol per day compared with none, an HDL cholesterol difference of 10 mg/dl, and an LDL cholesterol difference of 30 mg/dl. Other independent variables in the model are age, systolic blood pressure, cigarette smoking, BMI and high/low triglycerides. Adapted from Criqui et al (1987).

In 1987 we published two papers from the Lipid Research Clinics (LRC) Follow-Up Study employing such analyses. In one paper we investigated the degree to which the benefit of moderate alcohol consumption might be mediated by HDL cholesterol (Criqui et al 1987). The results are shown in Table 1. After adjusting the association between alcohol intake and CVD mortality for the confounding variables of age and cigarette smoking, we found a 20% decrease in the risk of CVD death in men for a 20 ml intake of ethanol per day ($\approx$1.5 drinks per day). Addition of HDL cholesterol to this model produced a sharp change in the alcohol association; the reduction in CVD mortality risk was reduced to only 9%, a 55% relative change from the model without HDL cholesterol. Results for CHD, and results in women, were similar. These results suggested that about half the benefit of alcohol's protective effect was mediated by HDL cholesterol. Addition of LDL cholesterol to these models produced little change in the alcohol coefficient.

In a second paper we used similar analyses to evaluate whether alcohol might exert a harmful effect on CHD/CVD through a blood pressure pathway (Criqui 1987). Separate models for CHD and CVD showed that addition of systolic blood pressure (SBP) to the model increased the apparent benefits of alcohol, indicating a hazard for CHD and CVD mortality from increases in blood pressure with alcohol consumption.

In 1992, we published similar analyses from a different population — the Honolulu Heart Study — using essentially the same methodology (Langer et al

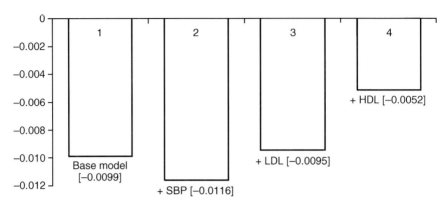

FIG. 1.   Coefficients for alcohol (ml/day) in sequential Cox proportional hazards models for CHD in men in the Honolulu Heart Program. (Adapted from Langer et al 1992.)

1992). In this study the endpoint was all-incident CHD, including both non-fatal and fatal events. Figure 1 shows the results. As in the LRC Follow-Up Study, the base model included alcohol, age and cigarette smoking. The coefficient for alcohol was −0.0099, the inverse coefficient indicating a protective effect, and was statistically significant ($P < 0.05$). Addition of SBP to the model made the coefficient larger (more inverse), a result similar to that obtained in the LRC Follow-Up Study above, indicating an alcohol hazard through increased SBP. Further addition of LDL cholesterol to the model reduced the size of the alcohol coefficient to essentially the baseline level, indicating a modest pathway for alcohol's benefit through lowered LDL cholesterol in this population, of about the same magnitude as the alcohol hazard through increased blood pressure. The next sequential model included the above variables, and in addition HDL cholesterol. The beta coefficient was reduced to −0.0052, a change of 45%. This result was strikingly similar to the LRC Follow-Up Study and again indicated that about half the benefit of alcohol consumption was mediated by increased HDL cholesterol.

At least two other publications have shown similar results. In the MRFIT Study, 45% of the benefit of moderate alcohol consumption in preventing CHD death appeared to be mediated by HDL cholesterol (Suh et al 1992). A case-control study of myocardial infarction, the Boston Area Health Study, found about 60% of alcohol's benefit was mediated by HDL cholesterol (Gaziano et al 1993). Table 2 outlines the similar findings in the LRC Follow-Up, Honolulu Heart Study, MRFIT and the Boston Area Health Study.

The finding that HDL mediates about half of alcohol's benefit in these studies, with a narrow range of 45–55%, is an unusually consistent finding for

TABLE 2   Alcohol, HDL and CHD/CVD in four epidemiological studies

	LRC Study	Honolulu Study	MRFIT Study	Boston Area Study
Study type	Cohort	Cohort	Cohort	Case-control
Baseline status	No CHD	No CVD	No CHD	MI/Controls
Endpoint	CVD death	Total CHD	CHD death	Non-fatal MI
Events/subjects	130/4105	124/1768	190/1688	340/680
Relative risk for alcohol				
Alcohol	0.80	0.83	0.89	0.60
+HDL	0.91	0.91	0.94	0.84
%Δ in alcohol coeff.	55%	47%	45%	60%

epidemiological studies of CVD. Despite this consistency, the results must be interpreted cautiously. First, these analyses usually evaluate light to moderate alcohol consumption as the independent variable. At light to moderate levels, the untoward cardiovascular effects of alcohol are minor compared to the benefit through increased HDL cholesterol. With heavier alcohol consumption, the elevation of blood pressure and direct toxic effects on the myocardium become increasingly important. Second, these statistical pathways do not prove causality, despite their reproducibility. It is possible that an as yet unknown variable, highly correlated with HDL cholesterol and protective for CHD/CVD, also increases with alcohol intake (Criqui 1995).

What about the one-half of alcohol's protective effect that is not explained by HDL cholesterol? There are several possibilities. First, it may be that the HDL pathway explains somewhat more than half of the effect, since some non-systematic misclassification is likely in epidemiological studies, and such misclassification would tend to underestimate the extent of an HDL pathway (Copeland et al 1977). Second, the Boston Area Health Study measured HDL subfractions HDL_2 and HDL_3, and apolipoproteins (Gaziano et al 1993). Adding apolipoproteins A_1 and A_2 to the multivariate risk equation indicated an additional substantial alcohol pathway through these variables. However, these measurements were done on only a subset of study subjects.

Third, the most likely candidates for additional mediators of alcohol's effect are haemostatic factors. Several such factors, including fibrinogen and measures of platelet aggregation, are related to alcohol consumption and associated with CHD/CVD (Meade et al 1979, Renaud et al 1992). Unfortunately, the studies noted above did not have measurements of haemostatic factors and thus could not evaluate such factors in pathway analyses. Tissue-type plasminogen activator (tPA) has been reported to be higher with greater alcohol consumption, and the investigators proposed this as a possible pathway (Ridker et al 1994). However, such a pathway seems problematic given that endogenous tPA levels are associated with greater CVD risk (Ridker et al 1993). Some population studies, such as the Atherosclerosis Risk In Communities (ARIC) study, have measured multiple haemostatic factors as well as lipids, lipoproteins and other standard CVD risk factors. Such studies could provide important information on pathways for the effect of alcohol.

Fourth, recent observations indicate both fasting and post-challenge insulin levels are inversely associated with alcohol intake, suggesting that alcohol intake might favourably modify insulin resistance (Razay et al 1992, Kiechl et al 1996). Interestingly, the Copenhagen Male Study reported that the benefit of alcohol consumption in reducing the risk of CHD was limited to the 9.6% of the population with the Lewis phenotype blood group marker Le(a$^-$b$^-$) (Hein et al 1993). This phenotype has been shown to be a marker for the insulin resistance syndrome, including higher body mass index, lower HDL cholesterol, higher serum triglycerides, and a higher prevalence of diabetes and hypertension.

Ecological studies have consistently reported that wine appears more beneficial for CHD protection then either beer or spirits (Renaud & de Lorgeril 1992, Artaud-Wild et al 1993, Criqui & Ringel 1994). Wine appears to have both antioxidant (Frankel et al 1993) and non-ethanol antithrombotic factors (Demrow et al 1995) which in theory might produce additional benefit for wine. However, in ecological studies, the unit of analysis is a group (typically a country), and other characteristics of wine drinking countries may be difficult to adjust for statistically. In a careful analysis of cohort studies, where the unit of analysis is the individual and 'cultural confounding' is much less likely, beer, wine, and spirits all appear to have roughly equal cardioprotective effects (Rimm et al 1996). Thus, the major cardioprotective component in alcoholic beverages appears to be ethanol, and ethanol likely influences risk through one or more of the cardioprotective mechanisms outlined above. Other substances in wine or other alcoholic beverages may in the future prove to have beneficial effects, but their role is likely to be minor compared to ethanol.

Alcohol for cardioprotection

Should we recommend the consumption of alcohol to reduce the occurrence of atherosclerotic diseases? Figure 2 is taken from a prospective study of 276 802 men and is representative of large population studies which have looked at the relationship of alcohol to mortality from different causes (Boffetta & Garfinkel 1990). There was no additional benefit in terms of coronary disease prevention

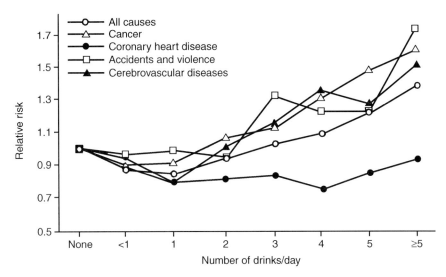

FIG. 2.   Alcohol consumption and relative risk of death over 12 years in American Cancer Society prospective study of 276 802 men aged 40–59. Mortality ratios are adjusted for age and smoking habits, and are for the four most common causes of death and death from all causes. (Adapted from Bofetta & Garfinkel 1990.)

beyond a single drink per day. However, at two drinks per day there were increases in each of the other major causes of mortality — cancer, cerebrovascular diseases, and accidents and violence — leading to an increase in all-cause mortality. With higher levels of drinking all-cause mortality continued to increase in a dose–response fashion. Thus recommendations to the public to consume alcohol for cardioprotection would need to have safeguards to limit consumption to about one drink per day. Such safeguards are not possible. The proportion of abuse in a population is a direct function of the mean consumption (Skog 1985, Rose 1991) and this correlation is difficult to disentangle, given the intoxicating nature of alcohol and the potential for addiction. One could speculate that if ethanol were a new pharmaceutical proposed to the US Food and Drug Administration for cardioprotection, review of trials in humans would reveal an increase in HDL cholesterol and possibly a reduction in LDL cholesterol, changes in selected thrombotic factors and perhaps improvement of insulin resistance. Such trials also might show benefit for short-term coronary atherosclerotic endpoints, such as coronary stenosis change assessed by quantitative coronary angiography. However, these trials would also reveal uniform dose-dependent intoxication and interference with coordination and cognition, along with increasing consumption leading to addiction in about 10% of study subjects. Such a drug would stand little chance of approval.

Careful evaluation of ethanol's diverse biological effects might allow development of pharmaceuticals with similar cardioprotective effects, but without intoxication or addiction potential.

References

Artaud-Wild SM, Connor S, Sexton G, Connor W 1993 Differences in coronary mortality can be explained by differences in cholesterol and saturated fat intakes in 40 countries but not in France and Finland. A paradox. Circulation 88:2771–2779

Boffetta P, Garfinkel L 1990 Alcohol drinking and mortality among men enrolled in an American Cancer Society prospective study. Epidemiology 1:342–348

Copeland KT, Checkoway H, McMichael AJ, Holbrook RH 1977 Bias due to misclassification in the estimation of relative risk. Am J Epidemiol 105:488–495

Criqui MH 1987 Alcohol and hypertension: new insights from population studies. Eur Heart J 8 (suppl B):19–26

Criqui MH 1994 Alcohol and the heart: implications of present epidemiologic knowledge. Contemp Drug Prob 21:125–142

Criqui MH 1995 Protective effects of moderate consumption of alcohol on the incidence of coronary heart disease. In: Gotto AM, Lenfant C, Catapano AL, Paoletti R (eds) Multiple risk factors in cardiovascular disease: vascular and organ protection. Kluwer Academic Publishers, Dordrecht, p 413–415

Criqui MH, Ringel BL 1994 Does diet or alcohol explain the French paradox? Lancet 344:1719–1723

Criqui MH, Cowan LD, Tyroler HA et al 1987 Lipoproteins as mediators for the effects of alcohol consumption and cigarette smoking on cardiovascular mortality. Results from the Lipid Research Clinics Follow-up Study. Am J Epidemiol 126:629–637

Demrow HS, Slane PR, Folts JD 1995 Administration of wine and grape juice inhibits *in vivo* platelet activity and thrombosis in stenosed canine coronary arteries. Circulation 91:1182–1188

Ettinger PO, Wu CF, De la Cruz C, Weisse AB, Ahmed SS, Regan TJ 1978 Arrhythmias and the 'holiday heart': alcohol associated cardiac rhythm disorders. Am Heart J 95:555–562

Frankel EN, Kanner J, German JB, Parks E, Kinsella JE 1993 Inhibition of oxidation of human low-density lipoprotein by phenolic substances in red wine. Lancet 341:454–457

Gaziano JM, Buring JE, Breslow JL et al 1993 Moderate alcohol intake, increased levels of high-density lipoprotein and its subfractions, and decreased risk of myocardial infarction. N Engl J Med 329:1829–1834

Haut MJ, Cowan DH 1974 The effect of ethanol on hemostatic properties of human blood platelets. Am J Med 56:22–33

Hein HO, Sorenson H, Suadicani P, Gyntelberg F 1993 Alcohol consumption, Lewis phenotypes and risk of ischaemic heart disease. Lancet 341:392–396

Kiechl S, Willeit J, Poewe W et al 1996 Insulin sensitivity and regular alcohol consumption: large, prospective cross sectional population study (Bruneck Study). Br Med J 313:1040–1044

Langer RD, Criqui MH, Reed DM 1992 Lipoproteins and blood pressure as biologic pathways for the effect of moderate alcohol consumption on coronary heart disease. Circulation 85:910–915

Meade TW, Chakrabarti R, Haines A, North WR, Stirling Y 1979 Characteristics affecting fibrinolytic activity and plasma fibrinogen concentrations. Br Med J 1:153–156

Mikhailidis DP, Jeremy JY, Barradas MA, Green N, Dandona P 1983 Effect of ethanol on vascular prostacyclin (prostaglandin I$_2$) synthesis, platelet aggregation, and platelet thromboxane release. Br Med J 287:1495–1498

Randin D, Vollenweider P, Tappy L, Jequier E, Nicod P, Scherrer U 1995 Suppression of alcohol-induced hypertension by dexamethasone. N Engl J Med 332:1733–1737

Razay G, Heaton KW, Bolton CH, Hughes AO 1992 Alcohol consumption and its relation to cardiovascular risk factors in British women. Br Med J 304:80–83

Renaud SC, de Lorgeril M 1992 Wine, alcohol, platelets, and the French Paradox for coronary heart disease. Lancet 379:1523–1526

Renaud SC, Beswick AD, Fehily AM, Sharp DS, Elwood PC 1992 Alcohol and platelet aggregation: The Caerphilly Prospective Heart Disease Study. Am J Clin Nutr 55:1012–1017

Ridker PM, Vaughan DE, Stampfer MJ, Manson JE, Hennekens CH 1993 Endogenous tissue-type plasminogen activator and risk of myocardial infarction. Lancet 341:1165–1168

Ridker PM, Vaughan DE, Stampfer MJ, Glynn RJ, Hennekens CH 1994 Association of moderate alcohol consumption and plasma concentration of endogenous tissue-type plasminogen activator. JAMA 272:929–933

Rimm EB, Klatsky A, Grobbee D, Stampfer MJ 1996 Review of moderate alcohol consumption and reduced risk of coronary disease: is the effect due to beer, wine or spirits? Br Med J 312:731–736

Rose G 1991 Ancel Keys lecture. Circulation 84:1405–1409

Skog OJ 1985 The collectivity of drinking cultures: a theory of the distribution of alcohol consumption. Br J Addict 80:83–99

Suh I, Shaten BJ, Cutler JA, Kuller LH 1992 Alcohol use and mortality from coronary heart disease: the role of high density lipoprotein cholesterol. Ann Intern Med 116:881–887

Urbano-Márquez A, Estruch R, Novarro-Lopez F, Grau JM, Mont L, Rubin E 1989 The effects of alcoholism on skeletal and cardiac muscle. N Engl J Med 329:409–415

Valimaki M, Taskinen MR, Ylikahri R, Roine R, Kuusi T, Nikkila EA 1988 Comparison of the effect of two different doses of alcohol on serum lipoproteins, HDL-subfractions and apolipoproteins A-I and A-II: a controlled study. Eur J Clin Invest 18:472–480

Veenstra J 1990 Alcohol and fibrinolysis. Fibrinolysis 4 (suppl 2):64–68

DISCUSSION

Keil: I think that the concept of years of life lost is an important one. In Germany we claim that 108 000 premature deaths per year occur because of smoking and 40 000 premature deaths per year because of alcohol, but this latter calculation takes into account only the detrimental effects of heavy drinking, not the beneficial effects of light drinking. Do you know of any study incorporating both and trying to balance the detrimental and beneficial effects of alcohol?

Criqui: No. There's a paper called 'Actual causes of death in the USA' (McGinnis & Foege 1990). This paper estimates that in 1990 there were 100 000 excess deaths per year due to alcohol, but I believe that calculation was done without considering the protection against CHD. In this paper the figure for smoking deaths was 400 000 per year.

Rehm: Recent economic cost studies on alcohol in Australia (English et al 1995) and Canada (Single et al 1996, Xie et al 1996) showed that in terms of mortality, alcohol 'saved' more lives through preventing CHD than it caused deaths through all the conditions it is adversely related to. However, if you switch from number of deaths to another epidemiological measure, number of life years lost, the picture reverses: in terms of life years lost, alcohol cost more than it saved. The reason is that alcohol mortality in these and other industrialized countries is related to a lot of premature deaths by accidents, whereas the protective effect on CHD only comes into play at later ages. Moreover, it should be said that the studies cited were based on the meta-analyses of English et al (1995) which do not take into account any upturn for CHD at any point — this is not realistic.

Anderson: The other study worth mentioning is the Global Burden of Disease study, which has looked at many different risk factors globally (Murray & Lopez 1996). The effect of alcohol depends on which part of the world you look at: whereas what Jürgen Rehm says may be true for European and North American populations, if you take African populations with low rates of heart disease then alcohol is clearly causing excess deaths due to violence.

Klatsky: There are a many assumptions and problems with this sort of balancing act. One of them is that for most of these conditions it's difficult to discern what proportion of the condition is related to alcohol in the first place at any level of alcohol drinking. The second is that in balancing benefit and harm from alcohol drinking, we are in a sense comparing apples and oranges. This is because we're comparing the effects of light to moderate drinking in the case of coronary disease with the effects of heavier drinking in the case of motor vehicle accidents, suicide, cirrhosis and certain cancers. It would be pertinent in scientifically based public health advice to stratify these estimates — and they are no better than estimates — in terms of effects of heavier drinking and effects of light to moderate drinking. I haven't seen that done, and if it is the results might come out quite differently.

Bondy: That does reflect the methodology for the English et al (1995) meta-analyses. Attributable risks were calculated on the basis of estimated relative risks, for various consequences, associated with four different levels of alcohol intake defined for each sex.

Rehm: Overall, the Australian meta-analysis (English et al 1995) identified around 20 conditions where alcohol would be detrimental in the case of mortality. Coronary heart disease was the only one in which alcohol is beneficial.

Klatsky: I still think there's a problem in comparing on the one hand what may be the preponderant effects of light to moderate drinking (on coronary and total mortality) and the preponderant effect of heavier drinking (which are adverse for practically everything else).

Criqui: It depends on the question, of course. For instance, when you use potential years of life lost, you differentially take into account the additional potential experience of younger people who have more years to live. Light to moderate drinking gives absolutely no benefit below the age of 40. On the other hand, in this age group heavy drinking poses enormous hazards, and young people also drink a lot more than older people.

Farrell: You raised the issue about the types of cohorts that are studied: that they tend to involve those who are more stable and middle class. To raise the issue of social and health inequalities, heavier drinkers in the general population may be poorer and exposed to multiple risks. How do we take account of this?

Criqui: In these cohort studies which show the benefit of moderate consumption, in a sense you get the best possible scenario because in fact people who participate in these studies tend to be more responsible than the population at large. Alcoholics are very poor at participating in these cohort studies. In our paper we published in the *Lancet* (Criqui & Ringel 1994) we looked at total mortality. As powerful as wine was at preventing coronary disease, there was absolutely no association between any alcoholic beverage and total mortality. In fact, the association with beer was positive. The only thing that was protective in the population was fruit, which suggests that the populations as a whole does not do well with alcohol. However, stable, responsible individuals who can handle alcohol — which is generally the group that participates in follow-up studies — do reasonably well.

Rehm: A couple of further comments on meta-analyses and cost studies. I agree that it's of no use to counterbalance those numbers against one another, and there is no formal economic analysis available to compare social costs and benefits. Also, you can reduce most of the costs associated with alcohol without losing any benefits by just moving the heavy drinkers and the harmful drinkers to moderate consumption. If we compare the costs and the differential effects of alcohol on mortality for different social strata, it is very illuminating to see that social class somewhat changes the alcohol–mortality relationship, making the detrimental effects of alcohol much worse for lower social classes. However, even the most detrimental effects of alcohol are in a range of relative risk that is much lower than the usual findings for social class, even in industrialized countries.

Bondy: Alcohol abuse is often an exclusion criteria from this type of epidemiological study. Consequently, we should be cautious about making generalizations from selected study populations to the population at large, which includes people at risk of abusing alcohol. We should also be careful before we say that certain types of beverage are better, because this might merely be a reflection of the fact that, for example, wine is consumed by a higher social class of people in a more moderate way or more regularly.

Wannamethee: Professor Criqui mentioned the effects of alcohol in the general healthy population. In our own population study of middle-aged men we have been looking at this not in terms of years of life lost, but in terms of probability of survival to age 65 years free of major cardiovascular events and diabetes. We find that smoking is by far the most critical factor, followed by physical activity and

BMI. If you lead a healthy life in terms of these three indicators, your probability of healthy survival is about 88%. If you drink lightly this increases to about 89%. If you look at the other extreme — fat, inactive smokers — the probability of healthy survival is only about 40%, and it is in this group that alcohol seems to have some benefit. But is it alcohol consumption we should be advocating or should we recommend that people stop smoking, lose weight and exercise? The protective role of alcohol must be put into proper perspective.

Farchi: It has been hypothesized, and preliminary data support the notion, that drinking patterns could have important influences in determining the health effects of alcohol.

It is interesting to note — also in the absence of definite epidemiological findings — that the recommendation if you 'drink alcoholic beverages, do so in moderation, with meals, and when the consumption does not put you or others at risk', is already included in the *Dietary Guidelines for Americans* (US Departments of Agriculture and Health and Human Services 1995).

In Italy, analysing the data from a large cohort of men and women, the Italian Risk Factor and Life Expectancy Pooling Project, we found evidence for an important effect of drinking pattern on health (M. Trevisan, E. Schisterman, A. Menotti, G. Farchi, S. Conti and the Risk Factor and Life Expectancy Research Group, unpublished data).

Among the 8980 men eligible for the analyses, 959 (11.1%) reported no consumption of alcoholic beverages, 56 950 (65.3%) reported drinking wine with meals, 600 (6.9%) reported drinking wine outside meals, and 1438 (16.7%) reported drinking wine and liquors. Among the 6669 women, 2195 (33.7%) reported no consumption of alcoholic beverages, while 4090 (62.6%) reported drinking wine only at meals, 38 (0.6%) reported consuming wine outside meals, and 198 (3.1%) reported drinking wine and liquors.

Men and women drinking wine outside of meals appeared to experience higher mortality rates compared with drinkers of wine at meals, while in men, drinking wine with meals is associated with lower mortality from all causes, CVD and CHD, compared with non-drinkers. In women, drinkers of wine with meals experience mortality rates from all- and non-CVD causes similar to non-drinkers. Results for cardiovascular mortality endpoints could not be analysed in women because of the limited number of events that occurred during the follow-up period.

The observed effects are independent from the possible confounding effects of age, smoking and from a number of well established cardiovascular risk factors. In addition, the excess risk in drinkers of wine outside meals compared with drinkers of wine with meals appears to be independent of the observed differences in the amount of alcohol consumed across the different drinking pattern categories. These results may explain why in Mediterranean countries, where the majority of people (about 65% in our study) drink wine during meals only, the minimum of the

J-shaped curve seems to be located at a very high level of alcohol consumption — about 50 g alcohol per day.

Criqui: I went into the literature on this subject, and there is not much known about it. However, we know that alcohol taken with a meal is absorbed at a slower rate and the blood alcohol level peaks at a lower level. Thus the blood alcohol curve is flatter. This is probably of benefit, because we think spikes of alcohol will lead to more intoxication and at least some behavioural and accident-type risks, if not to other diseases. Whether or not taking alcohol with food actually does something to the lipid composition or the absorption of nutrients is an interesting question. The limited data available suggest that postprandial lipaemia is aggravated rather than attenuated by alcohol consumption, but that's in the short term. Is there some sort of rebound later on where the metabolism is more efficient because it has been changed? Nobody knows.

Hendriks: One of the things we have studied in our controlled nutrition trials is the composition of HDL in the postprandial phase (van Tol et al 1995). Plasma contained higher triglyceride concentrations after moderate wine consumption as compared to water consumption. Also, triglyceride concentration may increase in HDL particles, as suggested by a decreased molar ratio of cholesterol esters over triglycerides in HDL after wine consumption as compared to water consumption. We thought that this composition change might fit in the sequence of lipid transfers between lipoproteins involved in reverse cholesterol transport.

Miller: I am unsure whether we're looking here at a pattern of consumption effect, or simply a confounder. Men who drink wine between meals regularly may represent a different group who possess other lifestyle factors that may be of importance. For instance, we might be talking about men who are divorced, or of a different social class. There may be other relevant factors that distinguish them as a group but which we are not measuring.

References

Criqui MH, Ringel BL 1994 Does diet or alcohol explain the French paradox? Lancet 344:1719–1723

English DR, Holman CDJ, Milne E et al 1995 The quantification of drug caused morbidity and mortality in Australia. Australian Government Publishing Service, Canberra

McGinnis JM, Foege WH 1993 Actual causes of death in the United States. JAMA 270:2207–2212

Murray CJL, Lopez AD 1996 The global burden of disease: a comprehensive assessment of mortality and disability from diseases, injuries, and risk factors in 1990 and projected to 2020. Harvard University Press, MA

Single E, Robson L, Xie X et al 1996 The costs of substance abuse in Canada. Canadian Center on Substance Abuse, Ottawa

US Department of Agriculture, US Department of Health and Human Services 1995 Dietary Guidelines for Americans, Fourth Edition van Tol A, Groener JEM, Scheek LM et al 1995 Induction of net mass lipid transfer reactions in plasma by wine consumption with dinner. Eur J Clin Invest 25:390–395

Xie X, Rehm J, Single E, Robson L 1996 The economic costs of alcohol, tobacco and illicit drug use in Ontario, 1992. Addiction Research Foundation (ARF Research Document Series No. 127), Toronto

The J-shaped curve and changes in drinking habit

A. G. Shaper and S. G. Wannamethee

Department of Primary Care and Population Sciences, Royal Free Hospital School of Medicine, London NW3 2PF, UK

Abstract. The accepted interpretation of the J-shaped curve relating alcohol intake to mortality or coronary heart disease is that the lowest point on the curve (light/moderate drinking) represents optimum exposure to alcohol and that the increased risk in non-drinkers reflects the consequence of sub-optimum exposure. However, non-drinkers, both ex-drinkers and lifelong teetotallers, consistently show an increased prevalence of conditions likely to increase morbidity and mortality compared with occasional or light drinkers. In addition, regular light drinkers tend to have characteristics extremely advantageous to health. Changes take place in alcohol intake in individuals over time, with a strong downward drift from heavy or moderate drinking towards non-drinking, affected to a considerable extent by the accumulation of ill health. Reduction in alcohol intake or giving up drinking is associated with higher rates of new diagnoses than remaining stable in alcohol intake and also with higher rates of both cardiovascular and non-cardiovascular mortality. The use of non-drinkers as a baseline, and failure or inability to adequately take into account the characteristics of subjects in the different alcohol intake categories, exaggerates the risk of coronary heart disease events and all cause mortality in non-drinkers and the benefits of light/moderate alcohol intake.

1998 Alcohol and cardiovascular diseases. Wiley, Chichester (Novartis Foundation Symposium 216) p 173–192

'*We ought to be strongly suspicious of ideas that are enormously comforting.*'
   Stephen J. Gould, 1990

A J-shaped or U-shaped curve is a common finding when exposure to a risk factor for a specific disease or for all cause mortality is examined (e.g body mass index [BMI], serum total cholesterol). The simplistic interpretation is that the lowest point on the curve represents the optimum exposure to the risk factor and that the increased risk preceding the optimum level of exposure reflects the consequence of inadequate (sub-optimum) exposure to the benefits of the risk factor.

The J- or U-shaped curves in relation to alcohol and coronary heart disease (CHD), cardiovascular disease (CVD) and all-cause mortality are well established, with non-drinkers having higher incidence and mortality rates than light or moderate drinkers and sometimes even higher rates than heavy drinkers. There are also well established mechanisms affecting high density lipoprotein (HDL) cholesterol, thrombosis and fibrinolysis which support the concept that alcohol at certain levels of intake may be beneficial to CHD in particular and to mortality in general (Lands 1996). However, as has been done for BMI and serum total cholesterol (Wannamethee & Shaper 1989, Wannamethee et al 1995), it seems reasonable to examine the characteristics of those who appear to have a sub-optimum exposure to alcohol in order to determine the extent to which their increased risk is due to their characteristics rather than to an inadequate exposure to the benefits of alcohol.

The British Regional Heart Study (BRHS)

This is a prospective study of cardiovascular disease involving 7735 men aged 40–59 years, selected at random from the age–sex registers of one group general practice in each of 24 towns in England, Wales and Scotland, and examined between January 1978 and July 1980 with a 78% response rate (Shaper et al 1981). Each man was administered a standard questionnaire (Q1) which included questions on frequency, quantity and type of alcohol intake. Five years later, a postal questionnaire (Q5) was completed by 98% of the available survivors and on this occasion information was obtained from non-drinkers about past drinking habits. In 1992, some 12–14 years after screening, a further postal questionnaire (Q92) obtained information on changes in alcohol intake from 91% of available survivors. On all these occasions, information was also obtained on smoking, physical activity, social class, BMI and medical history including regular medication. From the initial screening, all men were followed up for all-cause mortality and for cardiovascular morbidity (Walker & Shaper 1984). All major CHD (heart attacks) and stroke events (fatal and non-fatal) have been recorded and follow-up has been achieved for 99% of the men. Regular biennial reviews of the patients' General Practice records (including hospital and clinic correspondence) supplemented the information on death collected routinely through the 'tagging' procedures provided by the National Health Service registers.

Classification of drinking categories

Eight drinking categories were provided in the standardized questionnaire: non-drinkers, occasional drinkers (special occasions only and 1–2 drinks/month), weekend drinkers (1–2, 3–6, > 6 drinks/day) and men drinking daily or most days (1–2, 3–6, > 6 drinks/day). More than 6 drinks/day is an open-ended category. One drink (1 UK unit) = 8–10 g alcohol. Five years later (Q5) and at Q92 (mean of 11.8 years later), men were asked about past as well as current drinking habits, allowing separation of non-drinkers into lifelong teetotallers and ex-drinkers. For the purpose of comparison with other studies, regular drinkers were grouped into light, moderate and heavy categories: light, 1–15 units/week (= weekend 1–2, 3–6 and daily 1–2); moderate, 16–42 units/week (= daily 3–6 and weekend > 6); heavy, > 42 units/week (= daily > 6).

Men who do not drink

We have drawn attention to the fact that middle-aged men who do not drink have an increased prevalence of conditions likely to increase their morbidity and mortality rates (Wannamethee & Shaper 1988a). In Table 1 we show that at all three points of assessment (Q1, Q5 and Q92), non-drinkers consistently have higher rates of recall of CHD, hypertension, stroke, diabetes, and regular medication than light drinkers and for most of these conditions they have the highest rates of any alcohol intake category.

TABLE 1 Prevalence (%) of recall of doctor diagnoses and regular medication in non-drinkers and light drinkers at Q1, Q5 and Q92

	Q1		Q5		Q92	
	Non	Light	Non	Light	Non	Light
New diagnoses						
CHD	11.2	5.1	13.4	8.1	21.6	14.5
High blood pressure	14.6	12.3	17.4	13.9	28.0	24.8
Stroke	1.5	0.6	3.0	0.8	6.4	2.8
Diabetes	3.0	1.6	4.1	1.7	6.3	3.8
Gout	1.9	2.0	2.4	3.4	4.9	6.4
Gall bladder	2.2	2.2	3.9	1.8	3.8	3.1
Arthritis	10.5	8.9	14.8	11.9	27.5	24.7
Bronchitis	18.2	15.0	16.5	12.4	19.5	15.6
Asthma	4.3	3.7	4.7	3.4	6.2	7.7
Medication	40.8	26.3	43.7	28.3	58.1	47.2

Lifelong teetotallers and ex-drinkers

Non-drinkers include ex-drinkers and lifelong teetotallers (LLTTs) and the proportion of non-drinkers classified as LLTTs or ex-drinkers will depend to some extent upon the criteria used for classification and may vary depending upon the age of the subjects when the assessment is made. In the majority of studies, LLTTs consist of non-drinkers who claim at a single examination never to have drunk in the past. However, the consistency of this LLTT status has seldom been assessed and those who claim to be LLTTs may be found to be drinkers on later occasions, and *vice versa*.

LLTTs: consistency of reporting. Three separate reports of drinking patterns at Q1, Q5 and Q92 enable an examination of the consistency of self-reporting of lifelong abstinence. In summary, at Q5 and at Q92, over 90% of those claiming never to have drunk could be regarded as virtual LLTTs and had never been regular drinkers. About half were consistently non-drinkers and about half had been occasional drinkers, with a very small proportion having been light drinkers on one or other occasion. Middle-aged men who claim to be LLTTs may be accepted as never having been regular drinkers.

LLTTs in other studies. The proportion of LLTTs varies considerably between studies from 4.7% in the BRHS, to 7.2% in the Kaiser Permanente Study (Klatsky et al 1990), 17% in Japanese physicians (Kono et al 1986) and in US adults in the National Mortality Study (Li et al 1994) to 36% in the Honolulu Study of Japanese-Americans (Yano et al 1977). Clearly the proportion depends heavily upon the cultural pattern of the society but also on the availability of repeated assessments which enable a long-term view of drinking behaviour.

Definition of ex-drinkers. In the first BRHS report on non-drinkers, some 70% of non-drinkers were regarded as ex-drinkers as even those who were occasional drinkers at Q1 and who reported non-drinking at Q5, were categorized as ex-drinkers (Wannamethee & Shaper 1988a). However, it seems misleading to refer to non-drinkers who have been occasional or 'special occasions only' drinkers as ex-drinkers given the connotations of that term. The term 'ex-drinker' should probably be restricted to those who have been regular drinkers (light, moderate or heavy) in the past.

Distribution of LLTTs and ex-drinkers at Q5 and Q92

LLTTs are defined as men who at Q5 said they had never drunk and were non-drinkers or occasional drinkers at Q1. Also, men who at Q92 said that they had never drunk and were occasional or non-drinkers at Q1 and Q5. Ex-drinkers included those who said that they had drunk in the past or those who had been

TABLE 2   Distribution (% and *n*) in alcohol categories.

	Q5 *(n = 7168)*	*Q92* *(n = 5544)*
LLTT	4.7 (335)	6.0 (334)
Ex-drinker	5.1 (366)	11.3 (629)
Occ/light	66.9 (4793)	67.7 (3589)
Mod/heavy	23.3 (1674)	17.9 (992)

LLTT, lifelong teetotaller.

regular drinkers on the previous assessments. The proportion of non-drinkers increased from Q5 to Q92 (Table 2). At Q5, about half of the non-drinkers are ex-drinkers; by Q92 about two-thirds are ex-drinkers. The absolute number and proportion of moderate/heavy drinkers has considerably declined, possibly due to a combination of mortality and migration downward in alcohol intake.

Characteristics of LLTTs, ex-drinkers and drinkers at Q5 and Q92

The patterns of reported ill health according to alcohol category are similar at Q5 and Q92 although the absolute rates of disease for most conditions are higher at Q92. Table 3 shows these characteristics at Q5.

Ex-drinkers are older than drinkers, have a higher proportion of manual workers and non-married men, and a similar rate of current smoking to moderate/heavy drinkers. They have the highest rates of recall of doctor diagnoses of CHD, high blood pressure, stroke, diabetes, gall bladder disease, regular medication and self-assessment of poor/fair health.

LLTTs are also older than drinkers, have a higher proportion of manual workers than occasional/light drinkers and also have somewhat higher rates of CHD, diabetes, gall bladder disease, regular medication and self-assessment of poor/fair health. They are clearly not as healthy overall as occasional/light drinkers.

Changes in alcohol intake over time

Table 4 shows the changes in reported drinking habits over 12–14 years between Q1 and Q92 for the 5549 men available at Q92. By middle-age, most non-drinkers, occasional drinkers and light drinkers have become fairly stable in their habit, tending to remain at the same level of intake or lower over time. Only 1.4% of occasional drinkers and 10.8% of light drinkers moved to moderate or heavy drinking. Moderate and heavy drinkers progressively declined in reported intake; 21% of moderate drinkers and 11% of heavy drinkers had become

TABLE 3   Characteristics of lifelong teetotallers (LLTTs), ex-drinkers and drinkers at Q5

	LLTTs (335)	Ex-drinkers (366)	Occ/light (4793)	Mod/heavy (1674)
Mean age	56.4	56.6	55.1	54.4
% Manual	66.7	75.1	55.2	61.4
% Married	88.4	82.5	89.7	83.6
% Never smoked	39.5	15.6	26.9	15.6
% Current smoker	27.8	39.5	28.8	39.5
% CHD (604)	11.3	15.3	8.3	6.8
% High BP (1058)	13.1	21.3	13.8	16.4
% Stroke (92)	1.2	4.6	1.1	1.2
% Diabetes (152)	3.0	5.2	2.1	1.3
% Gout (281)	1.8	3.0	3.1	7.0
% Gall bladder (150)	2.4	5.2	2.1	1.4
% Arthritis (962)	13.7	15.6	12.4	15.9
% Bronchitis (996)	12.5	20.2	12.6	26.6
% Asthma (257)	5.1	4.4	3.4	3.5
% Medication (2267)	37.9	49.2	30.0	31.1
% Poor/fair health (1640)	26.3	44.8	20.6	24.0
% CVD => >1 (1845)	27.2	37.2	24.1	27.2
% Non-CVD = >1 (2308)	30.7	42.4	30.0	37.5

CHD, coronary heart disease; CVD, cardiovascular disease; BP, blood pressure.

occasional or non-drinkers. Only 20% of heavy drinkers at Q1 remained in that category at Q92. Data from the General Household Survey (England and Wales) around the Q1 to Q5 period support these findings (OPCS 1980). A far lower proportion of men over 65 were heavy drinkers than in the men aged 45–64 (4% vs. 16%), a lower proportion were moderate drinkers (7% vs. 14%) and non-drinkers had increased from 5% at 45–64 years to 11% in older men.

Changes in drinking habits and development of disease

We have previously shown that BRHS men who are moderate or heavy drinkers in middle-age are likely to reduce their alcohol intake as they grow older, and many do so in response to the development of disease (Wannamethee & Shaper 1988b). We have now examined changes in drinking habits from Q1 to Q5 and from Q5 to Q92 in order to determine whether those who change drinking habits differ from

TABLE 4   Alcohol intake at Q92 (% men in each category at Q1)

Q1	n (%)	Non	Occ	Light	Mod	Heavy
Non	306 (6)	79	14	5	2	0
Occ	1378 (25)	30	45	23	1	0.4
Light	1920 (35)	9	23	57	10	0.8
Mod	1381 (25)	7	14	48	26	4
Heavy	564 (10)	4	7	29	40	20

those who remain stable in their habit, in regard to their health status or their risk of future events. The men were classified into five groups:

(1)   Non-drinkers: non-drinkers at both Q1 and Q5 or Q5 and Q92.
(2)   Stable/increased: those drinkers who remained the same or increased their intake.
(3)   Minor reduction: down one drinking category but not to non-drinking status.
(4)   Major reduction: down two categories but not to non-drinking (heavy to light; moderate to occasional).
(5)   Given up: non-drinkers who were regular drinkers previously.

Table 5 shows the distribution of these categories in the two periods Q1 to Q5 and Q5 to Q92. In the first period, one-third of the men reduced their alcohol intake or gave up drinking. In the second period, one-quarter of the men did so.

   Table 6 shows the changes in drinking habits Q1 to Q5 (5 years) and the development of new diagnoses in that period. The data from Q5 to Q92 (not shown) revealed similar patterns. It is evident that those who reduced their alcohol intake had a greater rate of acquisition of new diagnoses, particularly cardiovascular disease and diabetes, and of regular medication than those

TABLE 5   Changes in drinking habits

	Q1 to Q5 (7165 men)	Q5 to Q92 (5495 men)
Non-drinkers	4.4% (313)	7.3 (400)
Stable/increased	60.0% (4282)	66.1 (3632)
Minor reduction	24.9% (1782)	14.7 (806)
Major reduction	5.6% (400)	1.9 (104)
Given up	5.4% (388)	10.1 (553)

TABLE 6   Changes in drinking habits from Q1 to Q5 (5 years) and new diagnoses (%)

	Non-drinkers (313)	Stable/ increased (4282)	Minor reduction (1782)	Major reduction (400)	Given up (388)
Mean age	56.8	54.9	54.9	55.1	56.3
CHD (300)	4.8	3.4	4.2	9.0	7.2
Diabetes (66)	1.0	0.4	1.3	0.8	2.8
Stroke (65)	2.6	0.6	0.9	1.3	2.3
HBP (501)	9.3	5.9	8.4	9.8	7.7
Medication (969)	12.8	12.0	15.2	19.3	17.8
CVD=>1 (1043)	16.9	12.9	15.8	21.0	19.1
Non-CVD=>1 (1027)	16.3	13.6	15.2	15.8	15.5
Poor/fair (1640)	34.8	19.5	24.3	30.3	36.9

HBP, high blood pressure; CHD, coronary heart disease; CVD, cardiovascular disease.

remaining on a stable alcohol intake. Non-drinkers also tend to have higher acquisition rates of illness/medication than stable drinkers. Non-cardiovascular disease did not appear to be as strongly associated with changes in alcohol intake as cardiovascular disease.

Changes in drinking habit and mortality

A further critical question relates to whether those who change their drinking habits differ in their mortality rates from those who remain stable.

Cardiovascular disease.   On short-term follow-up (5 years), non-drinkers and those who reduce or give up drinking show increased age-adjusted relative risks compared with those who remain stable, irrespective of the level at which stability is maintained. These increased relative risks are attenuated after adjustment for smoking, poor/fair health and regular medication. Increased drinking is associated with increased relative risk of cardiovascular mortality even after full adjustment. It appears that non-drinking status or reduction in alcohol intake is associated with an increased risk of cardiovascular mortality which is explained to a considerable extent by ill-health and smoking.

Non-cardiovascular disease.   The relationships were different in some respects. In non-drinkers and in those who reduce drinking, the relative risks remain significantly increased even after full adjustment. This suggests that the increased risk of non-cardiovascular disease is explained to a lesser extent by ill-health than it is for cardiovascular mortality (Fig. 1).

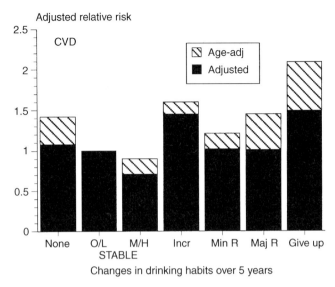

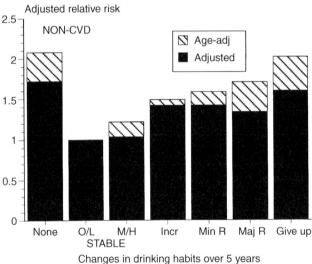

FIG. 1.   Changes in drinking habits (Q1 to Q5) and mortality on five year follow-up. Age-adjusted and adjusted for smoking, poor/fair health and regular medication.

Alcohol intake and mortality

A previous report on the BRHS men showed that even after all men with pre-existing CVD had been excluded, non-drinkers (LLTTs and ex-drinkers combined) had a somewhat higher risk of major CHD events than light or moderate drinkers, but a similar risk of all cause mortality to that of occasional and regular drinkers (Shaper et al 1994). In a subsequent report we have examined the risk of all-cause mortality and the incidence of major CHD events separately in LLTTs and ex-drinkers (Wannamethee & Shaper 1997). The report is concerned with 7167 men who completed the 5th year questionnaire and is based on 9.8 year follow-up. There were 929 deaths (472 cardiovascular, 457 non-cardiovascular) and 490 major CHD events (210 fatal, 280 non-fatal).

Ex-drinkers showed increased total, cardiovascular and non-cardiovascular mortality rates; LLTTs showed the lowest cardiovascular mortality but a significantly increased non-cardiovascular mortality. After adjustment for confounding variables and pre-existing disease (Fig. 2), the two non-drinking groups did not differ significantly in all-cause mortality from occasional and regular drinking groups but LLTTs still showed the lowest cardiovascular mortality and a significant increase in risk of non-cardiovascular deaths compared with occasional drinkers. LLTTs and ex-drinkers both showed similar increased risk of major CHD events compared with regular drinkers even after exclusion of men with a history of CHD/stroke. Regular drinkers (combined) showed about a 30% reduction in risk compared with non-drinkers (combined) and a 20% reduction compared to occasional drinking. The conclusion from this study was that although both LLTTs and ex-drinkers showed a significantly increased relative risk of CHD compared with regular drinkers, this risk reduction is small in absolute terms (about two to three major CHD events/1000 person-years) and there was no convincing evidence that light or moderate drinking has a protective effect on total or overall cardiovascular mortality in middle-aged British men.

Discussion

Alcohol consumption, similarly to other human behaviours, varies considerably over time. The development of physical illness, and particularly CVD, predisposes towards reduction in intake or giving up alcohol, leading to an accumulation of ill health and higher risks of morbidity and mortality in non-drinkers. Thus when non-drinkers are used as the baseline, any true benefits that might accrue from drinking alcohol will be exaggerated. Most alcohol-related studies are initiated in middle-aged or older subjects and by this time a considerable amount of health-related change in drinking behaviour has already taken place. Further changes towards non-drinking associated with ill health continue in later life, affecting moderate and heavy drinkers in particular. In addition, LLTTs in populations in which drinking is the norm, appear to be less healthy than occasional/light drinkers. That non-drinkers (ex-drinkers and LLTTs) have higher rates of morbidity and mortality than light/moderate drinkers is the most consistent finding in the vast literature related to alcohol and

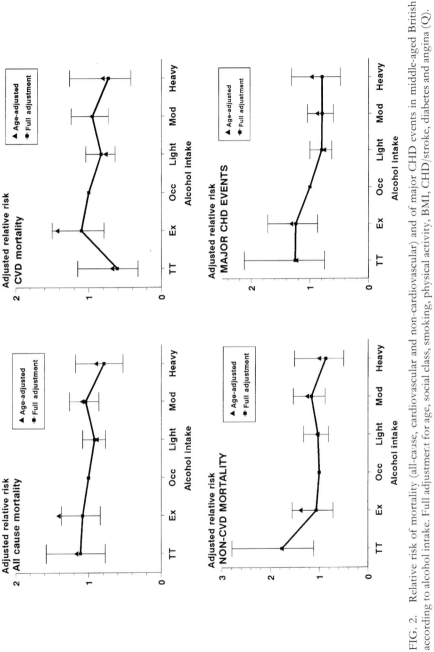

FIG. 2. Relative risk of mortality (all-cause, cardiovascular and non-cardiovascular) and of major CHD events in middle-aged British men according to alcohol intake. Full adjustment for age, social class, smoking, physical activity, BMI, CHD/stroke, diabetes and angina (Q).

health. This finding is more consistent than any relationship between the quantity of alcohol taken in and the risk of CHD or mortality and the lowest point of the curve varies considerably in position from study to study. It is the interpretation of the finding in non-drinkers that is the crucial issue in examining the effects of alcohol on CHD. If occasional drinkers are used as the baseline, the benefit of light/moderate drinking is diminished. In most studies, there is no consistent dose–response seen from light drinking to heavy drinking for CHD incidence or mortality, although many studies show increased risk in the heaviest drinkers. It is equally important to note that in most studies, the light drinking group i.e. 1–2 drinks/day on most days, has the lowest rates for all-cause mortality, cardiovascular mortality and for major CHD events. This is perhaps not surprising as in Great Britain at least, these men have the highest social class, the lowest prevalence of smoking, the lowest mean blood pressure and BMI and the highest levels of physical activity in leisure time. This must further exaggerate the differences in outcome observed between non-drinkers and light drinkers. In exploring the J-shaped curve, causality may lie as much in these characteristics as in the direct effects of alcohol.

Changes in alcohol intake over time

We have shown that men in the BRHS may change alcohol intake over time and that a proportion of moderate and heavy drinkers show a change towards non-drinking status. This is also a finding in other studies that have looked for the phenomenon. In the Busselton (Australia) study, 28% of drinkers reported non-drinking on a 9 year follow-up (Cullen et al 1993). A number of American studies indicate that with increasing age the prevalence of heavy drinking and alcohol-related problems decreases and movement out of the heavy drinking categories increases (Fillmore 1987). A Boston study on abstainers and drinkers showed that 21% of current abstainers had been heavy drinkers and that 40% of current abstainers had stopped drinking because of health reasons directly or indirectly related to their alcohol intake (Goldman & Najman 1984).

Change and mortality

It is evident that those who make major reduction or give up drinking often do so as a consequence of ill health and this is reflected in an increased mortality, particularly in those who have given up completely. This can obviously bias the alcohol–mortality relationship when follow-up is taken from alcohol intake at time of screening and when such changes have taken place before screening. The increased risk of CVD mortality in those who reduce their intake compared to those who remain stable is explained to a considerable extent by ill-health.

The Alameda Country study (Lazarus et al 1991) examined changes in reported alcohol intake in men and women over a nine year period (1965–74) and subsequent 11 year mortality and showed significantly higher risk of death from all causes and CHD in those who gave up drinking than in those who continued to drink. In men the excess mortality was related to the presence of chronic conditions associated with giving up drinking but this did not account for the excess mortality in women who gave up drinking. The reasons for the gender difference in the impact of giving up drinking are not apparent, but emphasise the need for sex-specific analyses.

Reverse causation — disproving the hypothesis

Men with ill health may move from regular drinking categories into lower or non-drinking categories. The concept of reverse causation ('sick quitters') implies that this migration explains *to some degree* the high rates of mortality from all causes or from CHD in non-drinkers (Shaper et al 1988). In recent years, several studies have addressed the reverse causation hypothesis, generally by exclusion or separation of subjects with a history of ill health in order to produce a group uncontaminated by the problems that might have led to changes in alcohol intake towards non-drinking status. These include the Nurses Health Study (Stampfer et al 1988, Fuchs et al 1995), American Cancer Society Prospective Study (Boffetta & Garfinkel 1990), Health Professionals Follow-up Study (Rimm et al 1991), British Doctors Study (Doll et al 1994), Kaiser Permanente Study (Klatsky et al 1990, 1992) and the Normative Aging Study (De Labry et al 1992). In general, these studies have still found lower rates of CHD events in light or moderate drinkers, as we have done in our own study which used occasional drinkers as baseline (Shaper et al 1994).

We are concerned about these studies, not because they all purport to show a protective effect for drinking, but because they use non-drinkers as a baseline group against which to compare the effects of alcohol. In many of these studies no trend was seen among the drinking categories, i.e. no dose–response relationship, with risk of mortality only raised in the non-drinking groups. In other studies, benefit has even accrued from very occasional drinking, and in this situation it is difficult to attribute this to mechanisms usually held responsible for the benefits of alcohol. Few of the studies cited have presented the detailed characteristics of non-drinkers and drinkers and most have relied on adjustment procedures to take account of any differences which may exist. Non-drinkers have characteristics which will inevitably increase their risk of mortality and exclusion of those with diagnosed disease may not necessarily leave the non-drinking group without an excess of factors likely to increase their risk. LLTTs are usually a small and self-selected group in most Western countries in which alcohol consumption is normal behaviour, and they tend to have characteristics which might increase their risk of mortality, particularly from non-CVD disease (Fillmore et al 1998). This is not to deny that alcohol at some level of intake may have a beneficial effect on the incidence of heart attacks, but to suggest that the degree of protection claimed will almost certainly be exaggerated by comparison with an inappropriate control group, and by the limited ability of adjustment procedures to take into account the characteristics of the various alcohol intake groups. This probably remains true even after the exclusion of subjects with manifest problems likely to increase their morbidity or mortality. Furthermore, moderate drinkers in almost all these studies includes the large group of regular light drinkers who are likely to have characteristics highly advantageous to health. Ferrence & Bondy (1994), in drawing attention to the limitations of data and design in studies of alcohol intake and health, maintain that eliminating respondents with pre-existing disease or adjusting for disease in the analysis may not be sufficient to solve the problem. Apart from producing a healthy group of subjects very dissimilar to the general population, bias may be introduced in other ways. For example, not everyone who becomes ill changes their alcohol intake. We know very little about why people choose to drink or abstain, and these determining factors may be of importance in the development of ill health (Fillmore et al 1998). Ferrence & Bondy (1994) also emphasize that lifelong abstainers constitute a deviant group in most Western societies where drinking is the norm.

The magnitude of any true protective effect of alcohol on CHD or mortality is further obscured in most studies by the presentation of data entirely in terms of relative risk, so that no estimate of absolute benefit is possible.

Conclusion

Non-drinkers, that variable mixture of LLTTs and ex-drinkers, are unsuitable as a baseline group in studies of the effects of alcohol on morbidity or mortality. LLTTs on their own are also unsuitable as a baseline, both because their proportion is usually small in most populations and because they have characteristics which affect their morbidity and mortality patterns in somewhat unpredictable ways. Despite the overwhelming consensus that alcohol protects against the risk of major CHD events, we remain concerned that the continuing use of non-drinkers as a baseline leads to exaggeration of any true benefit. In addition, the regular light drinkers have characteristics — socioeconomic, behavioural and physical — which are extremely advantageous to health, and this further exaggerates the benefit of light drinking compared with non-drinking. The problem lies not in the data but in their analysis and interpretation. We draw attention to the caveats already proposed for studies on the relationship between alcohol and ill health (Shaper 1995) and particularly to the need to describe fully the characteristics of the various alcohol intake groups. It may well be that occasional drinkers, a large and relatively stable group in most populations, constitute a more appropriate baseline for assessing the effects of alcohol in regular amounts on risk factors, on illness and on mortality.

Acknowledgements

The British Regional Heart Study is a British Heart Foundation Research Group. SGW is a British Heart Foundation Research Fellow.

References

Boffetta P, Garfinkel L 1990 Alcohol drinking and mortality among men enrolled in an American Cancer Society prospective study. Epidemiology 1:342–348

Cullen K J, Knuiman MW, Ward N J 1993 Alcohol and mortality in Busselton, Western Australia. Am J Epidemiol 137:242–248

De Labry LO, Glynn R J, Levenson MR, Hermos JA, Locastro JS, Vokonas PS 1992 Alcohol consumption and mortality in an American male population: recovering the U-shaped curve-findings from the Normative Aging Study. J Stud Alcohol 53:25–32

Doll R, Peto R, Hall E, Wheatley K, Gray R 1994 Mortality in relation to consumption of alcohol: 13 years' observations on male British doctors. Br Med J 309:911–918

Ferrence R, Bondy S J 1994 Limitations of data and design in studies on moderate drinking and health. Contemporary Drug Problems 21:59–70

Fillmore KM 1987 Prevalence, incidence and chronicity of drinking patterns and problems among men as a function of age: a longitudinal and cohort analysis. Br J Addict 82:77–83

Fillmore KM, Golding JM, Graves KL et al 1998 Alcohol consumption and mortality, I. Characteristics of drinking groups. Addiction 93:183–203

Fuchs CS, Stampfer M J, Colditz GA et al 1995 Alcohol consumption and mortality among women. N Engl J Med 332:1245–1250

Goldman E, Najman JM 1984 Life time abstainers, current abstainers and imbibers: a methodological note. Br J Addict 79:309–314

Gould S J 1990 If only things had been different... New Scientist 1705:64–65

Klatsky AL, Armstrong MA, Friedman GD 1990 Risk of cardiovascular mortality in alcohol drinkers, ex-drinkers and non-drinkers. Am J Cardiol 66:1237–1242

Klatsky AL, Armstrong MA, Friedman GD 1992 Alcohol and mortality. Ann Intern Med 117:646–654

Kono S, Ikeda M, Tokudome S, Nishizumi M, Kuratsune M 1986 Alcohol and mortality: a cohort study of male Japanese physicians. Int J Epidemiol 15:527–532

Lands WEM 1996 Alcohol and cardiovascular risk factors. In: Zakhari S, Wassef M (eds) Alcohol and the cardiovascular system. Bethesda, NIH Publication No. 96-4133, Research Monograph 31, p 359–368

Lazarus NB, Kaplan GA, Cohen RD, Diing-Jen L 1991 Change in alcohol consumption and risk of death from all causes and from ischaemic heart disease. Br Med J 303:553–556

Li G, Smith GS, Baker SP 1994 Drinking behaviour in relation to cause of death among US adults. Am J Public Health 84:1402–1406

Office of Population Censuses and Surveys (OPCS) 1980 General Household Survey 1978. HMSO, London

Rimm EB, Giovannucci EL, Willett WC et al 1991 Prospective study of alcohol consumption and risk of coronary heart disease in men. Lancet 338:464–468

Shaper AG 1995 Alcohol and coronary heart disease. Eur Heart J 16:1760–1764

Shaper AG, Pocock SJ, Walker M, Cohen NM, Wale CJ, Thomson AG 1981 British Regional Heart Study: cardiovascular risk factors in middle-aged men in 24 towns. Br Med J 283: 179–186

Shaper AG, Wannamethee SG, Walker M 1988 Alcohol and mortality in British men: explaining the U-shaped curve. Lancet ii:1267–1273

Shaper AG, Wannamethee SG, Walker M 1994 Alcohol and coronary heart disease: a perspective from the British Regional Heart Study. Int J Epidemiol 23:482–494

Stampfer MJ, Colditz GA, Willett WC, Speizer FE, Hennekens CH 1988 A prospective study of moderate alcohol consumption and the risk of coronary heart disease and stroke in women. N Engl J Med 319:267–273

Walker M, Shaper AG 1984 Follow-up of subjects in prospective studies in general practice. J R Coll Gen Pract 34:365–370

Wannamethee SG, Shaper AG 1988a Men who do not drink: a report from the British Regional Heart Study. Int J Epidemiol 17:307–316

Wannamethee SG, Shaper AG 1988b Changes in drinking habits in middle-aged British men. J R Coll Gen Pract 38:440–442

Wannamethee SG, Shaper AG 1989 Body weight and mortality in middle-aged British men: impact of smoking. Br Med J 299:1497–1502

Wannamethee SG, Shaper AG 1997 Lifelong teetotallers, ex-drinkers and drinkers: mortality and incidence of coronary heart disease events in middle-aged British men. Int J Epidemiol 26:523–531

Wannamethee SG, Shaper AG, Whincup PH, Walker M 1995 Low serum total cholesterol concentration and mortality in middle-aged British men. Br Med J 311:409–413

Yano K, Rhoads GG, Kagan A 1977 Coffee, alcohol and risk of coronary heart disease among Japanese men living in Hawaii. N Engl J Med 297:405–409

DISCUSSION

Peters: So is the 'beneficial effect' of alcohol all a ghastly artefact?

Criqui: Gerry Shaper's point about ex-drinkers and life-long non-drinkers is well taken. In all fairness, though, many studies have either gone to great lengths to exclude individuals with any evidence of CHD at baseline and have separated lifelong non-drinkers and ex-drinkers. In fact most studies using lifelong non-drinkers as a baseline still find a protective effect of alcohol.

Did you repeat the drinking questionnaires at the follow-ups?

Wannamethee: Yes, we did this at five years and 12 years after screening. In our recent data, looking at 5 or 10 years, the curve is inverse. The people at high risk have died, and of the healthy remainder there is a small minority of heavy drinkers: at 5 years this group was reduced from 10 to 4%, and at 12 years only 2% are still heavy drinkers.

Criqui: So the population sample is now composed of non-drinkers, light drinkers and a very resistant subset of heavy drinkers.

Wannamethee: I think we have migration problems at both ends of the scale, affecting both non-drinkers and heavy drinkers.

Fillmore: I am delighted to see more work that describes the characteristics of abstainers. Some of our work distinguishes cross-sectionally former drinkers from long-term abstainers (Fillmore et al 1998a,b, Leino et al 1998). We have a dataset at the University of California which consists of about 40 general population samples, for the most part longitudinal, from 16 different countries. We have some mortality data. I wanted to add our findings to your description differentiating former drinkers from a long-term abstainers. In nine general population studies (again these are cross-sectional analyses), adult male former drinkers across studies are significantly and consistently more likely than long-term abstainers to be heavier smokers, depressed, unemployed and of lower social class. Some of these findings are supportive of yours. Among females we find that adult former drinkers across studies are significantly and consistently and more likely than long-term abstainers to be heavier smokers, in poorer health, better educated (oddly enough), unmarried and not religious. Both types of abstainers are significantly and consistently more likely than light drinkers to be of lower socioeconomic status and in poor health among the males, and among the females they are more likely to be blue collar workers and overweight. Obviously, abstainers are not a homogenous group. It seems to me that the direction you're going in is the appropriate one. Also, in our studies, because they're all general population studies and they are longitudinal, we've looked at changes in drinking over time. People change their behaviour a lot with respect to drinking. This must be taken into account, particularly when you look at the interval between measurements. Therefore I think that studies that have multiple life measurement points are the most valuable.

Klatsky: We have struggled with the problem of which is the proper reference group over quite a few years. In fact, one of the reasons we basically started over again and designed a new database in the late 1970s, was because in our original studies we did not have the ability to separate ex-drinkers from lifelong abstainers, nor could we separate out various lighter drinking categories. We have a lot of information about the characteristics of lifelong abstainers and what I call 'special occasion only' drinkers. Certainly, the ex-drinkers have unfavourable traits compared to almost any other group. This is most striking in our California population in the group that's most similar to yours: middle-aged white men. The lifelong abstainers are a somewhat atypical group, although we're unable to determine that they have any important health differences from the special occasion only drinkers.

The atypicality of abstainers varies with the population being studied. It all depends to a large degree on race, sex and age group. Among women, for example, lifelong abstainers are much less atypical. Among Asian American women, lifelong abstainers are the majority, so they're hardly an atypical group. However, in your particular population lifelong abstainers are indeed an atypical group. One other thing that we have learned, and which I think your data support, is that the same people will define themselves at different times as lifelong abstainers or as special occasion only drinkers. I notice you had a larger proportion of lifelong abstainers in your follow up study than you did in your original study. We have found the same thing. There are a certain number of people who, probably not dishonestly, consider themselves at point A to be non-drinkers and at point B to be a person who takes a drink occasionally at a wedding or other special occasion. I think that's an important point. What we have often done is to lump the lifelong abstainers with the special occasion only drinkers. We have never found any significant difference in health outcomes between lifelong abstainers and the special occasion only drinkers.

Shaper: I wish I could explain to you why we find this increased non-cardiovascular mortality in lifelong teetotallers. It is a small group, but it seems to be quite a strong finding. They have low levels of cardiovascular risk factors. Even amongst occasional drinkers, Goya Wannamethee has observed that there are differences between people who are occasional drinkers, and those who are 'special occasion only'. It is clear that even within these categories, to the left of the so-called optimum level of alcohol intake, we are encountering a group that possibly ought to be ignored (like the non-drinkers) when we're trying to look at the overall benefits or otherwise of alcohol.

Wannamethee: We have always used occasional drinking, but I think there is some difference between people who say they only drink on special occasions, which can be once or twice a year, and people who drink occasionally, such as once or twice a month. In some studies these categories are combined.

Klatsky: We specifically use the term 'special occasion only' because there are a considerable number in the USA drink rather infrequently, and we take this to mean less than once per month.

Keil: Your statement that non-drinkers may be the wrong comparison group is well taken. I would buy that if the comparison group was a small one in which ex-drinkers or sick people may be playing a large role. When I look at our data from southern Germany, among males 13% claim that they didn't drink the previous week and categorize themselves as non-drinkers. When we compare this group with those who drink alcohol we see a 50% reduction in CHD and in total mortality. In women, we have 44% who say they do not drink, and therefore we are comparing 56% with 44% and we get the same reduction in total mortality, namely 50%. This control group of 44% can't all be deviants and sick people.

Shaper: I quite agree. Nevertheless, even with your 13% of men who say they didn't drink in the last week, you really cannot be sure of what category they fall into. That is a very limited view over time of their drinking behaviour. It may well be that you're either exaggerating or diminishing your effect. I'm not quite sure how it would turn out, but you need repeated assessments of alcohol to be able to know whether somebody who said 'I didn't drink last week' is a consistent abstainer. A good example is given by the Whitehall study (Marmot et al 1981), which shows U-shaped curves for mortality. However, when you look at their data, they only have data on alcohol intake in men between Monday and Friday: they have no weekend intake at all. In the British community that makes the data fairly meaningless. You have to be careful about what you are using as a baseline. We have learned from Dr Klatsky's group, which has varied their baseline category over the years, that using the lifelong teetotallers who are an abnormal group in any drinking society or the ex-drinkers is probably inappropriate. We ought to be using the very large group of occasional drinkers or even light drinkers as a baseline. Then I suspect that we will see a linear positive relationship between alcohol intake and mortality.

Miller: I want to refer very briefly to the questionnaire we used in our Trinidad study some years ago (Miller et al 1990)—the CAGE questionnaire (Ewing 1984). This provides another way of looking at the issues of alcohol and alcohol consumption, including changes in habit. We went to Trinidad because it has a very high coronary disease rate. There were two issues that interested us. The first concerned what I call the abstemious group (either total abstinence or the occasional drink). Their baseline pattern of ill health was described, including their slightly higher prevalence rate of cardiovascular disease in comparison with moderate drinkers. Was this excess a consequence of abstemiousness or vice versa? The CAGE questionnaire was useful, because it included the question, 'Have you ever felt in the past that you should cut down your drinking for whatever reason?' The worry with this inverse relationship between consumption and mortality has been that before the men came into the study they had been reducing their consumption because of subclinical ill health, and this explains the association we are picking up at baseline. But when we included the response to that question in the statistical analysis, it was found to contain no information whatsoever about risk for coronary events. The association between actual consumption reported at baseline and subsequent outcome was completely uninfluenced by whether the men had felt the need to reduce drinking. And a very significant number of men had felt the need to cut down before they had entered the study. Although it is common for people to reduce their drinking as they get older, we couldn't find any association between this behaviour and cardiovascular health.

References

Ewing JA 1984 Detecting alcoholism. The CAGE questionnaire. JAMA 252:1905–1907
Fillmore KM, Golding JM, Graves KL et al 1998a Alcohol consumption and mortality, I. Characteristics of drinking groups. Addiction 93:183–203

Fillmore KM, Golding JM, Graves KL et al 1998b Alcohol consumption and mortality, III. Studies of female populations. Addiction 93:219–229

Leino EV, Romelsjo A, Shoemaker C et al 1998 Alcohol consumption and mortality, II. Studies of male populations. Addiction 93:205–218

Marmot MG, Rose G, Shipley MJ, Thomas BJ 1981 Alcohol and mortality: a U-shaped curve. Lancet i:580–583

Miller GJ, Beckles GLA, Maude GH, Carson DC 1990 Alcohol consumption: protection against coronary heart disease and risks to health. Int J Epidemiol 19:923–930

Mechanisms of alcohol-related strokes

Matti Hillbom, Seppo Juvela* and Vesa Karttunen

*Department of Neurology, Oulu University Hospital, FIN-90220 and *Department of Neurosurgery, Helsinki University Hospital, Helsinki, Finland*

Abstract. Epidemiological investigations have shown a linear positive correlation between the risk of haemorrhagic stroke and level of alcohol consumption. Ischaemic stroke shows a weaker relationship, which is J-shaped, suggesting that regular light-to-moderate alcohol consumption may carry a decreased risk. Case reports and case-control studies indicate that heavy recent drinking, but not heavy former drinking, increases the risk for both types of stroke. Larger amounts of alcohol are needed to trigger aneurysmal subarachnoid haemorrhage than spontaneous intracerebral haemorrhage. The increased risk caused by recent heavy drinking may be partly due to elevated systolic blood pressure, but alcohol may also provoke cerebral arterial vasospasm, as observed in animal experiments. Alcohol-induced fluctuation in haemostatic and fibrinolytic factors has not been proved to precipitate alcohol-related strokes, but may contribute to both an increase and a decrease of the risk. Subtypes of ischaemic stroke associate differently with alcohol consumption. A recent series of patients with ischaemic brain infarction showed that of the victims having a high and medium risk for cardiogenic embolism, 50% and 45% were intoxicated, respectively. This suggests that cardiogenic embolism is a significant mechanism leading to ischaemic stroke during heavy drinking of alcohol.

1998 Alcohol and cardiovascular diseases. Wiley, Chichester (Novartis Foundation Symposium 216) p 193–207

There is a consensus that heavy drinking increases the risk of stroke (Bornstein 1994), particularly the risk of haemorrhagic stroke (Easton et al 1995). Epidemiological investigations have shown a linear positive correlation between alcohol consumption and the risk for haemorrhagic stroke, and a J-shaped (Fig. 1) correlation for ischaemic stroke (Camargo 1989, Sacco et al 1997). Heavy drinkers of alcohol show more frequent recurrences of ischaemic stroke than other drinkers (Sacco et al 1994) and they also seem to be stricken at an earlier age (Walbran et al 1981). Former heavy drinking has not been proved to increase the risk for stroke, whereas recent heavy drinking associates with the onset of stroke (Hillbom & Juvela 1996). Carotid atherosclerosis is a frequent cause of ischaemic stroke. However, regular light-to-moderate consumption of alcohol associates with the absence of prominent carotid atherosclerosis (Kiechl et al 1994).

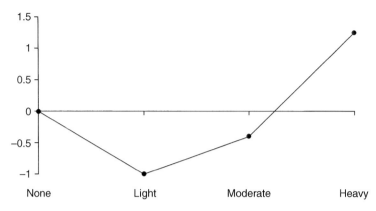

FIG. 1.   The J-shaped risk curve showing the relationship between alcohol consumption and ischaemic stroke (Sacco et al 1997).

Because it is obvious that recent heavy drinking increases the risk for stroke, it is of interest to identify the mechanisms by which the alcohol-related strokes are triggered. Some actions of alcohol, such as the effects on heart rate and rhythm, the effect on blood pressure, the effect on cerebral arterial tone and the effects on haemostatic and fibrinolytic systems, could be important. In order to illuminate this matter, we thoroughly investigated the aetiology of strokes among young adults and people of working age, and simultaneously gathered detailed data on their drinking habits and recent alcohol consumption. This paper will present new clinical data to suggest the mechanisms by which recent heavy alcohol intake could precipitate different types of stroke. Points which seem to be relevant to the other papers in this book and to experimental observations will be discussed.

Methods

The methods of the previously published investigations cited in this paper can be found in the original publications. The protocol applied in the present patient series was basically as follows. The first step included routine laboratory tests and electrocardiograms, and differentiated between haemorrhagic and ischaemic stroke on the basis of head computed tomography (CT) performed in each individual within 24 h of the onset of stroke. The second step included duplex imaging of the carotid and vertebral arteries and/or an aortic arch angiogram by means of an intra-arterial digital subtraction technique, and these investigations were made in the first four days after the onset of stroke. The third step took place at the end of the first week and included cardiac imaging by transesophageal and/or transthoracic echocardiography. Finally, if these steps did not reveal the precise aetiology of the index stroke, special laboratory tests were tailored to establish the rare haematological and other abnormalities possibly predisposing to stroke. This protocol made it possible to classify the patients into aetiological categories of acute ischaemic stroke.

We excluded patients with acute brain infarction precipitated during a surgical operation or angiography as well as those who were incompletely evaluated. We did not have any patients with vasculitides or blood dyscrasias in this series. We had 88 patients who could be classified to the following seven categories, the diagnostic criteria of which were proposed by Adams et al (1993): (1) large-artery atherosclerosis; (2) cardioembolism with a high-risk source; (3) cardioembolism with a medium-risk source; (4) small-artery occlusion (lacune); (5) stroke of other determined aetiology; (6) stroke with two or more causes identified; and (7) cryptogenic stroke. Altogether we had nine patients with large-artery atherosclerosis, 32 with cardioembolism (10 having a high-risk source), 15 with small-artery occlusion, eight with cervicocerebral arterial dissection, eight with two or more causes identified, and 16 with a negative evaluation (cryptogenic stroke).

Recent drinking was estimated by asking the patient or control subject how many drinks of alcohol they had consumed during the 24 h preceding the onset of the first symptoms of stroke. Heavy drinkers included subjects whose recent mean weekly alcohol intake had regularly exceeded 300 g of ethanol, or who were classified as problem drinkers by using the short CAGE questionnaire (Mayfield et al 1974).

We compared the patients with control subjects who had been admitted to the emergency department of the Helsinki University Hospital because of acute appendicitis, nephrolithiasis, dyspnea, viral meningitis and cholecystitis. These medical emergencies were not considered to accumulate among either heavy drinkers or teetotallers. Altogether we had 270 controls with complete risk factor data.

The data were analysed using the BioMedical Data Package statistical programs (1993 version by BMDP Statistical Software Inc., Los Angeles, CA). The categorical variables were compared using Fisher's exact two-tailed test or the Pearson χ^2 test. Odds ratios, as estimates of multivariate relative risks, and 95% confidence intervals before and after adjustment for possible confounding variables were calculated by logistic regression. Hypotheses were tested and 95% confidence intervals determined using standard error estimates for the logistic coefficients.

Results and discussion

Very few epidemiological studies have aimed to determine whether different drinking habits influence stroke morbidity or stroke mortality. In a Swedish

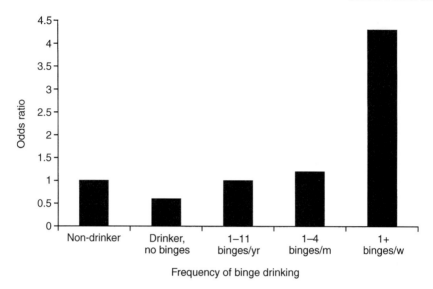

FIG. 2. Risk of subarachnoid haemorrhage in relation to frequency of binge drinking (Longstreth et al 1992). Yr, year; M, month; W, week.

cohort study, however, the men who reported binge drinking showed a significantly elevated risk of mortality from ischaemic stroke, whereas the women who reported no binge drinking had a reduced risk of dying from ischaemic stroke compared with lifelong abstainers (Hansagi et al 1995). Despite this, the relative risks of haemorrhagic stroke mortality among both men and women with different drinking habits were similar to those of lifelong abstainers.

The role of drinking habits has been investigated in several case-control studies. Two studies have addressed drinking habits and the risk for aneurysmal subarachnoid haemorrhage (Longstreth et al 1992, Juvela et al 1993). Longstreth et al (1992) reported that frequent binge drinking significantly increased the risk for aneurysmal subarachnoid haemorrhage, whereas infrequent binge drinking did not (Fig. 2). Binge drinking was defined as consumption of five or more drinks during a 24 h period. The association remained clear even after cigarette smoking, history of hypertension, education and the use of stimulant drugs had been accounted for. Interestingly, drinkers who did not report binge drinking had a lower risk for subarachnoid haemorrhage than non-drinkers.

Juvela et al (1993) investigated alcohol consumption during the week immediately preceding the onset of aneurysmal subarachnoid haemorrhage. Adjustments were made for age, sex, hypertension and smoking status. Light drinking did not significantly influence the risk, but the risk was elevated by moderate and heavy drinking (Fig. 3). A dose-response effect was also found

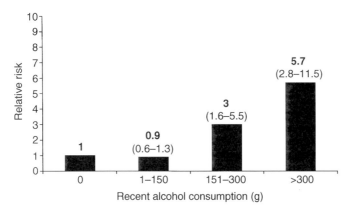

FIG. 3.   Relative risk of aneurysmal subarachnoid haemorrhage by consumption of alcohol in
the week before the onset of illness (Juvela et al 1993).

when the consumption of alcohol within the 24 h preceding the onset of illness was
investigated (Fig. 4). However, light drinking seemed to decrease the risk for
aneurysmal subarachnoid haemorrhage. Whether the latter observation was
associated with regular or occasional light drinking was not separately studied.

Similar observations were later reported concerning spontaneous intracerebral
haemorrhage (Juvela et al 1995). Unlike in the case of subarachnoid haemorrhage,
the risk for this disease was elevated by even light drinking within the index week
before onset of the stroke, excluding alcohol consumption within the last 24 h
(Fig. 5). However, the consumption of alcohol within the 24 h preceding the onset
of illness showed relative risks similar to those for aneurysmal subarachnoid
haemorrhage, i.e. a risk significantly lowered by light drinking (Fig. 6). Former

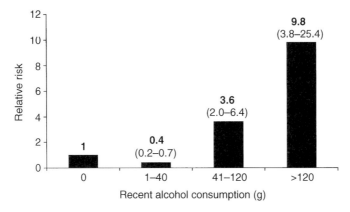

FIG. 4.   Relative risk of aneurysmal subarachnoid haemorrhage by consumption of alcohol in
the 24 h preceding the onset of illness (Juvela et al 1993).

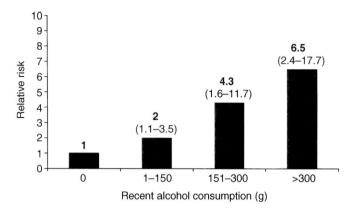

FIG. 5.   Relative risk of spontaneous intracerebral haemorrhage by consumption of alcohol in the week before the onset of illness (Juvela et al 1995).

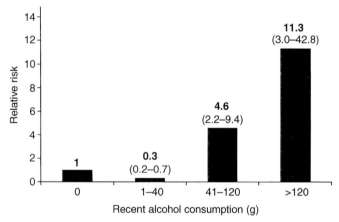

FIG. 6.   Relative risk of spontaneous intracerebral haemorrhage by consumption of alcohol in the 24 h preceding the onset of illness (Juvela et al 1995).

heavy drinking of alcohol did not seem to increase the risk. Taken together, the data (Juvela et al 1993, 1995) suggest that larger amounts of alcohol may be needed to trigger aneurysmal subarachnoid haemorrhage than spontaneous intracerebral haemorrhage.

The mechanisms of alcohol-related haemorrhagic strokes have not been investigated by clinical methods. However, episodic heavy drinking seems to increase blood pressure more than regular heavy drinking (Marmot et al 1994). This finding could explain the positive association between the elevated risk of aneurysmal subarachnoid haemorrhage and frequent binge drinking (Longstreth et al 1992). Although the risk was reported to be independent of hypertension, the latter may still play a significant role. The studies cited above did not take into account occasional peaks in systolic blood pressure (Kannel et al 1981), but did acknowledge the history of hypertension, when adjusting for confounding factors.

Another interesting alternative to explain the mechanism by which heavy drinking could precipitate cerebral bleeding involves the effect of alcohol on tone in cerebral arteries (Altura & Altura 1984). Vasoconstriction of cerebral cortical arteries resulting in haemorrhage, precipitated by amounts of alcohol comparable to heavy intoxication, has been demonstrated in living experimental animals via a cranial window (Altura et al 1983, Mayhan & Didion 1995) and by *in vitro* methods (Gordon et al 1995). The phenomenon may be due to magnesium depletion (Altura et al 1995). However, a corresponding effect of alcohol on human cerebral arteries is still to be demonstrated.

The relationship between alcohol consumption and ischaemic stroke is a complex one. Regular light-to-moderate consumption of alcohol seems to protect against the development of large-artery atherosclerosis and associated stroke (Stampfer et al 1988, Rodgers et al 1993, Palomäki & Kaste 1993, Sacco et al 1995). Since, however, lifelong abstainers have been used as reference material and since occasional drinkers, regular non-heavy drinkers and ex-drinkers do not differ significantly in their risk of stroke, the protective effect of alcohol has been questioned (Wannamethee & Shaper 1996). On the other hand, heavy alcohol consumption may exert an increase of the risk of ischaemic brain infarction by as yet unknown mechanisms.

In a case–control study, we found that recent light-to-moderate drinking of alcohol (< 40 g ethanol within 24 h or < 150 g ethanol within 1 week) before the illness did not increase the risk for acute brain infarction (Haapaniemi et al 1997). However, the relative risk of brain infarction was elevated by heavier consumption of alcohol. Stepwise logistic regression showed that alcohol intake (41–120 g ethanol within the 24 h preceding the onset of illness) increased the risk in both men and women (Table 1). The relative risks shown in the table have been adjusted for age, body mass index, hypertension, cardiac disease, diabetes, current smoking, history of migraine and current use of oral contraceptives in women.

Our most recent series of patients (Table 2) confirms the finding that recent heavy drinking of alcohol ($P < 0.001$) elevates the risk for ischaemic brain infarction among people of working age. Other significant risk factors were hypertension ($P < 0.001$), diabetes mellitus ($P < 0.001$) current smoking ($P < 0.05$) and cardiac disease (not shown in the table). This series includes patients who have been thoroughly investigated for the cause of acute brain infarction. Accordingly, we have also been able to investigate the relationship of recent alcohol consumption to different aetiological subtypes of ischaemic stroke.

TABLE 1   Relative risk (RR) of brain infarction in men and women of working age by alcohol consumption (Haapaniemi et al 1997)

Recent alcohol consumption (g ethanol/24 h)	Men		Women	
	RR	95% CI	RR	95% CI
1–40	1.09	0.60–1.96	0.68	0.35–1.32
41–120	3.74	1.91–8.12	5.68	1.75–18.48
>120	7.57	1.97–29.10		

CI, confidence intervals.

TABLE 2   Baseline characteristics in 88 patients with acute brain infarction and 270 control subjects

Characteristic	Case	Control
Number of patients	88	270
Sex (male/female)	66/22	160/110
Mean ± SD age (y)	52.2 ± 12.0	44.7 ± 12.5
Mean ± SD body mass index (kg/m^2)	27.6 ± 5.2	25.8 ± 4.2
Hypertension (%)	48 (55)	54 (20)
Diabetes mellitus (%)	18 (20)	17 (6)
Hyperlipemia (%)	9 (10)	24 (9)
Migraine (%)	16 (18)	42 (16)
Current smoking (%)	46 (52)	99 (37)
Heavy drinking (%)	35 (40)	40 (15)
Recent alcohol consumption(%)	Within 24 hours	
0 g	46 (52)	192 (71)
1–40 g	3 (3)	57 (21)
41–120 g	25 (28)	18 (7)
>120 g	14 (16)	3 (1)
	Within 1 week	
0 g	24 (27)	117 (43)
1–150 g	26 (30)	126 (47)
151–300 g	16 (18)	16 (6)
>300 g	10 (11)	11 (4)

TABLE 3   Number of subjects with heavy recent alcohol consumption by subtype of acute ischaemic stroke among 88 consecutive patients

Subtype of stroke	Total number of subjects (n = 88)	With alcohol intake ≥ 60 g/24 hours (36/88)	With alcohol intake ≥ 300 g/week (16/76)
Cardioembolism high risk	10	5	3
Cardioembolism medium risk	22	10	5
Large artery atherosclerosis	9	3	1
Small-vessel occlusion (lacune)	15	6	4
Cervicerebral arterial dissection	8	3	0
Two or more causes identified	8	4	2
Cryptogenic stroke	16	5	1

The crude data (Table 3) suggest that quite a few of the subjects with high and medium risks for cardiogenic embolism had, in fact, been drinking heavily immediately before the onset of stroke. Half of the patients with high-risk sources and 45% of those with medium-risk sources reported such drinking. After combining these two groups, we had a total of 32 subjects with cardiogenic embolism. A comparison with 270 control subjects showed that the relative risk of developing cardiogenic embolism of the brain was significantly increased by consumption of 151–300 and ≥ 300 g alcohol within the preceding week (Table 4). Similar observations were made when recent alcohol consumption was measured as grams of alcohol consumed within the preceding 24 h. Before drawing any firm conclusions, however, the findings should be confirmed in sufficiently large series of unselected patients.

If recent heavy drinking increases the risk for cardiogenic embolism of the brain, the underlying mechanism could be increased heart rate and cardiac arrhythmias or both. These effects of acute heavy drinking may contribute to the propagation of existing thrombi from the heart. One may also speculate that alcohol-induced arrhythmias could predispose to intracardiac thrombus formation. Periodic heavy drinking may also cause fluctuation in haemostatic (Rubin & Rand 1994, Renaud & Ruf 1996) and fibrinolytic (Hendriks et al 1994) activities, and such effects may either increase or decrease thrombus formation. We have recently reported that alcohol-induced thrombocytopenia and rebound thrombocytosis are both often seen at the onset of brain infarction in patients who are heavy alcohol drinkers (Numminen et al 1996).

The number of subjects with the other subtypes of acute ischaemic stroke was so small that multiple logistic regression analysis could not be used. However, heavy

TABLE 4   **Multivariate relative risks (RRs) of cardiogenic embolism to the brain**

Variable	RR	95% CI
Migraine	2.49	0.79–7.84
Hypertension	2.10	0.75–5.85
Diabetes mellitus	1.36	0.36–5.16
Heavy drinking	1.17	0.31–4.41
Current smoking	0.91	0.29–2.88
Recent alcohol consumption (g/week)		
1–150	1.38	0.47–4.06
151–300	10.5[a]	2.11–52.0
> 300 g	13.0[b]	1.60–106

CI, confidence interval. RRs are adjusted for other variables listed and for age, sex, body mass index and hyperlipemia; they represent comparisons with patients without a risk factor.
[a] $P < 0.01$.
[b] $P > 0.05$.

recent drinking was also seen in the other groups. Large-artery atherosclerosis and lacunar syndromes occurred in about one-third of the cases in association with recent heavy drinking. The mechanism which leads to the onset of acute brain infarction in a subject with marked large-artery atherosclerosis during a drinking bout could be brain emboli arising from the arterial system. The alcohol-induced increase in heart rate speeds up circulation, which could dispatch emboli from the existing thrombi attached to atherosclerotic arterial walls.

Qureshi et al (1995) have reported a high frequency of hypertension, hypertensive intracerebral haemorrhage, and lacunar infarctions among young black patients who were also often heavy drinkers of alcohol. Although lacunar infarctions are not specific to small-vessel disease, most of them result from characteristic vascular lesions of the penetrating cerebral arteries. Alcohol has been shown to provoke vasospasm in cerebral arteries and arterioles of experimental animals (Altura et al 1983). If a similar phenomenon occurs in humans, this could explain the triggering of small deep infarctions in the brain during heavy drinking of alcohol.

Recent heavy alcohol drinking may also trigger the onset of ischaemic stroke due to cervicocerebral arterial dissection. This subtype of stroke frequently associates with cervical trauma. The trauma may occur during alcoholic intoxication. The association of alcohol drinking with the trauma should be known, because the resulting brain infarction sometimes occurs later on. In other words, in case of a traumatic dissection one should ask about alcohol consumption preceding both the onset of trauma and the onset of stroke.

In conclusion, the role of alcohol drinking as a risk factor for ischaemic stroke has been contradictory in previous papers. However, very few studies have taken into account the great variability of drinking habits. Epidemiological studies have usually categorized people dichotomously into alcohol drinkers and non-drinkers. It is not surprising that in such studies drinkers and non-drinkers have shown an equal risk for brain infarction. More reliable data can be obtained by case histories and case-control studies. Each individual patient should be carefully evaluated to identify the real cause of stroke, and the relationship of each subtype of stroke to drinking habits should be investigated.

References

Adams HP, Bendixen BH, Kappelle LJ et al 1993 Classification of subtype of acute ischemic stroke: definitions for use in a multicenter clinical trial. Stroke 24:35–41

Altura BM, Altura BT 1984 Alcohol, the cerebral circulation and strokes. Alcohol 1:325–331

Altura BM, Altura BT, Gebrewold A 1983 Alcohol-induced spasms of cerebral blood vessels: relation to cerebrovascular accidents and sudden death. Science 220:331–333

Altura BM, Gebrewold A, Altura BT, Gupta RK 1995 Role of brain [Mg^{2+}] in alcohol-induced hemorrhagic stroke in a rat model: a ^{31}P-NMR *in vivo* study. Alcohol 12:131–136

Bornstein NM 1994 Lifestyle changes: smoking, alcohol, diet and exercise. Cerebrovasc Dis 4:59–65

Camargo CA 1989 Moderate alcohol consumption and stroke: the epidemiological evidence. Stroke 20:1611–1626

Easton JD, Kaste M, Orgogozo JM, Aichner F, Gorelick PB 1995 Does alcohol prevent or cause stroke? Cerebrovasc Dis 5:375–380

Gordon EL, Nguyen T-S, Ngai AC, Winn HR 1995 Differential effects of alcohols on intracerebral arterioles. Ethanol alone causes vasoconstriction. J Cereb Blood Flow Metab 15:532–538

Haapaniemi H, Hillbom M, Juvela S 1997 Lifestyle-associated risk factors for acute brain infarction among persons of working age. Stroke 28:26–30

Hansagi H, Romelsjö A, Gerhardsson de Verdier M, Andréasson S, Leifman A 1995 Alcohol consumption and stroke mortality 20-year follow-up of 15,077 men and women. Stroke 26:1768–1773

Hendriks HFJ, Veenstra J, Velthuis-te Wierik EJM, Schaafsma G, Kluft C 1994 Effect of moderate dose of alcohol with evening meal on fibrinolytic factors. Br Med J 308:1003–1006

Hillbom M, Juvela S 1996 Alcohol and risk for stroke. In: Zakhari S, Wassef M (eds) Alcohol and the cardiovascular system. Baltimore, NIAAA research monograph No. 31:63–83

Juvela S, Hillbom M, Numminen H, Koskinen P 1993 Cigarette smoking and alcohol consumption as risk factors for aneurysmal subarachnoid hemorrhage. Stroke 24:639–646

Juvela S, Hillbom M, Palomäki H 1995 Risk factors for spontaneous intracerebral hemorrhage. Stroke 26:1558–1564

Kannel WB, Wolf PA, McGee DL, Dawber TR, McNamara P, Castelli WP 1981 Systolic blood pressure, arterial rigidity and risk of stroke. JAMA 245:1225–1229

Kiechl S, Willeit J, Egger G, Oberhollenzer M, Aichner F 1994 Alcohol consumption and carotid atherosclerosis: evidence of dose-dependent atherogenic and antiatherogenic effects. Results from the Bruneck Study. Stroke 25:1593–1598

Longstreth WT, Nelson LM, Koepsell TD, van Belle G 1992 Cigarette smoking, alcohol use, and subarachnoid hemorrhage. Stroke 23:1242–1249

Marmot MG, Elliott P, Shipley MJ et al 1994 Alcohol and blood pressure: the INTERSALT study. Br Med J 308:1263–1267

Mayfield D, McLeod G, Hall P 1974 The CAGE questionnaire: validation of a new alcoholism screening instrument. Am J Psychiatry 131:1121–1123

Mayhan WG, Didion SP 1995 Acute effects of ethanol on responses of cerebral arterioles. Stroke 26:2097–2102

Numminen H, Hillbom M, Juvela S 1996 Platelets, alcohol consumption, and onset of brain infarction. J Neurol Neurosurg Psychiatry 61:376–380

Palomäki H, Kaste M 1993 Regular light-to-moderate intake of alcohol and the risk of ischemic stroke. Is there a beneficial effect? Stroke 24:1828–1832

Qureshi AI, Safdar K, Patel M, Janssen RS, Frankel MR 1995 Stroke in young black patients. Risk factors, subtypes, and prognosis. Stroke 26:1995–1998

Renaud SC, Ruf J-C 1996 Effects of alcohol on platelet functions. Clin Chim Acta 246:77–89

Rodgers H, Aitken PD, French JM, Curless RH, Bates D, James OFW 1993 Alcohol and stroke. A case-control study of drinking habits past and present. Stroke 24:1473–1477

Rubin R, Rand ML 1994 Alcohol and platelet function. Alcohol Clin Exp Res 18:105–110

Sacco RL, Shi T, Zamanillo MC, Kargman DE 1994 Predictors of mortality and recurrence after hospitalized cerebral infarction in an urban community: the Northern Manhattan Stroke Study. Neurology 44:626–634

Sacco RL, Kargman DE, Gu Q, Zamanillo MC 1995 Race-ethnicity and determinants of intracranial atherosclerotic cerebral infarction. The Northern Manhattan Stroke Study. Stroke 26:14–20

Sacco RL, Lin IF, Boden-Albala B et al 1997 Alcohol and the risk of ischemic stroke: verification of a J-shaped relationship from the Northern Manhattan Stroke Study. Stroke 28:250 (abstr 93)

Stampfer MJ, Colditz GA, Willett WC, Speizer FE, Hennekens CH 1988 A prospective study of moderate alcohol consumption and the risk of coronary disease and stroke in women. N Engl J Med 319:267–273

Walbran BB, Nelson JS, Taylor JR 1981 Association of cerebral infarction and chronic alcoholism: an autopsy study. Alcohol Clin Exp Res 5:531–535

Wannamethee SG, Shaper AG 1996 Patterns of alcohol intake and risk of stroke in middle-aged British men. Stroke 27:1033–1039

DISCUSSION

Bondy: I have a question about the acute effects. I have looked in the literature for information about the level of alcohol intake that leads to cardiac arrhythmias in experimental studies (e.g. Regan et al 1981). The published studies show tolerance to the effects of alcohol in these outcomes, so if you look at light drinkers and you administer alcohol, you would measure cardiac arrythmias at blood alcohol levels that cause subjective mild intoxication. Yet when you get alcoholics into the lab you have to get them intoxicated before you start to see arrhythmias. Thus there is a tolerance to the cardiac effect as well as the intoxicating effect. Would the same hold for heart rate and would you agree with the hypothesis that special occasion only drinkers who drink heavily would therefore be at exceptionally high risk of stroke?

Hillbom: The problem is still unresolved. There are only a few case reports that address this issue. Rather small amounts of alcohol have been reported to provoke cardiac arrhythmias.

Puddey: The rising star on the risk factor stage — probably more so for stroke than for coronary heart disease — is, of course, homocysteine. It may well be worth considering this in relation to the association between alcohol and stroke. There have been two studies so far that I'm aware of, both reporting higher homocysteine levels in alcoholics on a case-control basis (Hultberg et al 1993, Cravo et al 1996). This phenomenon has a logical pathophysiological basis, given the folate antagonism of alcohol.

Gorelick: There may be a counterbalance in those who are heavy alcohol users. This is liver disease and the associated coagulation problems. I am managing a number of patients with liver disease and hyper-homocysteinaemia, but they also have abnormalities of coagulation parameters which tend to act as a counterbalance.

Shaper: We have studied this and there's no doubt that homocysteine is a risk factor for stroke (Perry et al 1995).

Urbano-Márquez: In our experience, many heavy drinkers have cerebral atrophy. Do you think it is possible that cerebral haemorrhages may be related to cerebral atrophy?

Hillbom: Not in my opinion, but I didn't mention traumatic subarachnoid haemorrhage which was described long ago by both British and Danish investigators (Simonsen 1963, 1984, Harland et al 1983). Particularly in the Danish paper it seems that almost all of those who die because of this rare disease are heavily intoxicated. When they are heavily intoxicated they get into fights and fall down: these rapid movements of the head cause laceration of the vertebral artery against bony processes in the neck. This is the mechanism behind the disease.

Shaper: You stated that regular light-to-moderate intake causes a lower degree of stroke. When one looks at the figures you showed, there is a progressive increase of strokes from light-to-moderate drinking towards heavier; in other words, heavier drinkers do worse. Are you basing that statement on the fact that the non-drinkers have somewhat higher risks in many of those studies? If you are, you haven't told us anything about the characteristics of those non-drinkers.

Gorelick: I recently served as a member of the American Heart Association stroke risk factor panel. We had to wrestle with this issue. If you study the data, there is good consistency for the so-called linear relationship of haemorrhagic stroke and alcohol consumption. But when the ischaemic stroke data are carefully studied, one does not find consistency across prospective studies for the alcohol–ischaemic stroke relationship. Thus, you cannot conclude that for ischaemic stroke there is a J-shaped curve. Gerry Shaper's point is very well taken about the sick-quitter hypothesis as ex-drinkers may be included in the non-drinking group in these stroke studies. The epidemiological data on alcohol and stroke are not as advanced as those on alcohol and coronary heart disease. That is why I believe that Arthur Klatsky's on-going prospective epidemiological study on alcohol and stroke is going to be so exciting. Appropriate methodology will help to better define the alcohol–stroke J-shaped relationship. With regard to stroke, preliminarily it does not appear that mild or moderate drinking is harmful as there are relatively few haemorrhagic strokes compared with ischaemic strokes. If alcohol consumption affords protection from ischaemic stroke, the number of ischaemic strokes that are saved should be far greater than the number of haemorrhagic strokes that occur at mild to moderate alcohol consumption levels.

Shaper: This takes us back to 1926, and our friend Raymond Pearl: the point he was trying to make is that light to moderate drinking does not do most people any harm. However, this is not the issue we are arguing about at this meeting. We are concerned with whether low level drinking is actually beneficial. My assertion is that until you know the characteristics of your non-drinking population and have shown that they are not a group with increased risk, your J-shaped curves do not indicate a benefit.

Puddey: I had occasion last year to review the studies that have used duplex Doppler ultrasound to look at extracranial vasculature. There are about seven studies of varying quality that have looked at alcohol intake either as a primary predictor of interest or as one of a variety of risk factors (Sutton-Tyrell et al 1993, Fine-Edelstein et al 1994, Kiechl et al 1994, Demirovic et al 1993, Jungquist et al 1991, Szirmai et al 1993, Bogousslavsky et al 1990). Interestingly, the overall picture is one of a pro-atherosclerotic effect for the extracranial vasculature with heavy drinking. Most of the studies were case-control with heavy drinkers, looking at either intima-medial thickness or the presence or absence of plaque. In the first of the two large-scale population studies, the Atherosclerosis Risk in Communities Study, there was no overall relationship, but a subset analysis in women showed increasing intima-medial thickness (Demirovic et al 1994). In the second, the Framingham study, there was a positive relationship between alcohol intake and intima-medial thickness (Fine-Edelstein et al 1994). There may well be a difference between the cerebral vasculature and the coronary vasculature in the effects of alcohol on atherosclerosis.

Gaziano: There's another area where the two vascular beds seem to be different, and that is with cholesterol. In the Framingham and many other studies, total cholesterol seems to be a less important predictor for cerebral vascular events than it is for coronary disease. But we have to keep in mind that the study of coronary disease is largely a study of one disease process, whereas the study of cerebral vascular diseases involves three processes: embolic events from the heart, atherosclerotic disease and haemorrhagic disease. We have to distinguish carefully between the types of disease that we are talking about. Recently we did two meta-analyses. In the first we took all the cholesterol-lowering trials and showed absolutely no effect for stroke prevention. We had reverse results when we published another meta-analysis looking at all the statin trials and we saw a stroke-reduction effect. However, we don't know whether that's truly a cholesterol effect on atherosclerosis or whether we are preventing heart disease and thus embolic events.

Klatsky: With respect to the large subset of ischaemic strokes that are cardio-embolic, there are multiple heart conditions involved here, some of which may be related to alcohol and some not. All this has nothing to do with the vascular disease in the brain or in the carotid arteries. It becomes very complicated.

References

Bogousslavsky J, van Melle G, Despland PA, Regli F 1990 Alcohol consumption and carotid atherosclerosis in the Lausanne stroke registry. Stroke 21:715–720

Cravo ML, Gloria LM, Selhub J et al 1996 Hyperhomocysteinemia in chronic alcoholism: correlation with folate, vitamin B12 and vitamin B6 status. Am J Clin Nutr 63:220–224

Demirovic J, Nabulsi A, Folsom AR et al 1993 Alcohol consumption and ultrasonographically assessed carotid artery wall thickness and distensibility. The Atherosclerosis Risk in Communities (ARIC) Study Investigators. Circulation 88:2787–2793

Fine-Edelstein JS, Wolf PA, O'Leary DH et al 1994 Precursors of extracranial carotid atherosclerosis in the Framingham study. Neurology 44:1046–1050

Harland WA, Pitts JF, Watson AA 1983 Subarachnoid haemorrhage due to upper cervical trauma. J Clin Pathol 36:1335–1341

Hultberg B, Berglund M, Andersson A, Frank A 1993 Elevated plasma homocysteine in alcoholics. Alcohol Clin Exp Res 17:687–689

Jungquist G, Hanson BS, Isacsson SO, Janzon L, Steen B, Lindell SE 1991 Risk factors for carotid artery stenosis: an epidemiological study of men aged 69 years. J Clin Epidemiol 44:347–353

Kiechl S, Willeit J, Egger G, Oberhollenzer M, Aichner F 1994 Alcohol consumption and carotid atherosclerosis: evidence of dose dependent atherogeniogenic and antiatherogenic effects. Results from the Bruneck study. Stroke 1994 25:1593–1598

Perry IJ, Refsum H, Morris RW, Ebrahim SB, Veland PM, Shaper AG 1995 Prospective study of serum total homocysteine concentration and risk of stroke in middle-aged British men. Lancet 346:1395–1398

Regan TJ, Ahmed SS, Ettinger PO 1981 Cardiovascular consequences of acute and chronic ethanol use. In: Israel Y, Glaser FB, Kalant H, Popham RE, Schmidt W, Smart RG (eds) Research advances in alcohol and drug problems. Vol 6. Plenum, New York, p 217–254

Simonsen J 1963 Traumatic subarachnoid haemorrhage in alcohol intoxication. J Forensic Sci 8:97–116

Simonsen J 1984 Fatal subarachnoid haemorrhages in relation to minor injuries in Denmark from 1967 to 1981. Forensic Sci Int 24:57–63

Sutton-Tyrell K, Alcorn HG, Wolfson SK, Kelsey SF, Kuller LH 1993 Predictors of carotid stenosis in older adults with and without isolated systolic hypertension. Stroke 24:355–361

Szirmai IG, Kamondi A, Magyar H, Juhasz C 1993 Relation of laboratory and clinical variables to the grade of carotid atherosclerosis. Stroke 24:1811–1816

The French paradox and wine drinking

S. Renaud and R. Gueguen*

INSERM *(Institut National pour la Santé et la Recherche Médicale), Unit 330, Université Bordeaux 2, 146 rue Léo Saignat, 33076 Bordeaux Cedex, and *Centre de Médecine Préventive, 2 Avenue du Doyen Parisot, B.P. 7, 54501 Vandoeuvre les Nancy Cedex, France*

Abstract. Despite a high level of risk factors such as cholesterol, diabetes, hypertension and a high intake of saturated fat, French males display the lowest mortality rate from ischaemic heart disease and cardiovascular diseases in Western industrialized nations (36% lower than the USA and 39% lower than the UK). By contrast, mortality from all causes is only 8% lower than in the USA and 6% than in the UK, owing to a high level of cancer and violent deaths. In a recent study of 34 000 middle-aged men from Eastern France with a follow-up of 12 years we have observed that for 48 g of alcohol (mostly wine) per day as the mean intake, mortality from cardiovascular diseases was lower by 30%, all-cause mortality was reduced by 20%, but mortality by cancer and violent death was increased compared with abstainers. Thus the so-called 'French Paradox' (a low mortality rate specifically from cardiovascular diseases) may be due mainly to the regular consumption of wine.

1998 Alcohol and cardiovascular diseases. Wiley, Chichester (Novartis Foundation Symposium 216) p 208–222

The first scientific observation of the 'French Paradox' seems to have been reported by Ducimetière et al (1980) in the Parisian protective study on 7434 subjects. They observed that, for the same level of the main risk factors (cholesterol, smoking, hypertension, diabetes), the incidence of coronary heart disease (CHD) was lower (by 36–55%) than in the Pooling Project (Pooling Project Research Group 1978) or in the Seven Country Study (Keys 1970) Considering the most recent statistics of World Health Organization (1995), the reduction in the mortality rate form CHD in France as compared to the USA was 61% for men and 69% for women. As compared to the UK, the reduction was 68% for men and 71% for women. As we emphasized elsewhere (Renaud & de Lorgeril 1992, 1993) these differences do not seem to be due to unreliable statistics since the French paradox has been confirmed by the MONICA Project (World Health Organization 1989). The number of premature deaths of men (35–64 years) from CHD in the three MONICA centres in France were 78 in Toulouse, 102 in Strasbourg and 105 in Lille, compared with 182 in Stanford and 380 in Glasgow. This difference is despite the fact that average serum cholesterol in the French centres (233 mg/dl) is intermediate between that of

Stanford (209 mg/dl) and of Glasgow (244 mg/dl). The prevalence of smoking and the fat intake are also similar in France and many other centres. Hypertension, especially in Lille and Strasbourg, are among the highest of the 43 MONICA centres investigated throughout the world (World Health Organization 1989).

Is the paradox real?

To explain this paradox, it has been emphasized that some fatal events (sudden death) categorized as unclassifiable in France and a few other countries would be considered as coronary death in most countries with a high incidence of CHD (Tunstall-Pedoe et al 1994). In that case, the rates in France would be similar to those of southern populations such as Italy, Switzerland and Spain. The conclusion of Tunstall-Pedoe et al (1994) was that compared with elsewhere, French CHD mortality remains relatively low even after such correction. This is also confirmed by the rate of non-fatal definite myocardial infarction which is, in France, the lowest of the MONICA centres after China and Catalogna in Spain. The paradox is not that the mortality rate from CHD is low in France, but that it is low despite the high level of risk factors. As an example, in the MONICA centres, average serum cholesterol (mg/dl) was 239 in France, 227 in Italy, 223 in Spain and 231 in Switzerland. Average systolic blood pressure (mm Hg) was 142 in France, 138 in Italy, 123 in Spain and 133 in Switzerland. But none seems to be as convincing as the intake of saturated fats, especially dairy products, the richest in saturated fatty acids. As shown in Fig. 1, the average daily consumption of dairy products in France (590 kcal) is much higher than in Spain (253 kcal), Italy (346 kcal) and even the USA (399 kcal) or the UK (469 kcal). In Fig. 1, France does not appear to follow the trend shown by the other countries, namely a strong positive relationship between CHD mortality and the intake of dairy products.

In addition, when looking at the most recent World Health Organization statistics (World Health Organization 1995), it is not only CHD mortality which is lower in France but also total cardiovascular death (Table 1). As a matter of fact, France has the lowest cardiovascular mortality of Western industrialized countries. By contrast, mortality from all causes is lower in Greece. The reason why France is not the lowest in mortality from all causes is that the mortality from cancer (as high as in Scotland) and violent death is higher than expected. Thus, the French pattern of mortality is characterized by a mortality rate low from cardiovascular diseases but high from cancer and accidents. Could this pattern be due to a factor specific to France? It does not seem that this factor could be genetic in origin since numerous studies have shown that the risk of CHD in population is mostly due to environmental factors rather than to heredity (Renaud & de Lorgeril 1989).

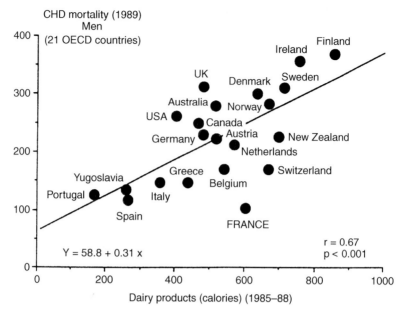

FIG. 1.   Relationship between the mortality rate from CHD in 1989 in humans as reported by
World Health Organization (1995), and the mean consumption of dairy products (per person/
day) in the 21 most industrialized Western countries of the Organization for Economic Co-
operation and Development (OECD 1991). As shown, the positive relation is highly
significant ($P < 0.001$) only France being at distance from regression line.

TABLE 1   **Age standardized death rate for men in 1992–1994 per 100 000 of the
standard population**

	Cardiovascular	*Cancer*	*Cirrhosis*	*Violent death*	*All causes*
France	254	293	23	148	909
Japan	233	228	17	100	768
Spain	316	258	28	101	923
Italy	354	278	30	98	921
Greece	378	219	19	95	841
USA	399	248	15	125	993
UK	417	262	8	62	947
Germany	452	266	31	101	1028

Adapted from World Health Organization (1995).

Vegetables and the French paradox

It has been emphasized by Artaud-Wild et al (1993) that a higher consumption of vegetable foods could explain the protection of France from CHD as compared with Germany, the UK or Finland. In our duplication of the protective effects of the Cretan diet, the patients consumed more vegetables and fruits (de Lorgeril et al 1994, Renaud et al 1995) in addition to changes in the intake of dietary fatty acids. Cardiac death as well as non-fatal myocardial infarction were reduced by 76%. Nevertheless, the question is whether it is the consumption of vegetables and fruit that can explain the French protection against CHD. For this purpose, we examined the relationship between the intake of vegetables, vegetable fats, fruits and the mortality from CHD in the 21 most industrialized Western countries. We observed (Fig. 2) a significant exponential inverse correlation ($r = -0.49$, $P < 0.05$), suggesting a protective effect from vegetables. Nevertheless, it can be noted that Greece, Italy and Spain consume far larger amounts of vegetables without benefiting from the protection from CHD seen in France. France does

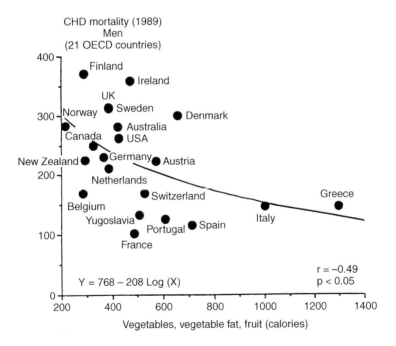

FIG. 2.   Relationship between the mortality rate from CHD as in Fig. 1 and the consumption of vegetables, vegetable fats and fruit (OECD 1991). An inverse relation is observed, the regression being exponential ($P < 0.05$).

not have a larger consumption of vegetables and fruit than countries such as Austria or Denmark which have a much higher mortality rate from CHD.

There is no doubt that vegetable consumption is a healthy dietary habit associated with a protection from CHD and cancer (Phillips et al 1978). However, it does not seem that this habit can explain the French paradox, i.e. a low mortality rate from CHD but a high mortality from cancer and accidents.

Alcohol and the French paradox

An inverse relationship between CHD mortality and the consumption of alcohol has been repeatedly observed since 1979 (St Leger et al 1979). In the last 10 years, studies on a total of close to one million subjects have consistently shown that alcohol drinking was associated with a 20–60% lower risk of CHD (Renaud et al 1993). In the largest prospective study ever performed in this field, on 276 802 men followed for 12 years (Boffetta & Garfinkel 1990), not only was CHD mortality reduced by 20% over a large range of alcohol consumption, but mortality from all causes was also lower by at least 10% with alcohol intake of up to 24 g per day.

Wine and the French paradox

Most alcohol consumption in the USA is of beer and spirits (89% of alcohol drunk), whereas in France the major drink is wine (63%). The early studies performed in the USA did not observe differences in protection offered by wine, beer or spirits on CHD mortality (Hennekens et al 1979). In addition, a systematic review of epidemiological studies concluded that at least for the benefit on CHD mortality, all alcoholic drinks seem to be equivalent (Rimm et al 1996). However, it could be different with cardiovascular diseases in general, and France has the lowest mortality rate from cardiovascular diseases.

Klatsky et al (1992) in California have shown in 128 934 adults, that wine drinkers had a 30% to 40% lower risk for cardiovascular death compared with liquor drinkers. Beer did not show similar protective effects to wine. These results have been confirmed by a prospective study in Denmark on more than 12 800 subjects followed for 12 years (Grønbæk et al 1995). Those who drank three to five glasses of wine per day had a reduction of 49% in the mortality rate from cardiovascular diseases, compared to those not drinking wine. It can be emphasized that each of the two studies above, with more than 1200 deaths from cardiovascular diseases, had the statistical power to evaluate precisely the respective roles of the different alcoholic beverages. Nevertheless, for evaluating the effect of wine on mortality and its role in the French paradox, studies in France are necessary. To this end we have recently completed a prospective study on 34 000 middle-aged men from Eastern France.

TABLE 2 Average daily alcohol consumption (g/day) according to social classes in men aged 40–60 from eastern France

Social classes (number)	Wine	Beer	Aperitifs and liqueurs	Total alcohol
Tradesmen (1633)	47.6	7.2	4.0	58.0
High-level managers (4228)	36.2	5.3	3.8	45.0
Middle-level managers and foremen (10 572)	41.2	5.8	3.6	50.1
Employees (2797)	41.8	5.6	3.6	50.2
Workers (14 801)	48.9	7.1	3.0	58.1
Total %	82.0	11.6	6.4	100

Adapted with permission from Renaud et al (1998).

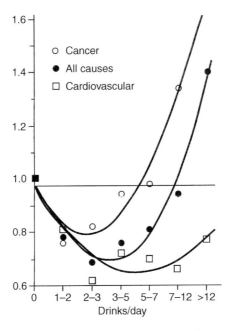

FIG. 3.   Relative-risk of mortality from cancer, all causes and cardiovascular diseases in relation to the intake of alcohol, 82% being wine. (One drink = 10.5 g alcohol.) Relative-risk evaluated by Cox model adjusted for age, education, smoking, systolic blood pressure, serum cholesterol and body mass index. Reference (1.0) is the group of non-drinkers. Polynomial regression curves. Adapted with permission from Renaud et al (1998).

The cohort was a representative sample of active men, 40–60 years of age, with 418 068 person-years of follow-up. In all social classes (Table 2) wine was the main alcoholic beverage, i.e. 82% of alcohol consumption. The mean total alcohol intake was 48 g/day at the beginning of the study (1978–1983).

Compared with abstainers, mortality rate from CHD in those consuming two or more glasses of wine per day was lower by 30–39%, after adjusting the model for six confounding factors (Renaud et al 1998). Independent of the type of alcohol consumed, cardiovascular mortality in those consuming two to seven drinks per day was 30–40% lower than in abstainers (Fig. 3). Mortality from cancer was significantly reduced by 20%, and mortality from all causes reduced by 30%, but only for those consuming 2–3 drinks per day. No protection on total death compared to abstainers was seen in those consuming more than seven drinks per day. For 12 drinks per day a 40% increased risk of death was seen, due to more than a 60% higher risk of cancer. Violent death was higher in each category of alcohol intake (Renaud et al 1998).

On average, the drinkers in the present cohort consumed approximately five drinks per day. For that level of intake, cardiovascular mortality was lower by 35%, all cause mortality was lower by 20%, but there was no reduction in mortality from cancer and an increased risk of violent death (5–77%).

The mechanism behind the protective effect of wine

Several studies have shown that the intake of alcohol is beneficial for health only when consumed regularly and moderately (Gordon & Kannel 1983, Rimm et al 1991). Binge drinking is harmful. The only study that has shown an increased mortality at all levels of alcohol consumption was in Finland (Suhonen et al 1987), most of the fatal events being sudden death. In that study, 60% of the subjects drank spirits for intoxication.

If alcohol drinking is only beneficial when used moderately and regularly, this pattern corresponds exactly to the way wine is normally consumed. In Mediterranean countries, wine is used mostly at meals, as a foodstuff.

In addition, wine contains antioxidant substances that have been shown to increase the antioxidant activity of plasma (Maxwell et al 1994) and to be more efficient than vitamin E to protect low density lipoproteins (LDLs) from peroxidation (Frankel et al 1993). However, since the protective effect of alcohol is essentially on myocardial infarction (Renaud et al 1993) — i.e. coronary thrombosis (De Wood et al 1980) — we therefore had to investigate the effect of wine on platelet aggregation (Renaud & Ruf 1996), one of the earliest steps in coronary thrombosis. In the rat we have observed that red wine, owing to the antioxidant polyphenols it contains, is not associated with the rebound effect on blood platelet aggregation reported with alcohol drinking (Ruf et al 1995). The occurrence of this rebound effect, which has also been observed in humans, might explain stroke (Hillbom 1987) and sudden death associated with episodes of drunkenness. The platelet rebound effect to thrombin has also been observed in moderate drinkers of beer and spirits (Renaud et al 1992) but not in French wine drinkers. Therefore, since platelet function seems to be closely related to CHD, as demonstrated by the 50% reduction in coronary events induced by aspirin (a specific inhibitor of platelet aggregation)(Fuster et al 1989), the more efficient protective effect of wine on platelets compared with other alcoholic beverages could also be observed in regular drinkers not necessarily binge drinking.

Conclusion

The French paradox — a low mortality rate from CHD and cardiovascular diseases despite a high level of risk factors — has been documented by several studies in addition to the World Health Organization statistics. The evaluation from the MONICA Project (Tunstall-Pedoe et al 1994) indicates that if the mortality rate from CHD in France is not the lowest in the world, it is amongst the lowest, as also confirmed by the rate of hospitalized non-fatal myocardial infarction.

The moderate consumption in France of fresh vegetables, fruit and vegetable fats, could contribute to the healthy effects of the French diet. Nevertheless, the French paradox is also associated with a higher mortality from cancer and accidents that cannot be explained by the intake of vegetables.

As shown by our prospective study on 34 000 middle-aged French men, consumption of at least two drinks (mostly wine) per day was associated with a 30–40% lower mortality rate from cardiovascular diseases. Nevertheless, that level of alcohol was related to a higher mortality from violent death and, at levels above five drinks per day, from cancer. Thus the so-called 'French paradox' appears to be mainly explained by the regular consumption of wine. Finally, provided wine is used with moderation (two to three glasses per day for men), it may be associated with a lowering of mortality from cancer (-20%) and all causes (-30%) in adults.

The use of wine at meals, an essential part of the Mediterranean civilization, may be a healthy dietary habit owing to the presence in wine of both alcohol and antioxidants.

Acknowledgements

The research was supported in part by INSERM, the Ministry of Agriculture, the Technical Institute of Wine and Danone Group.

References

Artaud-Wild SM, Connor S, Sexton G, Connor WE 1993 Differences in coronary mortality can be explained by differences in cholesterol and saturated fat intakes in 40 countries but not in France and Finland. A paradox. Circulation 88:2771–2779

Boffetta P, Garfinkel L 1990 Alcohol drinking and mortality among men enrolled in an American Cancer Society prospective study. Epidemiology 1:342–348

de Lorgeril M, Renaud S, Mamelle N et al 1994 Mediterranean alpha-linolenic acid-rich diet in secondary prevention of coronary heart disease. Lancet 343:1454–1459

De Wood MA, Spores J, Notske R et al 1980 Prevalence of total coronary occlusion during the early hours of transmural myocardial infarction. N Eng J Med 303:897–902

Ducimetière P, Richard L, Cambien F, Rakotovas R, Claude JR 1980 Coronary heart disease in middle-aged Frenchmen. Comparisons between Paris Prospective Study, Seven Countries and Pooling Project. Lancet 1:1346–1350

Frankel EN, Kanner J, German JB, Parks E, Kinsella JE 1993 Inhibition of oxidation of human low-density lipoprotein by phenolic substances in red wine. Lancet 341:454–457

Fuster V, Cohen M, Halpern J 1989 Aspirin in the prevention of coronary disease (editorial). N Engl J Med 321:183–183

Gordon T, Kannel WB 1983 Drinking habits and cardiovascular disease. The Framingham Study. Am Heart J 105:667–673

Grønbæk DA, Deis A, Sørensen TIA, Becker U, Schnohr P, Jensen G 1995 Mortality associated with moderate intake of wine, beer or spirits. Br Med J 310:1165–1169

Hennekens CH, Willet W, Rosner B et al 1979 Effects of beer, wine, and liquor in coronary death. JAMA 242:1973–1974

Hillbom ME 1987 What supports the role of alcohol as a risk factor for stroke? Acta Med Scand 717 (suppl):93–106

Keys A 1970 Coronary heart disease in seven countries. Circulation 41 (suppl 1):1–211

Klatsky AL, Armstrong MA, Friedman GD 1992 Alcohol and mortality. Ann Intern Med 117:646–654

Maxwell S, Cruickshank A, Thorpe G 1994 Red wine and antioxidant activity in serum. Lancet 344:193–194

Organization for Economic Co-operation and Development (OECD) 1991 Food consumption statistics. OECD, Paris

Phillips RL, Lemon FR, Beeson WL, Kuzma JW 1978 Coronary heart disease mortality among seventh-day adventists with differing dietary habits: a preliminary report. Am J Clin Nutr 31 (suppl):191–198

Pooling Project Research Group 1978 Relationship of blood pressure, serum cholesterol smoking habit, relative weight and ECG abnormalities to incidence of major coronary events: final report of the Pooling Project. J Chron Dis 31:201–306

Renaud S, de Lorgeril M 1989 Dietary lipids and their relation to ischaemic heart disease: from epidemiology to prevention. J Intern Med 225:39–46

Renaud S, de Lorgeril M 1992 Wine, alcohol, platelets and the French Paradox for coronary heart disease. Lancet 339:1523–1526

Renaud S, de Lorgeril M 1993 The French paradox: dietary factors and cigarette smoking-related health risks. Ann N Y Acad Sci 686:299–309

Renaud S, Ruf JC 1996 Effect of alcohol on platelet functions. Clin Chim Acta 246:77–89

Renaud S, Beswick AD, Fehily AM et al 1992 Alcohol and platelet aggregation: the Caerphilly prospective heart disease study. Am J Clin Nutr 55:1012–1017

Renaud S, Criqui MH, Farchi G, Veenstra J 1993 Alcohol drinking and coronary heart disease. In: Verschuren PM (ed) Health issues related to alcohol consumption. ILSI Press, Washington DC, p 81–123

Renaud S, de Lorgeril M, Delaye J et al 1995 The Cretan Mediterranean diet for prevention of coronary heart disease. Am J Clin Nutr 61(Suppl):1360S–1367S

Renaud S, Gueguen R, Schenker J, d'Houtand A 1998 Alcohol and mortality in middle-aged men from Eastern France. Epidemiology, in press

Rimm EB, Giovannucci E, Willett WC et al 1991 Alcohol and mortality. Lancet 338:1073–1074

Rimm EB, Klatsky A, Grobee D, Stampfer M J 1996 Review of moderate alcohol consumption and reduced risk of coronary heart disease: is the effect due to beer, wine or spirits? Br Med J 312:731–736

Ruf JC, Berger JL, Renaud S 1995 Platelet rebound effect of alcohol withdrawal and wine drinking in rats. Relation to tannins and lipid peroxidation. Arterioscler Thromb Vasc Biol 15:140–144

St Leger AS, Cochrane AL, Moore F 1979 Factors associated with cardiac mortality in developed countries with particular reference to the consumption of wine. Lancet 1:1017–1020

Suhonen O, Aromas A, Reunanen A, Knekt P 1987 Alcohol consumption and sudden coronary death in middle-aged Finnish men. Acta Med Scand 221:335–341

Tunstall-Pedoe H, Kuulasmaa K, Amonyel P, Arveiler D, Rajakangas AM, Pajak A 1994 Myocardial infarction and coronary deaths in the World Health Organization MONICA Project. Circulation 90:583–612

World Health Organization 1989 World Health Statistics Annual. World Health Organization, Geneva

World Health Organization 1995 World Health Statistics Annual. World Health Organization, Geneva

DISCUSSION

Rehm: The Global Burden of disease study (Murray & Lopez 1997) has found that there are fundamental differences in how coronary heart disease is diagnosed in different countries. France seems to be one of the countries which underdiagnoses coronary heart disease. I'm not trying to say that the French paradox is just an artefact of diagnosis, but this has often been cited as one of the main reasons for it.

You explained the French paradox by wine drinking and you showed the recent data from France. What is suspicious about those data is that they show a protective effect of moderate drinking on cancer, which has not been found in any of the meta-analyses so far carried out, and which to my knowledge has no potential mechanism. This makes one wonder whether part of the explanation is really in the abstainers which are used as a baseline.

Renaud: It is true that in France sudden death is not necessarily included in cardiac death. But even if you take account of all the sudden deaths, which we did in our trial, the paradox still shows up. Secondly, if you look at the French data on morbidity from coronary disease, which are probably more reliable because in France all people with myocardial infarction are hospitalized, the coronary morbidity in France is among the lowest in the world.

Concerning your second point, our baseline is the abstainers plus the occasional drinkers. Yesterday, we saw data from the American Physicians Study showing exactly a 20% reduction in the mortality rate from cancer at the same intake of alcohol as in our study. This is one of the first times this reduction in cancer has been shown, but it is not the first time. Up to now it was mostly a global evaluation of alcohol drinking that was done in relation to the mortality by cancer. Similarly, in our French middle-aged men, when the totality of the drinkers are compared to abstainers it is an increased risk of cancer that is observed.

Peters: What is the possible mechanism behind the reduced risk of cancer in individuals consuming small amounts of alcohol?

Renaud: Resveratrol, which is a substance contained in wine, has been shown to inhibit the three main steps of carcinogenesis. This is one possibility.

Klatsky: Dr Renaud correctly cited our findings about cardiovascular mortality, in that people who preferred wine had lower mortality compared with those who preferred liquor, and people who preferred beer were intermediate. We have re-done a study of coronary disease not using mortality as an endpoint but rather hospitalization (Klatsky et al 1997). We looked at 3900 persons hospitalized with coronary disease, excluding lifelong non-drinkers, ex-drinkers and very infrequent drinkers. We didn't use preference definitions because we had found that such definitions exaggerated the user differences. We included all information about use of wine, liquor and beer. Our beverage choice variable represents roughly drinks per day of the beverage. For example, a 0.8 relative risk represents the diminution in relative risk per glass of wine per day in a multivariate analysis which was not controlled for total alcohol. To cut a long story short, in the analyses not controlled for total amount of alcohol, each beverage type showed statistically significant reductions in risk per glass per day of the beverage (Table 1 [*Klatsky*]). It was strongest for beer and weakest for liquor, but each one was statistically significant. When we control for total alcohol, all statistically significant differences disappear, except for beer drinking in men. As another method of control for amount of alcohol, we did the analysis only on those who reported one or two drinks per day. This is the most specific drinking category in our sample and it is the category at which coronary risk is lowest. Among these one-to-two per day drinkers, only beer appears to show weakly statistically significant independent protection.

We also broke down wine as to the type of wine. The definition involved four mutually exclusive subsets: 'red' means they take only red table wine, 'white' means they take only white table wine, 'red and white' means both (and we don't know the proportions), and 'other' means that they failed to specify or they take fortified wines. As you can see in Table 2 (*Klatsky*), the red wine only group does not appear to be better protected. We also did a statistical test comparing these groups to each other and there were no differences. We concluded that the major effect appears to be of alcohol, because in this analysis as in every other that we've done there's a nice inverse relation to total alcohol. Type of beverage is a minor

TABLE 1   (*Klatsky*) Adjusted relative risk of hospitalization for CHD by wine, liquor and beer

Group	Wine[a]	Liquor[a]	Beer[a]
Total alcohol not controlled			
Both sexes	0.8[c]	0.9[c]	0.7[d]
Men	0.9	0.9	0.7[d]
Women	0.7[c]	0.9	0.7
Total alcohol controlled			
Both sexes	1.0	1.0	0.9
Men	1.0	1.0	0.8[b]
Women	0.9	1.3	1.0

[a]Proxy variable representing drink/day of type.
[b]$P < 0.05$.
[c]$P < 0.01$.
[d]$P < 0.001$.
Adapted from Klatsky et al (1997).

TABLE 2   (*Klatsky*) Adjusted relative risk of hospitalization for CHD by type of wine

Group	Red[a]	White[a]	Red and white[a]	Other[a]
Total alcohol not controlled				
Both sexes	1.0	0.9	0.7[c]	0.9
Men	1.2	1.0	0.8[b]	0.9
Women	0.6	0.7	0.5[b]	0.7
Total alcohol controlled				
Both sexes	1.1	1.0	0.8	0.9
Men	1.3	1.1	0.8	0.9
Women	0.8	1.0	0.6[b]	0.7

[a]Proxy variable representing drink/day of type.
[b]$P < 0.05$.
[c]$P < 0.01$.
Adapted from Klatsky et al (1997).

factor, but, if anything, beer drinking particularly in men appears to be the most protective, and perhaps wine drinking was the most protective in women.

Shaper: What is the control group?

Klatsky: This analysis only includes people who drink more than once per month, so the relative risk is per glass per day: there's no specific control group.

The control group is people who don't get hospitalized for coronary disease, if you will. The analysis involves the entire 80 000 people who report drinking.

Renaud: The problem with comparing wine to all alcoholic beverages is as follows. In our study on middle-aged French men we have observed that for a similar intake of alcohol, if this is made up of 10% beer and 90% wine, it is associated with the same all-cause mortality as 100% wine. This is also true if 40% of the alcohol is taken in the form of beer. It is only when the intake consists of more than 50% beer or spirit that the specific effect of beer or spirits can be seen, at least in our study. One possible explanation is that the wine supplies the polyphenols needed to counteract the prooxidant effect of other alcoholic beverages.

Shaper: Once again, I am concerned about the magnitude of the effect. I accept that something is going on with alcohol in cardiovascular disease that is not going on in all the other causes of mortality. Alcohol appears to be beneficial for coronary heart disease, but it is the magnitude of that effect that concerns me. Whether you use non-drinkers or very light drinkers as a baseline, there still appears to be an effect—this is most marked if you use non-drinkers. I'm worried about who those non-drinkers are: you have told us nothing about their characteristics, and in your adjustment you have made no mention of pre-existing ill health, medication or self assessment of ill health.

Renaud: First of all, that control group had the lowest cholesterol, lowest blood pressure, lowest triglyceride levels and lowest γ-glutamyl transferase. If the people dying in the first two years of recruitment are discarded, then you get exactly the same result. Consequently, those who remained were not sick when they joined the study. This study was done in a centre for preventive medicine, more or less similar to Kaiser-Permanente where Dr Klatsky works. Thus it was mostly healthy people that were recruited, the sick people being referred to hospitals.

Shaper: That's an answer, but not an adequate answer. I would suggest that you look at the characteristics of that non-drinking group to see whether in any respects, particularly reporting of ill health, there may be characteristics that make them different. Almost all studies show that the non-drinking groups include a proportion of people who have stopped drinking and this may prejudice the measurement of magnitude.

Grønbæk: I would like to comment on the issue raised by several of the speakers regarding effects of beer, wine and spirits. In my view, you could ask two questions with regard to the different types of alcoholic beverages in coronary heart disease. One would be, is there an effect of ethanol, or is the effect due to a co-factor in wine? The other question would be to ask whether there is an effect of ethanol *and* an additional effect of one or several co-factors in wine? The very heavily quoted review by Dr Rimm, Dr Klatsky and colleagues (Rimm et al 1996) answers the first question, and shows that there is an effect of ethanol itself with regard to coronary heart disease. However, of the 10 prospective studies reviewed in that paper, very few of them were able to compare the three types of beverages, and if you want to answer the question in a prospective cohort study you have to be able to include drinkers of all three types. To date the only studies that have been able to compare the three types of beverages all point to wine as the most beneficial, which indicates that there may be an additional effect of wine apart from the effect of ethanol that we have all agreed upon.

Anderson: The southern European countries have in a sense become an interesting experiment. These are countries that traditionally have had the highest levels of alcohol consumption, but they're are also countries which over the last 10–20 years have had the most rapid decrease in alcohol consumption. It would be very interesting to do some time series analysis relating per capita alcohol consumption with coronary heart disease deaths. At a crude level, in all of these countries coronary heart disease deaths are also decreasing, but a formal statistical time series analyses would be very interesting.

Hendriks: The data that Serge Renaud showed on the effects of alcohol on platelet aggregation were of course *ex vivo* data. These data may not be representative for the *in vivo* situation. For instance, with the oxidation studies on LDL, clear effects are seen *in vitro* but not *in vivo*.

Renaud: Working with platelets is difficult. None the less, our results on the effect of alcohol drinking on *ex vivo* platelet aggregability in 1600 subjects in Wales (Renaud et al 1992) suggest that the tests used were closely related to the risk of CHD. In addition, these tests have shown clearly the protective effect of alcohol on platelets. Finally, as we have observed previously (Renaud et al 1986), platelet aggregability evaluated in this way is closely related to the level of other risk factors such as smoking and intake of saturated fats. Thus we are confident of the close relationship between *ex vivo* platelet aggregability and CHD.

Keaney: There is an *in vivo* model of platelet function which was published by John Folts (Folts et al 1976). He has given wine and grape juice to dogs while he creates this model where platelets are deposited on the coronary artery that is denuded of endothelium. He can show clearly that red wine, white wine and grape juice all inhibit platelet activity both *in vivo* (in this model) and *ex vivo*. More importantly, he's also shown that this effect is probably not due to the anti-oxidant activity *per se*, but rather quercetin and rutin, two polyphenolic compounds that are both phosphodiesterase inhibitors, raise the cyclic nucleotide levels in platelets and cause long lasting prevention of platelet aggregation (Demrow et al 1995). In addition, the model that was presented by Dr Renaud, where platelet activity increases after 18 h of abstinence, fits well with Dr Criqui's comments about withdrawal. We know that 18 h after people are off alcohol their catechol levels are quite high, which sensitizes their platelets to stimuli such as thrombin. This therefore makes a reasonably consistent story.

Puddey: It would be nice to see these experiments that have been done in rats and dogs reproduced in humans.

I was quite intrigued to see your graph of increasing plasma vitamin E levels with increasing red wine consumption. Vitamin E is quite tightly correlated with total cholesterol and LDL cholesterol. I don't know whether you corrected for total or LDL cholesterol. If you do, do you still see that same relationship?

Renaud: If we correct for cholesterol the relationship is not completely lost, but it is much lower.

Puddey: Shouldn't you be presenting the vitamin E data corrected for cholesterol?

Renaud: We present them in both ways. There are many circumstances in which the plasma level of vitamin E increases along with that of cholesterol or LDL. Could it be more important to have that ratio of vitamin E to LDL increased, or might the total amount of vitamin E be as important? Perhaps the total amount of vitamin E is just as important as the ratio of vitamin E to LDL.

References

Demrow HS, Slane PR, Folts JD 1995 Administration of wine and grape juice inhibits *in vivo* platelet activity and thrombosis in stenosed canine coronary arteries. Circulation 91:1182–1188

Folts JD, Crowell EB, Rowe GG 1976 Platelet aggregation in partially obstructed vessels and its elimination with aspirin. Circulation 54:365–370

Murray CJL, Lopez AD 1997 Mortality by cause for eight regions of the world: Global Burden of Disease Study. Lancet 349:1269–1276

Klatsky AL, Armstrong MA, Friedman GD 1997 Red wine, white wine, liquor, beer and risk for coronary artery disease hospitalization. Am J Cardiol 80:416–420

Renaud S, Morazain R, Godsey F, Dumont E, Thevenon C 1986 Dietary fats, platelet functions and composition in nine groups of French and British farmers. Atherosclerosis 60:37–48

Renaud S, Beswick AD, Fehily AM et al 1992 Alcohol and platelet aggregation: the Caerphilly prospective heart disease study. Am J Clin Nutr 55:1012–1017

Rimm EB, Klatsky A, Grobee D, Stampfer MJ 1996 Review of moderate alcohol consumption and reduced risk of coronary heart disease: is the effect due to beer, wine or spirits? Br Med J 312:731–736

Alcohol and all-cause mortality: an overview

J. Rehm and S. Bondy

Addiction Research Foundation, 33 Russell Street, Toronto, Ontario M5S 2S1, Canada

Abstract. The relationship between alcohol consumption and all-cause mortality is J-shaped in most industrialized countries. The J-shape is the result of the combination of adverse and beneficial effects of alcohol consumption. Adverse effects include several types of cancer (oropharyngeal, oesophageal, liver, laryngeal and breast cancer), other diseases of the aerodigestive tract, diseases of the heart (alcoholic cardiomyopathy, haemorrhagic stroke, arrhythmia, hypertension), addiction-related mental disorders, and accidents and injuries. Beneficial effects are for ischaemic heart disease and ischaemic stroke. The exact shape of the all-cause mortality curve in a given region depends upon the proportion of the population consuming alcohol at different levels, especially heavy consumption, and on the prevalence of the disorders named above. Thus regions with a relatively low prevalence of ischaemic cardiovascular disease show almost no benefits of consumption, and an all-cause mortality curve which is almost exponential. Females experience a minimum mortality risk at a level of alcohol intake which is lower than that associated with the minimum risk for men. Similarly, an upturn in mortality risk occurs at lower intake levels for women than for men. At present, there is no satisfactory explanation for the observation that the shape of the mortality curve varies with the consumption level of the cohort under study. Heavier-drinking cohorts tend to display their minimum risk at relatively higher levels of alcohol intake than cohorts with lower alcohol consumption.

1998 Alcohol and cardiovascular diseases. Wiley, Chichester (Novartis Foundation Symposium 216) p 223–236

What is the exact shape of the curve between average level of alcohol consumption and all-cause mortality for both genders?

The answer to this seemingly simple question in fact requires one to answer each of the following ones as well. However, several comprehensive overviews have been written which make direct comparisons across various studies in terms of the relationship between multiple levels of average alcohol intake and incidence of mortality (Anderson et al 1993, Beaglehole & Jackson 1992). The overall mortality curve has often been described as U-shaped or J-shaped (e.g. Shaper

1990, Marmot & Brunner 1991), implying that abstainers and heavy drinkers have a relatively high mortality risk, but that moderate drinkers are relatively protected. Precisely this pattern of association has been found in some studies for both men and women (Camacho et al 1987, Grønbæk et al 1994, Klatsky et al 1992), or men alone (Doll et al 1994), or in specific age categories (Rehm & Sempos 1995a). However, this dose–response curve is not consistently described in all studies. Results closer to a simple positive association between alcohol intake and mortality have also been reported (Andréasson et al 1991), as have simple protective effects (Cullen et al 1993, Paunio et al 1994).

The most consistent observation across these studies is that subjects in the lowest categories of non-zero alcohol intake have lower mortality risk than abstainers, even after separating out former drinkers from this group, and making lifetime abstainers the basis of comparison. Deviation over the rest of the curve has been attributed to large differences in levels of intake reported by Beaglehole & Jackson (1992), and to characteristics of the population under study (Rehm & Sempos 1995a,b, Andréasson et al 1991; see also below).

Although others may be pending, just one meta-analysis has been published for alcohol and all-cause mortality, based on 16 cohort studies (English et al 1995). Significant J-shaped curves were found for both men and women, with the lowest observed risk found for an average of 10 g of alcohol per day for men, and less for women. For women, an average intake of 20 g per day was associated with a significantly increased risk, which increased thereafter, reaching a 50% increased risk over abstinence at an average of 40 g per day. For males, the risk curve was slightly attenuated. Those who average 30 g per day had the same mortality as abstainers while a significant increase was found for 40 g per day or higher.

Another meta-analysis (Duffy 1995) failed to control for age, but demonstrated the use of regression modelling to try to identify the so-called optimum level of drinking. Attempting to define the point in the dose–response curve at which the risk is lowest is a challenging task (Goetghebeur & Pocock 1995). There is no readily available and widely accepted technique for estimating the optimum point in a U-shaped risk curve. In unpublished work by the authors, estimates of the optimum level depend on the method of estimation being used (including parametric and non-parametric models). Also, when generalized linear modelling is used to estimate the shape of the relationship, the results are influenced by widely spaced observations at the higher levels of consumption, and more generally by the positive skew found in most consumption data.

What do we know about the mix of underlying causes?

The harmful effects and benefits of alcohol with regard to mortality have different shapes of risk curve. The following four areas of causes of mortality have been related negatively to alcohol consumption: cancer, chronic physical and mental disorders which include a reference to alcohol as part of the diagnostic definition (e.g. alcoholic psychosis), accidents and injuries, and certain cardiovascular conditions. All individual causes which are part of these areas will be listed below with International Classification of Diseases (ICD) 9 codes in parentheses.

There is ample evidence for oropharyngeal (ICD 141, 143–146, 148, 149), oesophageal (ICD 150), liver (ICD 155), laryngeal (ICD 161) and breast cancer (ICD 174), and limited evidence for colorectal cancer (ICD 153/154; for overviews see English et al 1995, Alcohol Health and Research World 1997, Longnecker 1995, Verschuren 1993; for breast cancer specifically see Longnecker 1994). The risk curves are often linear but with quite different slopes (Longnecker 1995), with colorectal and breast cancer having the smallest linear effects.

Causes of death for which the diagnosis requires an explicit link to alcohol are trivially related to alcohol as well (for an overview, see English et al 1995). Except for alcohol dependence and abuse, ICD 9 categorizes these conditions by adding the word 'alcoholic' in front of psychiatric or chronic physical health consequences. Mental disorders include in this category alcoholic psychosis (ICD 291), alcohol dependence (ICD 303) and alcohol abuse (ICD 305.0). Chronic physical health conditions related to alcohol, include alcoholic polyneuropathy (ICD 357.5), alcoholic cardiomyopathy (ICD 425.5), alcoholic gastritis (ICD 535.3), alcohol-related pancreatitis (ICD 577.0, 577.1) and alcoholic liver cirrhosis (ICD 571.0–571.3). Their risk curves are often exponential (e.g. cirrhosis, see Anderson 1995) due to the fact that a sustained pattern of heavy drinking is necessary to initiate these diseases. It should be noted that the diagnosis of most of these diseases as cause of mortality does not require a parallel diagnosis of alcohol dependence or abuse.

In addition, the area of accidents and injuries is clearly related to alcohol. English et al (1995) found sufficient evidence in their meta-analyses for a link between alcohol and the following conditions: road injuries (ICD E810–819), alcoholic beverage poisoning (ICD E 560.0), fall injuries (ICD E880–888), fire injuries (ICD E890–899), drowning (ICD E910), occupational and machine injuries (ICD E919–920), and suicide (ICD E950–959). There are other conditions such as assault (ICD E960, 965, 966, 968, 969) or child abuse (ICD E967) which are alcohol-related but are not picked up in individual risk curves because mortality is to others rather than the person consuming. Traditional epidemiological risk curves are quite rare in this area, as most of the evidence comes from emergency room studies and accident statistics. For motor vehicle crashes there is some evidence that the relationship between blood alcohol and risk of collision is exponential (Hurst et al 1994). Alcohol-related mortality in the area of accidents and injuries is different from the other areas, as mortality results here primarily from an acute condition or intoxication, and is not necessarily a consequence of long-term drinking habits (Rehm & Fischer 1997, Rehm et al 1996).

Finally, cardiovascular conditions such as haemorrhagic stroke (ICD 430–432), arrhythmia (ICD 427.0, 427.2, 427.3) or hypertension (ICD 401,405) have been linked to heavy alcohol consumption (Zakhari 1997).

In terms of causes for mortality on which alcohol has beneficial impact, sufficient evidence is available for two conditions: ischaemic heart disease (IHD) (ICD 410–414) and ischaemic stroke (ICD 433–434) (English et al 1995, Zakhari 1997). The risk curves are not clear at this point. Whereas Maclure (1993) has found an L-shaped curve for myocardial infarction with a drop in risk for small amounts of average alcohol consumption which stays low for heavy consumption, Rehm et al (1997) find for females an elevated risk of IHD mortality for average consumption of four drinks a day and more.

Using attributable fractions, the beneficial effects of alcohol outweigh the negative effects. Thus, recent studies have estimated more deaths prevented than caused by alcohol in industrialized countries such as Australia (English et al 1995) or Canada (Single et al 1996). If other measures of impact are used, such as lost life years or disability-adjusted life years, alcohol is seen to cause more harm than benefit. This has to do with the fact that many alcohol-related deaths, especially traumatic deaths, happen quite early in life, whereas the beneficial effect of alcohol on IHD comes into effect only later (e.g. Single et al 1996, Single 1997).

The different cause-specific alcohol–mortality risk curves tend to combine into a J-shape relationship between consumption and all-cause mortality (see above). The actual shape of the J is mainly determined by the relative importance of IHD as a cause of death in a society. In societies with relatively low levels of heart disease, the curve will look almost exponential. However, it should be noted that IHD is often miscoded in countries with apparently low rates (Murray & Lopez 1997a) and, as a result, the protective effect of alcohol can be falsely estimated (e.g. overestimated in France).

How do age and ethnicity influence the shape of the curve?

As the underlying causes mentioned above are distributed unevenly across age and ethnicity, the actual risk curves differ with age and ethnicity. For industrialized countries, up to ages where IHD does not play a role in total mortality (e.g. 40–50) the risk function between alcohol and all-cause mortality should be linear, and this prediction has been confirmed in respective studies (Andréasson et al 1991, 1988, Rehm & Sempos 1995a). For older persons, the curve is more U-shaped, as IHD becomes more and more important and the relative importance of accidents and injuries diminishes.

With respect to ethnicity, there is no reason to believe that there are effects of ethnicity that cannot be explained as a consequence of the differential effect of alcohol on different causes of death. Thus, to predict the influence of alcohol on different ethnicities, the mix of causes of death has to be known. It should be taken into account, however, that social inequality is strongly linked to both mortality (Marmot et al 1984) and ethnicity in many countries, so that apparent effects of alcohol could be explained by this factor.

The cultural role also is influenced by the mix of causes of deaths, as well as by drinking patterns (see below, and also Bondy 1996, Walsh & Rehm 1996). Countries where individuals display patterns of infrequent drinking with high consumption per occasion are predicted to have higher alcohol-related mortality than those in which individuals drink smaller amounts more frequently, even if the alcohol consumption is the same. The biological mechanisms behind the protective effect of alcohol on IHD may require regular drinking patterns (Goldberg et al 1995). In this sense, in countries where individuals display infrequent heavy drinking habits, alcohol is unlikely to have many protective effects.

The Global Burden of Disease study (Murray & Lopez 1997b) contributed detailed calculations on the role of alcohol in different cultures and regions for mortality, and for disability-adjusted life years lost. At this point, the influence of alcohol on these factors is more pronounced in developed than non-developed countries.

How does the consumption level in a cohort influence the shape of the curve?

If a uniform, underlying J-shaped relationship between alcohol consumption and mortality risk truly exists, then the observed relationship in a study will be highly dependent on the levels of intake in the study sample, or less directly on the adequacy of the sample size to describe the mortality risk at higher levels of intake with any real precision (such as is obtained through meta-analysis). Data for a population with high levels of intake by international standards is provided in the rural Italian cohorts of the Seven Countries Study (Farchi et al 1991), in the French Nancy cohort (Renaud & Gueguen 1998, this volume) or from two German cohorts recently reported (Brenner et al 1997, Keil et al 1997). All of these studies also find a curvilinear shape of the risk curve between alcohol consumption and all-cause mortality. However, it seems that in all four studies the nadir is pushed to the right, e.g. compared with other studies, higher consumption is still protective. Thus, Farchi et al (1991) found that the third quintile with an average consumption of about eight standard drinks per day was still showing less risk than abstainers, Brenner et al (1997) estimated a relative risk of 0.75 for a similar group of persons drinking between 50 and 99 g alcohol/day (the equivalent of five to 10 standard drinks), and in Keil et al (1997) only the highest drinking category (on average more than 80 g pure alcohol or the equivalent of more than eight standard drinks) displayed an all-cause mortality rate similar to abstainers. However, there are not enough studies on heavy drinking cohorts to generalize these results further.

Some simple inverse relationships between alcohol intake and mortality could be explained by very low levels of intake in a study population, such as the Nurses' Health Study (Fuchs et al 1995). In many cohort studies, the highest quintiles or other categories of reported consumption are defined by levels of absolute alcohol intake equal to the lower to middle quartiles of the Italian cohorts.

What do we know about patterns of drinking and all-cause mortality?

Groups of drinkers, both within and across cultures, do not all consume alcohol in the same manner. However, the vast majority of published mortality studies were simply never designed to address the effects of different drinking patterns. In most of the cohort studies reviewed, alcohol is but one of many dietary components studied, and intake is measured merely by one or two simple criteria. The most typical instruments are food-frequency records, yielding an estimate of average intake (serving size by frequency of use). However, it is also not uncommon for alcohol intake to have been measured using a single ordinal scale which combines frequency of drinking and heavy use (examples of such responses are 'less than once per month' through 'five or more drinks per day'). Such single-item measures are sometimes, more correctly, identified as frequency measures (Ridker et al 1994).

Cohort studies of relatively homogeneous populations of light drinkers further hamper our ability to study the effects of different patterns of drinking. Study criteria, such as the exclusion of subjects with prior drinking problems, also reduce the generalizability of the findings on all-cause mortality. In fact, arguably, many of the important epidemiological studies on average alcohol intake and mortality could be reinterpreted as studies of the influence of the frequency of drinking in the absence of problem drinking, in selected populations.

The role of various drinking patterns on overall mortality can be studied directly or indirectly, or by extrapolation from clinical and biochemical studies (Bondy 1996). Accidents and other injuries are an important cause of death related to alcohol, and risk of death due to injury or external cause is more closely associated with intoxication than volume. In contrast, increasing evidence suggests that more frequent, smaller amounts of alcohol may enhance beneficial cardiovascular effects, including short-lived anti-clotting effects (Goldberg et al 1995), and lower the risk of myocardial infarction (McElduff & Dobson 1997). A moderate intake spread over the week and taken with meals may also be most beneficial for lipid profiles and levels of atherosclerosis (Gruchow et al 1982, Veenstra et al 1990). It is not clear whether the same frequent moderate drinking also increases the risk of some cancers (Blackwelder et al 1980).

The effect of various styles of drinking on overall mortality risk will again depend on the age of the population and the relative prevalence of various diseases. More detailed study of the timing of alcohol use, size of acute dose, and presence of other carcinogens may be of interest in studying aetiology of some cancers directly attributable to alcohol. However, unlike cardiovascular disease and injury, these rarer events have little impact on total mortality rates.

Finally, even the limited measures in existing epidemiological data can be used to greater effect through the desegregation of measures of average alcohol intake into their various component parts. An example of this approach is found in a case control study of myocardial infarction (McElduff & Dobson 1997) in which usual frequency of drinking and usual quantity per occasion are examined separately. A similar analysis has shown the pattern of drinking to determine the relative proportion of deaths attributable to injury as opposed to other causes (Li et al 1994). However, none of the major cohort studies of alcohol and mortality have to date reported on secondary data analyses, which separate alcohol intake into meaningful component parts.

What are the most urgent research questions in the field?

There is enormous demand from the public, as well as from public health and medical bodies and industry, for a definition of the various levels of alcohol intake associated with lowered and elevated mortality risk (UK Inter-Departmental Working Group 1995, Anderson 1996).

One priority area is the development and application of studies to define more closely the minimum amount of alcohol required for cardiovascular benefit, and thresholds of risk. Statistical techniques for identifying inflexion points in dose–response curves should be applied to this task. In addition, further meta-analytic study and the application of non-parametric modelling represent great opportunities for contributing to this field.

Information about beneficial and harmful patterns of drinking and what determines the risk/benefit balance for the individual is also important. Research on the timing and acute quantity of alcohol intake are important aspects of this (McElduff & Dobson 1997, Jackson et al 1992). Among the first questions that should be addressed are whether we can establish the most important measure of drinking patterns in terms of their ability to predict relevant public health consequences, and how we should incorporate such measures into current and future epidemiological research.

References

Alcohol Health and Research World 1997 Alcohol's effect on organ function. Alcohol Health Res World 21:1–96

Anderson P 1995 Alcohol and risk. In: Holder H, Edwards G (eds) Alcohol and public policy: evidence and issues. Oxford University Press, Oxford, p 82–113

Anderson P 1996 WHO working group on population levels of alcohol consumption. Addiction 91:275–283

Anderson P, Cremona A, Paton A, Turner C, Wallace P 1993 The risk of alcohol. Addiction 88:1493–1508

Andréasson S, Allebeck P, Romelsjø A 1988 Alcohol and mortality among young men: longitudinal study of Swedish conscripts. Br Med J 296:1021–1025

Andréasson S, Romelsjø A, Allebeck P 1991 Alcohol, social factors and mortality among young men. Br J Addict 86:877–887

Beaglehole R, Jackson R 1992 Alcohol, cardiovascular diseases and all causes of death: a review of the epidemiological evidence. Drug Alcohol Rev 11:275–290

Blackwelder WC, Yano K, Rhoads GG, Kagan A, Gordon T, Palesh Y 1980 Alcohol and mortality: the Honolulu Heart Study. Am J Med 68:164–169

Bondy S 1996 Overview of studies on drinking patterns and their reported consequences. Addiction 91:1663–1674

Brenner H, Arndt V, Rothenbacher D, Schuberth S, Fraisse E, Fliedner T 1997 The association between alcohol consumption and all-cause mortality in a cohort of male employees in the German construction industry. Int J Epidemiol 26:85–91

Camacho TC, Kaplan GA, Cohen RD 1987 Alcohol consumption and mortality in Alameda County. J Chronic Dis 40:229–236

Cullen K, Knuiman MW, Ward NJ 1993 Alcohol and mortality in Busselton, Western Australia. Am J Epidemiol 137:242–248

Doll R, Peto R, Hall E, Wheatley K, Gray R 1994 Mortality in relation to consumption of alcohol: 13 years' observation on male British doctors. Br Med J 309:911–918

Duffy JC 1995 Alcohol consumption and all-cause mortality. Int J Epidemiol 24:100–105

English D, Holman D, Milne E et al 1995 The quantification of drug caused morbidity and mortality in Australia. Commonwealth Department of Human Services and Health, Canberra

Farchi G, Fidanza F, Mariotti S, Menotti A 1991 Alcohol and mortality in the Italian rural cohorts of the Seven Countries Study. Int J Epidemiol 21:74–82

Fuchs C, Stampfer MJ, Colditz GA et al 1995 Alcohol consumption and mortality among women. N Engl J Med 332:1245–1250

Goetghebeur EJT, Pocock SJ 1995 Detection and estimation of J-shaped risk-response relationships. J R Statist Soc 158:107–121

Goldberg DM, Hahn SE, Parkes JG 1995 Beyond alcohol: beverage consumption and cardiovascular mortality. Clin Chim Acta 237:155–187

Grønbæk M, Deis A, Sørensen TIA et al 1994 Influence of sex, age, body mass index, and smoking on alcohol intake and mortality. Br Med J 308:302–306

Gruchow HW, Hoffman RG, Anderson AF, Barboriack JJ 1982 Effects of drinking patterns on the relationship between alcohol and coronary occlusion. Atherosclerosis 43:393–404

Hurst PM, Harte WJ, Firth WJ 1994 The Grand Rapids dip revisited. Accid Anal Prev 26:647–654

Jackson R, Scragg R, Beaglehole R 1992 Does recent alcohol consumption reduce the risk of acute myocardial infarction and coronary death in regular drinkers? Am J Epidemiol 136:819–824

Keil U, Chambless LE, Döring A, Filipiak B, Stieber J 1997 The relation of alcohol intake to coronary heart disease and all-cause mortality in a beer-drinking population. Epidemiology 8:150–156

Klatsky AL, Armstrong MA, Friedman GD 1992 Alcohol and mortality. Ann Intern Med 117:646–654

Li G, Smith G, Baker S 1994 Drinking behavior in relation to cause of death among US adults. Am J Public Health 84:1402–1406

Longnecker MP 1994 Alcoholic beverage consumption in relation to risk of breast cancer: meta-analysis and review. Cancer Causes Control 5:73–82

Longnecker MP 1995 Alcohol consumption and risk of cancer in humans: an overview. Alcohol 12:87–96

Maclure M 1993 Demonstration of deductive meta-analysis: ethanol intake and risk of myocardial infarction. Epidemiol Rev 15:328–351

Marmot M, Brunner E 1991 Alcohol and cardiovascular disease: the status of the U-shaped curve. Br Med J 303:565–568

Marmot MG, Shipley M, Rose G 1984 Inequalities in death—specific explanations of a general pattern. Lancet 1:1003–1006

McElduff P, Dobson A 1997 How much alcohol and how often? Population-based case-control study of alcohol consumption and risk of major coronary event. Br Med J 314:1159–1164

Murray C, Lopez A 1997a Mortality by cause for eight regions of the world: Global Burden of Disease study. Lancet 349:1269–1276

Murray C, Lopez A 1997b Global mortality, disability, and the contribution of risk factors: Global Burden of Disease study. Lancet 349:1436–1442

Paunio M, Heinonen O, Virtamo J et al 1994 HDL cholesterol and mortality in Finnish men with special reference to alcohol intake. Circulation 90:2909–2918

Rehm J, Sempos CT 1995a Alcohol consumption and all-cause mortality. Addiction 90:471–480

Rehm J, Sempos CT 1995b Alcohol consumption and all-cause mortality—questions about causality, confounding and methodology. Addiction 90:493–498

Rehm J, Fischer B 1997 Measuring harm: implications for alcohol epidemiology. In: Plant M, Single E, Stockwell T (eds) Alcohol: minimizing the harm. What works? Free Association Books Ltd, London, p 248–261

Rehm J, Ashley M J, Room R et al 1996 On the emerging paradigm of drinking patterns and their social and health consequences. Addiction 91:1615–1621

Rehm JT, Bondy S J, Sempos CT, Vuong CV 1997 Alcohol consumption and CHD morbidity and mortality. Am J Epidemiol 146:495–501

Renaud S, Gueguen R 1998 The French paradox and wine drinking In: Alcohol and cardiovascular diseases. Wiley, Chichester (Novartis Found Symp 216) p 208–222

Ridker PM, Vaughan DE, Stampfer M J, Glynn R J, Hennekens CH 1994 Association of moderate alcohol consumption and plasma concentration of endogenous tissue-type plasminogen activator. JAMA 272:929–933

Shaper AG 1990 Alcohol and mortality: a review of prospective studies. Br J Addict 85:837–847

Single E 1997 The concept of harm reduction and its application to alcohol: the 6th Dorothy Black lecture. Drugs: education, prevention and policy 4:7–16

Single E, Robson L, Xie X, Rehm J 1996 The costs of substance abuse in Canada. Canadian Centre on Substance Abuse, Ottawa

UK Inter-Departmental Working Group 1995 Report on sensible drinking. Department of Health, London. Crown Copyright: 3647 IP 5R December

Veenstra J, Ockhuizen T, van de Pol H, Wedel M, Schaafsma G 1990 Effects of a moderate dose of alcohol on blood lipids and lipoproteins postprandially and in the fasting state. Alcohol Alcohol 25:371–377

Verschuren P 1993 Health issues related to alcohol consumption. ILSI Press Europe, Brussels

Walsh G, Rehm J 1996 Daily drinking and harm. Contemp Drug Prob 23:465–478
Zakhari S 1997 Alcohol and the cardiovascular system: molecular mechanisms for beneficial and
     harmful action. Alcohol Health Res World 21:21–29

DISCUSSION

Grønbæk: Denmark is one of the countries with a high level of alcohol intake per
capita. Nevertheless, in the Copenhagen City Heart Study we found a nadir with
regard to all-cause mortality at around one drink per day.

   Another factor that may cause some of the differences in the shape of the U-curve
from country to country is not only the potential misclassification of intake, which
may vary between countries, but also the fact that alcohol is a cofactor in the
development of many of these diseases. Physical activity, smoking and diet are a
few of the many factors attributable to risk of coronary heart disease. The shape of
the curve will therefore also be dependent on the distribution of these component
causes in the actual country under study.

   Peters: Another point of interest is the nadir in men and women: is there a general
shift to the left?

   Rehm: Yes, for all-cause mortality it is clear that the nadir for males is higher than
for females, and this is entirely due to chronic diseases. For some reason we find that
in the blood alcohol level and accident studies, contrary to all the biological
plausibility, the risks of males and females to run into the same problem with the
same blood alcohol level is about equal (Midanik et al 1996). However, the risk for
liver cirrhosis or cancer begins to be elevated much earlier for females than for
males (e.g. English et al 1995).

   Anderson: The nadir also must be age-related. Where is the cut-off when you
move from a straight line to the J-shaped curve?

   Rehm: The work on the nadirs is something I wanted to present here in a
workshop-type atmosphere. I believe that there's no biological reason for those
nadirs, and I think it must have something to do with questionnaire answering
and culture.

   Shaper: What worries me is that in almost all the studies you've shown, you are
using some measure of volume and frequency to give a weekly total intake. If we
move from that, we go back to the way we originally collected our data. We
separated the men into those who were predominantly daily drinkers, i.e. those
that drank throughout the week, and those who were weekend drinkers. The
problem was that we could not go on presenting them in that way as we could
not compare our findings with anybody else! Are you suggesting that we ought
to be presenting the data by the pattern of drinking rather than amount taken in
during an average period?

Bondy: This is something that we are also struggling with in doing things such as our regular cross-sectional surveys. We also include a generic quantity/frequency measure: we use it a lot because we know that it's directly comparable to other data. If your underlying hypothesis about the cause and effect deals with volume of drinking or total dose, I don't believe that you do need to separate things out, or do anything other than what you are doing now, measuring volume, because that is what you are biologically interested in. However, I think that we are at a point with a number of these specific effects we're studying where we do want to tease out mechanisms and we want to look at differences in drinking pattern. We would then make hypotheses about how different drinking patterns would have a differential effect. I think it's also important to look at pattern in terms of trying to generalize this information to the general public; for instance, to obtain information that may be generalized to populations that have an element of binge drinking. That's precisely the type of information that people come to the public health agencies for. Physician groups come to public health agencies and specifically ask us to describe the patterns of drinking which are hazardous: it is a tall order to do this, and it would be nice if more of this information were available from the studies. I would like people to use measures that allow one to tease out patterns for additional analysis.

Shaper: This will lead to much more complex presentations of material, where we present the detailed alcohol intake patterns and also try to present data that can be more generally comparable. I suspect that referees and editors of journals would be unreceptive.

Bondy: There are a couple of papers I have recently come across where a specific point of the article has been to discuss differences in drinking pattern. McElduff & Dobson (1997) talk about the difference between regular small amounts versus larger amounts less frequently, specifically in relation to cardiovascular disease. Also, Gruchow et al (1982) took differences in drinking pattern and compared that to coronary artery occlusion. I can also think of a couple of articles, one by Ridker et al (1994), where they identified what would typically be called a volume measure as a frequency measure. I don't think that every paper needs to cover all these aspects, just what is relevant to the hypothesis being tested.

Peters: It's very interesting that you are advocating a reductionist view. Those of us who look after people with alcohol problems go into great detail as to when, how, where and why people consume alcohol. We also put great emphasis on the time of day, ambience etc. in which individuals drink.

Rehm: On the question of costs related to alcoholism versus costs related to alcohol, that is, alcohol-related costs stemming from persons who would not qualify for a diagnosis of alcohol abuse or dependence. If you look at all alcohol-related costs in Ontario, Canada, only 50% are associated with behaviours of non-alcoholics (Rehm 1998). This ratio should always be taken into account when planning for research or setting health priorities. However, most research on alcohol, and the overwhelming majority of the biological models, only deal with addiction and not with the wider range of alcohol-related problems.

Anderson: In many countries, rates of coronary heart disease deaths, alcohol consumption and cigarette smoking are all coming down: if we think about this whole issue of alcohol and heart disease in that context, does it raise any questions in relation to the future design of studies?

Keil: The Global Burden of Disease projections for the year 2020 are that ischaemic heart disease will be on top of the list in practically all countries of the world. This would suggest that alcohol may have a greater role to play in the future as a protective regimen against ischaemic heart disease.

Klatsky: Does the difference between the amount of alcohol that people report on surveys and the amount sold differ by beverage? In other words, is a larger proportion of the beer and wine sold reported in terms of the survey data than for distilled spirits?

Fillmore: I don't think this has been analysed.

Peters: In multicultural societies, if the nadir differs among ethnic groups this will cause enormous problems for public health messages. Are there prospects of people doing more work in this field?

Rehm: Together with the Alcohol Research Group, we are currently working on a NIAAA grant to examine the effects of race on the alcohol–mortality relationship. It is a three group comparison: whites versus blacks versus hispanics. At this point we do not have the full dataset, but based on what the overall statistics say, it seems that the shape of the curve is not much related to the ethnicity once you control for social class. This is important: we have found that in a lot of our work, social class effects mask alcohol effects. If you look at ethnicity in the USA there is a clear social class gradient between hispanics, blacks and whites.

Klatsky: Our study populations are multiracial, with 60% white/Caucasian, 30% African American and 10% Asian American. The alcohol–CHD relationship and the alcohol–total mortality relationship are quite similar in these ethnic groups. These data are of course controlled for educational attainment, which is our marker for social class.

Criqui: I guess my comments are a bit provincial because they apply only to the USA, but we have a substantial African American population and a dramatically growing Latino population. We have a fair amount of information on cardiovascular disease epidemiological differences in those groups. In African Americans there is a predominance of hypertensive disease, and they have higher HDL levels at baseline and more problems with stroke. One might think that the trade-off between some of the cerebrovascular hypertensive-related things might be a little different in that group. The Latino population tends to disproportionately have more trouble with diabetes and syndrome X (low HDL, high triglyceride), so one might speculate that alcohol may have somewhat different effects in this group. We really need data on this subject before talking about any kind of inventions or public health issues within the USA.

Farrell: In the North American and UK data, moderate drinking is more associated with middle-class males. Serge Renaud, is moderate drinking more evenly spread across the French population?

Renaud: Yes, at least in our eastern France study, moderate drinking is more evenly distributed across the population. As a matter of fact, the workers drank slightly more wine than the other social classes. Therefore it is in France that we have to look for the effects of wine on health, since its consumption is not clustered primarily in the higher social classes. One study in Edinburgh (Jepson et al 1995) has shown that there was an inverse association between wine drinking and peripheral atherosclerosis. When these data were adjusted for social class, the inverse association was lost. In France, adjustment for social class obviously does not change the inverse relationship between wine drinking and cardiovascular mortality.

Shaper: I hesitate to talk again about non-drinkers, but in your meta-analysis you showed a very slight J-shaped curve, and in discussing the non-drinkers you almost casually said that they don't really matter. As you don't have any information on the characteristics of those non-drinkers, and all the rest of your curve is linear, could you just say something more about why you were so casual about those non-drinkers?

Bondy: I wouldn't say I was casual about them: I can't do much about this at this point. This was a meta-analysis conducted by English and Holman in Australia (English et al 1995), and it is the only one published on all-cause mortality to date.

Shaper: So it cannot take into account the possibility that the non-drinkers may be an unhealthy group.

Rehm: In another cohort, we've done several analyses on the curve with different definitions of the abstainer group. If you exclude the former drinkers, who tend to be sicker, the J-shape remains and the upturn tends to be way steeper (Rehm & Stempos 1995).

Shaper: Presumably the benefit then diminishes?

Rehm: Even with lifetime teetotallers, who were not in anyway more unhealthy, as a comparison group, there was a beneficial effect.

Shaper: It is smaller?

Rehm: Yes.

References

English D, Holman D, Milne E et al 1995 The quantification of drug caused morbidity and mortality in Australia. Commonwealth Department of Human Services and Health, Canberra

Gruchow HW, Hoffmann RG, Anderson A J, Barboriak J J 1982 Effects of drinking patterns on the relationship between alcohol and coronary occlusion. Atherosclerosis 43:393–404

Jepson RG, Fowkes FGR, Donnan PT, Housley E 1995 Alcohol intake as a risk factor for peripheral arterial disease in the general population in the Edinburgh Artery Study. Eur J Epidemiol 11:9–14

McElduff P, Dobson A 1997 How much alcohol and how often? Population-based case-control study of alcohol consumption and risk of major coronary event. Br Med J 314:1159–1164

Midanik LT, Tam TW, Greenfield TK, Caetano R 1996 Risk functions for alcohol-related problems in a 1988 US national sample. Addiction 91:1427–1437

Rehm J 1998 Ökonomische Aspekte von Substanzmißbrauch. In: Gaspar, Mann, Rommelspacher (eds) Stoffliche Suchterkrankungen. Thieme Verlag, Stuttgart, in press

Rehm J, Sempos CT 1995 Alcohol consumption and all-cause mortality: questions about causality, confounding and methodology. Addiction 90:493–498

Ridker PM, Vaughan DE, Stampfer MJ, Glynn RJ, Hennekens CH 1994 Association of moderate alcohol consumption and plasma concentration of endogenous tissue-type plasminogen activator. JAMA 272:929–933

Alcohol, cardiovascular diseases and public health policy

Peter Anderson

Lifestyles and Health Unit, World Health Organization, 8 Scherfigsvej, 2100 Copenhagen Denmark

Abstract. Public health policy should aim to reduce the harm done by alcohol use, whilst recognizing its real and perceived benefits. The reduced risk of coronary heart disease (CHD) with the consequent reduction of mortality for some people in older age is one such benefit. The increased risk of sudden coronary death from acute alcohol intoxication is one such harm. A number of policies have been demonstrated to be effective in the reduction of the harm done by alcohol use, at least in industrialized countries. These are: enforcement of a minimum drinking age; drink–drive deterrence; enforced prevention of intoxication in public drinking places; controls on access to alcohol, including restrictions on numbers of licensed premises and hours and days of sale; and taxation policy to regulate the affordability of alcohol. Many of these strategies seem unlikely to have a direct effect on drinking relevant for reduced risk of CHD, but are likely to have a direct beneficial effect on drinking relevant for sudden coronary death. The level of alcohol consumption associated with the lowest mortality rate for a population will vary depending on patterns of ill health and causes of death. In countries with high rates of CHD the per capita level may be in the order of about three litres of absolute alcohol per year among drinking adults. In countries with low rates of CHD, the level is likely to be substantially lower. Many countries in which alcohol is readily available are consuming at a level substantially above three litres per capita of drinking adults per year and in these countries public health policy should continue to advise action to reduce per capita consumption.

1998 Alcohol and cardiovascular diseases. Wiley, Chichester (Novartis Foundation Symposium 216) p 237–257

Alcohol is used in many, although not all, cultures. The meaning of drinking varies in different contexts — from cultures where traditional patterns are occasional and celebratory to those in which alcohol has played a role as part of the diet.

Alcohol can bring both benefit and harm to the individual. These effects can occur in both the short and the long term. Most of the scientific evidence about benefit as well as harm derives from industrialized countries and cultures where alcohol consumption is largely accepted. Any possible benefit from alcohol should therefore be considered in its sociocultural context and cannot be projected onto those cultures and societies where drinking is not acceptable and abstention is the norm.

Alcohol has significant adverse effects on the health of individuals, families and communities. The effects are diffuse and costly and are not confined to a minority of easily identified heavier drinkers. In all cultures in which alcohol has been freely available, policies, both formal and informal, have been developed to reduce the harm associated with its use.

Alcohol and ill health

Alcohol can adversely affect a number of aspects of drinkers' lives, including harm to health, happiness, home life, friendships, work, studies, employment opportunities and finances (Room et al 1995). These self-reported adverse effects increase with increasing alcohol consumption, although their frequency is affected by different patterns of drinking.

Alcohol is a dependence-producing drug and this dependence is associated with an increased risk of morbidity and mortality. Survey data show a positive relationship between self-reported levels of alcohol consumption and reports of dependence indicators such as withdrawal, tolerance, craving and impairment of control over drinking (Midanik et al 1996).

Alcohol and frequency of heavy drinking are associated with an increased risk of accidents, including road traffic accidents, intentional violence both towards self and others, suicide, family violence, violent crime, engaging in criminal behaviour, and victimization, including robbery and rape. The association increases with increasing levels of alcohol consumption and is influenced by patterns of drinking (Romelsjö 1995).

Alcohol and mortality

In research conducted both at the societal and individual level, alcohol has been found to increase the risk of death from a number of specific causes, including injury from traffic accidents and other trauma, violence, suicide, liver cirrhosis, cancers of the upper aerodigestive tract, cancer of the liver, breast cancer, haemorrhagic stroke, alcoholic psychosis, alcohol dependence and pancreatitis (Edwards et al 1994, English et al 1995).

The risk of coronary heart disease (CHD) is, however, reduced by alcohol use. The reduced risk of CHD is associated with reported alcohol consumption at a range of from one drink every other day to up to six drinks per day (Maclure 1993). Much of the reduction in risk occurs by reported consumption levels of about one drink every other day. The reduction in risk is not dose responsive, resulting in an L-shaped curve, with no substantial further reduction in risk occurring beyond reported consumption of about one to two drinks a day. The mechanisms underlying the reduced risk of CHD from alcohol are likely to be an elevation of HDL cholesterol and interference in coagulation mechanisms. Alcohol's impact on coagulation mechanisms is likely to be immediate and since lipid modification in older age groups produces significant benefit, the impact mediated through elevation of HDL cholesterol can probably be achieved by alcohol consumption in middle and older age (Criqui 1994).

When the relationship between alcohol consumption and total mortality is examined, the shape of the curve depends on the distribution of causes of death amongst the population studied and on the level and patterns of alcohol consumption within the population (World Health Organization 1995). At younger ages deaths from traffic accidents and violence (which are increased by alcohol consumption) predominate, while CHD deaths (which are reduced by alcohol consumption) are rare. The position is reversed at older ages.

There is a positive, largely linear relationship between reported usual alcohol consumption and total mortality in populations or groups with low CHD rates (which includes younger people everywhere). On the other hand there is a J or, among older populations, a U shaped relationship between reported usual alcohol consumption and total mortality in populations with high rates of CHD. The exact age when the relationship changes from linear to a J or U shape will depend on the distribution of causes of death, but in most industrialized countries this probably occurs at about an age of death of 50 to 60 years (Rehm & Sempos 1995).

In the relationship between alcohol consumption and total mortality, a number of potential confounders could influence the shape of the curve, the size of the effect and the level of alcohol consumption associated with the lowest risk of mortality. Differences in psychosocial characteristics between abstainers and lighter drinkers are potentially relevant confounders (Fillmore 1995).

Few studies have been able to address the issue of social integration, which can itself be related to the risk of mortality. This is likely to be lower in both abstainers and heavier drinkers relative to lighter drinkers. In analyses which fail to control adequately for this influence there will be an exaggeration of the size of the protective effect of alcohol on CHD and a bias towards a reduced risk at higher consumption levels (Skog 1995).

Inaccuracies in alcohol consumption measures, misclassification of abstainers and the temporal instability of alcohol consumption could all affect the observed relationship between benefit and harm at different consumption levels.

In societies with relatively low levels of violence, the number of deaths from alcohol-related causes in the younger sector of the population is low relative to alcohol's contribution to mortality in the older age groups. However, when looked at in terms of the numbers of preventable potential years of life lost the societal impact is seen more clearly.

Estimates of alcohol-related mortality in Australia compared the impact of higher levels of alcohol use with lower levels of drinking (English et al 1995). Aetiologic fractions were calculated for alcohol use of more than 40 g of absolute alcohol per day for men and more than 20 g for women. The decision to compare higher with lower levels of alcohol consumption meant that the impact of alcohol on CHD was not included in the estimates as there was inadequate evidence that the marginal exposure between lower and higher alcohol intake had an impact on CHD. It was estimated that in 1992, consumption of alcohol above the 20 and 40 g per day levels contributed to 2.9% of all deaths and 7.3% of all person years of life lost.

Societal-level data provide a complementary way of assessing the relationship between alcohol and mortality (Norström 1995). Societal estimates have the advantage of not being subject to selection bias and provide information about the impact of alcohol at the population level. There have been a number of aggregate level analyses which have examined this relationship using time-series analysis. A positive relationship between alcohol consumption and all-cause mortality has been found in France (1885–1958), in Prussia (1875–1918) and in Sweden (1860–1913). According to these findings, a one litre change in adult consumption was associated with a 1% change in mortality among middle-aged men. During these years CHD was not as common a cause of death as it has been in recent decades.

Other aggregate analyses have demonstrated alcohol's impact on mortality from specific causes. For example in an analysis of alcohol-related mortality which included liver cirrhosis, alcoholic psychosis, alcoholism, pancreatitis and cancers of the upper digestive tract and of the pancreas, there was a positive relationship found between male mortality from these causes and aggregate alcohol consumption of alcohol in Norway, Sweden and Denmark (see Norström 1995). A one litre change in alcohol consumption was associated with a 20–40% change in mortality. The estimate of the attributable fraction of these alcohol-augmented diseases in a country with a consumption of six litres of absolute alcohol per capita was 70%.

Fatal injury, much of which was from traffic accidents, has been found to have a positive relationship with alcohol in Sweden. The attributable fraction for fatal injury in the context of a country with six litres of absolute alcohol per capita was 40% (see Norström 1995).

Suicide is a cause of death which has also received attention in aggregate-level analyses (see Edwards et al 1994). Two US studies reported positive relationships between consumption and suicide rates temporally and cross sectionally. Significant relationships have also been established in a fairly large number of time-series studies (see Norström 1995). These analyses, which have been performed in a standardized way to facilitate comparisons, include Denmark,

Finland, France, Hungary, Norway, Sweden and Portugal. There is a general pattern from these studies which suggests that the higher the alcohol consumption in society, the weaker the alcohol effect on suicide (Norström 1995). A one litre change in per capita alcohol consumption was associated with a 10% change in suicide rates for Norway and Sweden. A one litre change was associated with a 3–4% change in suicide rates for France and Portugal. The estimates suggest an attributable fraction of about 45% for a consumption level of six litres of absolute alcohol per capita.

Of particular interest is the unprecedented sharp increase in mortality that occurred in most of the countries of the former Soviet Union during the first half of the 1990s, particularly in 1992–1994 (Fig. 1). For example, male life expectancy in the Russian Federation decreased from 64.9 years in 1987 to 57.6 years to 1994. The increase in mortality from cardiovascular diseases and external causes of death in the middle-aged population were responsible for about three quarters of this decline in life expectancy (World Health Organization 1997). As these changes in mortality and life expectancy coincided with the initial phase of transition to a free market economy, it is natural to attribute this health deterioration to the effect of the economic difficulties of the transition.

However, when describing the mortality trends during the transition, it is also necessary to account for the sharp improvement in mortality which occurred in

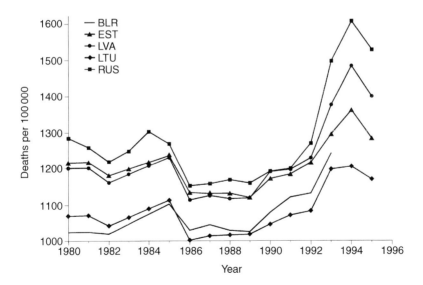

FIG. 1.   Trends in overall standardized death rates, selected countries of eastern Europe, from 1980 to the latest available year. BLR, Belarus; EST, Estonia; LVA, Latvia; LTU, Lithuania; RUS, Russia. Source: data from the WHO Regional Office for Europe.

1985–1986, as the result of the strict anti-alcohol campaign launched in the former Soviet Union in June 1985. The campaign caused an immediate and sharp decline in alcohol consumption and an associated reduction in the number of fatal accidents, suicide and homicide. With time and perestroika, the strict anti-alcohol measures were lifted and alcohol consumption increased sharply during the 1990s. At the same time, mortality from external causes started to increase, particularly during 1993–1994.

The role of alcohol in mortality from external causes is generally understandable. However, it is more difficult to accept that changes in alcohol consumption had a similar detrimental effect on mortality from diseases of the circulatory system (Fig. 2). Premature cardiovascular mortality trends in most countries of the former Soviet Union show a typical sharp decline in 1986, followed by a gradual increase until about 1991–1992 when it reached the pre-campaign levels of 1984–1985. For 1993–1994 it shows a further sharp increase as in the case of mortality from external causes.

There is some evidence indicating that a large proportion of the initial decrease (during 1985–1986) and the subsequent increase in cardiovascular mortality between 1986 and 1994 can be attributed to sudden cardiac deaths (pre-hospital

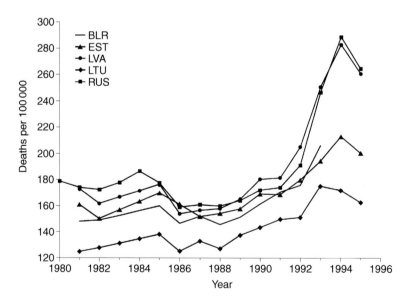

FIG. 2. Trends in standardized death rates from diseases of the circulatory system, age 0–64, selected countries of eastern Europe, from 1980 to the latest available year. BLR, Belarus; EST, Estonia; LVA, Latvia; LTU, Lithuania; RUS, Russia. Source: data from the WHO Regional Office for Europe.

and/or within 24 hours of the onset of symptoms) (World Health Organization 1997). According to data from the MONICA project centre in Moscow, the share of routinely registered sudden coronary deaths in total mortality from ischaemic heart disease among males aged 25–64 years increased from 43% in 1987 to 69% in 1993. Twenty per cent of these sudden coronary deaths resulted from alcohol intoxication, with blood alcohol concentrations of 3.5 g/l or higher. Another 10–30% of deaths which show postmortem alcohol concentration of less than 3.5 g/l could also be caused by alcohol intoxication prior to death. Further, the number of sudden cardiovascular deaths which were caused by alcohol poisoning increased during 1992–1993, as compared to previous years. During the period 1985–1991, 4741 sudden cardiovascular deaths were registered in the project area among population of age 25–64 (autopsy rate 65%). The registered cause of death, i.e. cardiovascular disease (CVD), was not confirmed by autopsy data in 15% of the cases, including about 6% which should be re-classified to alcohol poisoning (post-mortem blood alcohol exceeded 3.5 g/l). In the period 1992–1993, 1611 sudden CVD deaths were registered in the same area (average 805 per year or about 20% increase, as compared to the previous period). According to autopsy data, about 20% of these deaths should now be reassigned to other, non-CVD causes, including 14% attributable to alcohol poisoning. It means that approximately 56% of the increase in sudden 'CVD' deaths between the two above-mentioned periods should be attributed to alcohol poisoning. It is also very likely that in a large number of the remaining cases, i.e. those with post-mortem blood alcohol below the 3.5 g/l level, alcohol intoxication was also a triggering factor.

Taking into consideration that sudden CVD deaths account for close to half of total CVD mortality among males before the age of 65, it can be estimated that about one-quarter to one-third of the observed recent increase in the registered CVD morality among adult males in Moscow should actually be attributed to alcohol intoxication. There are no reasons why this proportion could not be applicable to CVD mortality also in other parts of the Russian Federation or neighbouring countries which are in a similar situation in respect of mortality trends and alcohol consumption.

J-shaped functions at the aggregate level

It is important to consider what kind of relationship one would get at the aggregate level, if the individual level relationship is J-shaped. What would happen to population mortality rates if the aggregate consumption level increased? This would depend to a large extent on the distribution of drinking within the population. If those who consumed less than the minimum risk level increased their intake, while those who consumed in excess of the minimum risk level cut back, the mortality rate must decrease. However, this is not a likely outcome, for it would imply that everybody adjusted their alcohol intake so as to maximize life expectancy. On the contrary, one could argue that if a substantial fraction of the population (the light drinkers) started to drink more heavily, then those who already drank above the minimum risk level might be induced to drink more, since they would find themselves living in an environment with more opportunities to drink.

In setting public health policies in the presence of a J-shaped risk function, it is crucial to make a distinction between the minimum risk level of intake for the individual and for the population. Due to the long tail of the consumption distribution, it is likely that the mean minimum risk consumption level for a population will be considerably lower than that for an individual. How much lower will depend on the shape of the risk function and on changes in the distribution of alcohol consumption as the consumption level of the population changes. In not too unrealistic circumstances (proportional changes in consumption), the minimum risk consumption level for the population could be less that that for an individual drinker by a factor of as much as five (Skog 1992). In countries with high rates of CHD the per capita level associated with minimum risk for mortality may be in the order of about three litres of absolute alcohol among drinking adults. In countries with low rates of CHD, the level is likely to be substantially lower. This would imply that most developed countries are already consuming in excess of the minimum risk level for populations. If this is the case, then an overall increase in intake that is triggered by the prospects of health benefits for light drinkers could in fact result in an overall increase in the mortality rate. However, a substantial change in the whole distribution of alcohol could, if it occurred simultaneously for example through alcohol rationing, theoretically prevent this from happening (Edwards et al 1994).

Implications for alcohol policies

Policy development is a process of resolving conflicting demands (Casswell 1995). In the alcohol field the conflicting demands include those of the market and those of the public good. They also involve finding a balance between the perceived benefits and enjoyment of drinking and the costs associated with alcohol use. Perception of the balance between risks and benefits will differ depending on what aspects are considered. Is attention focused only on delayed mortality among the older population or on potential years of life lost and alcohol's impact on community and family safety and well being?

The precise nature of the dose–response relationships found between alcohol and different aspects of harm is also relevant to policy development. Some relationships, such as that between alcohol and liver cirrhosis, show an exponential curve with no effect on the pattern of drinking. In response to this kind of dose–response relationship the targeting of effective strategies at heavier consumers only would result in a reduction of harm, since the heavier drinkers contribute a much larger fraction of all cases than the light and moderate drinkers.

Other relationships show more linear risk functions such as those between alcohol intake and both suicide and trauma injuries. The majority of these kinds of negative experiences are found among lighter and more moderate drinkers, when characterized by volume of drinking over time, because the majority of all instances of drunkenness, which underlies these harms, are found among these groups (Stockwell et al 1996, Skog 1995). In relation to alcohol-related harm of this sort the targeting of prevention strategies only at heavier drinkers, even if effectively applied, would not succeed in minimizing the harm.

Effective strategies which affect the drinking population more generally will, however, influence alcohol-related harm when the risk function is both moderately and very curved. This is because they have the potential to affect all of the drinkers who contribute to the experience of alcohol-related harm. If they could be effectively applied, preventive strategies targeted at occasions of harmful alcohol consumption would minimize harm resulting from episodes of intoxication.

Appropriate response strategies should be related to an assessment of their likely effectiveness. In general there are two differing approaches to the reduction of alcohol-related harm. The first attempts to persuade the individual to drink in a certain way by the provision of information and advice. The second attempts to change the drinker's environment to help shape the drinking patterns and contexts.

Educational programmes, when conducted in isolation in schools or via the mass media, have been found to be ineffective in changing drinking behaviour (Montonen 1995). With far fewer resources alcohol education has had to compete with messages about alcohol from commercial producers. The latter contradict the emphasis of the educational efforts and are likely to reinforce the cultural and social patterns of drinking. Compared with the messages from the public health field the educational messages of the vested interest groups are likely to resonate more strongly with the target group of heavy and potentially heavy consumers, given that advertising does not try to change their beliefs about alcohol but to support and uphold it.

The power of the media working on behalf of the alcohol beverage industry is illustrated by the aftermath of a CBS *60 minutes* documentary 'The French Paradox' which was broadcast to 21 million US homes in 1991, giving information about the reduced risk of CHD associated with alcohol use. It is reported that eight months after the 'heart-friendly red wine story' was broadcast sales of red wine had increased by 45% (See Casswell 1995).

In contrast to educational strategies, a number of strategies concentrating on the drinker's environment have been shown to have an effect on the experience of alcohol-related harm. These are: enforcement of minimum drinking age; drink–drive deterrence, particularly the use of random breath testing; prevention of intoxication in public drinking places; restricting access to alcohol; and taxation policy (Edwards et al 1994).

In the light of findings of the reduced risk of CHD it is relevant to examine the various environmental strategies for reducing harm in order to assess the likelihood of them influencing drinking which might reduce the risk of CHD among the older sector of the population. Many of the environmental strategies seem unlikely to have a major direct effect on drinking relevant for reduced risk of CHD. For instance, taxation policy has a disproportionate effect on younger and heavier drinkers.

There remains, however, the possibility that even without a direct effect on drinking patterns that reduce the risk of CHD, any decrease in heavier drinking amongst the population could have an indirect effect on lighter-drinking older consumers. The extent to which a pattern of light drinking for 'medicinal' reasons among older people at risk of CHD might emerge independent of the usual social network influences on drinking is not known.

In large part, continued commitment to the population-level policies is based on their effectiveness in contrast to the ineffectiveness of the alternative strategies available. This effectiveness is related to the greater direct impact of shaping the collective environment to make healthy choices easier choices, compared with attempts to persuade individuals to change their drinking while leaving the environmental influences unchanged.

Any impact of the effective available environmental strategies on the drinking of older people which might reduce the risk of CHD must be interpreted within the perspective of the competing policy goals in the alcohol arena. In the final analysis this may be a comparison between an increase in the life expectancy of the older sectors of the population by a few years and the loss of many years of potential life of the younger heavy drinkers who are killed in traffic accidents or as a result of alcohol-related violence. Another comparison has to be drawn with the effects of heavier drinking on the family, friends and work environment of the drinker, in particular the effect on women and children of alcohol-related family violence.

Conclusion

While the evidence of an association between alcohol use and reduced risk of CHD has introduced an important new element into the policy equation, the conclusion to be drawn is that the CHD data do not provide an argument against the use of population level policies known to be effective to reduce alcohol-related harm.

Even in those jurisdictions in which CHD is a major contributor to premature mortality, the significance of these strategies for reducing the totality of alcohol-related harm suggests that they remain a priority for effective public health policy.

Thus, whilst evidence on the protective effect of drinking on CHD is conclusive at the level of association, and most likely conclusive at the level of causation, it is not on present analysis significant at the policy level. Any attempt to put about a message which encourages drinking on the basis of hoped-for gains in CHD prevention, would be likely to result in more harm to the population than benefit.

Acknowledgements

This paper is an updated version based on the report of a WHO working Group, on Alcohol and Health — Implications for Public Health Policy, held in Oslo, 9–13 October 1995 (World Health Organization 1995). The data on alcohol, cardiovascular diseases and countries of eastern Europe are taken from the Report on the Third Evaluation of Progress towards Health for All in the European Region of WHO (1996–1997) (World Health Organization 1997).

References

Casswell S 1995 Health and alcohol policy. Paper presented at the WHO working group on alcohol and health — implications for public health policy, Oslo, 9–13 October 1995. ICP ALDT94 02 MT12/19

Criqui MH 1994 Alcohol and the heart: implications of present epidemiologic knowledge. Contemp Drug Prob 21:125–142

Edwards G, Anderson P, Babour TF et al 1994 Alcohol policy and the public good. OUP, Oxford

English D, Holman D, Milne E et al 1995 The quantification of drug caused morbidity and mortality in Australia. Commonwealth Department of Human Services and Health, Canberra

Fillmore K 1995 Alcohol, mortality and psychosocial confounders. Paper presented at the WHO working group on alcohol and health — implications for public health policy, Oslo, 9–13 October 1995. ICP ALDT94 02 MT12/11

Maclure M 1993 Demonstration of deductive meta-analysis: ethanol intake and risk of myocardial infarction. Epidemiol Rev 15:328–351

Midanik LT, Tam TW, Greenfield TK, Caetano R 1996 Risk functions for alcohol-related problems in a 1988 US national sample. Addiction 91:1427–1437

Montonen M 1995 Alcohol and the media. WHO regional Office for Europe, Copenhagen (European Series No. 62)

Norström T 1995 The aggregation relationship between alcohol consumption and harm. Paper presented at the WHO working group on alcohol and health — implications for public health policy. Oslo, 9–13 October 1995. ICP ALDT94 02 MT12/17

Rehm J, Sempos CT 1995 Alcohol consumption and all-cause mortality. Addiction 90:471–480

Romelsjö A 1995 Alcohol consumption and unintentional injury, suicide, violence, work performance, and intergenerational effects. In: Holder H, Edwards G (eds) Alcohol and public policy — evidence and issues. Oxford Medical Publications, Oxford

Room R, Bondy S, Ferris J 1995 The risk of harm to oneself from drinking, Canada 1989. Addiction 90:499–513

Skog O-J 1992 Epidemiological and biostatistical aspects of alcohol use, alcoholism, and their complications. In: Erickson PG, Kalant H (eds) Windows on science. Addiction Research Foundation, Toronto, p 3–35

Skog O-J 1995 Public health consequences of the J-shaped curve. Paper presented at the WHO working group on alcohol and health — implications for public health policy, Oslo, 9–13 October 1995. ICP ALDT94 02 MT12/18

Stockwell T, Hawks D, Lang E, Rydon P 1996 Unravelling the preventive paradox. Drug Alcohol Rev 15:7–15

World Health Organization 1995 Report of a WHO working group on alcohol and health — implications for public health policy, Oslo, 9–13 October 1995. World Health Organization Regional Office for Europe, Copenhagen

World Health Organization 1997 Report on the third evaluation of progress towards health for all in the European region of WHO (1996–1997). World Health Organization Regional Office for Europe, Copenhagen

DISCUSSION

Criqui: What exactly happened in Russia? In terms of policy it is interesting to be able to study a country where traditionally drinking levels have been high, then a control policy is instituted and death rates go down, and finally a social change occurs resulting in a higher rate of drinking and then increased mortality.

Anderson: There's a large literature on the programme that reduced alcohol consumption in Russia, which was introduced by Gorbachev in the 1980s. It wasn't a quite a prohibition programme but it was a tough top–down programme involving controls of access and availability, coupled with measures such as the decimation of vineyards. There is no doubt that this campaign had a dramatic impact on people's lives: even taking into account all the illegal production of alcohol, the best estimates still showed quite marked reductions in alcohol use. However, it was bound to fail because it didn't have the support of the people. The whole thing got bound up with the whole transformation process, and was seen by the people as part of the previous political regime, which led to its abandonment. Then with the economic liberalization, the whole place became an unregulated 'wild west', if you like. When you went to these Soviet Union countries immediately after the transformation you saw three things on the streets that were not there before: prostitutes, imported drinks and imported cigarettes. I think what one is seeing is complete unregulation. There is also the importation and production of very dangerous products. I know the chief narcologist who is responsible for alcohol services in St Petersburg, and during this time he refused to buy any alcohol in the Soviet Union. He didn't even trust what appeared to be imported brands, because he felt they could have been illegally made bottles with counterfeit labels. Another contributing factor is that in Russia alcohol is incredibly cheap compared with basic foodstuffs. However, consumption is now beginning to fall: for the sake of the economy the government is finally trying to get a grip on this problem.

Peters: The interesting thing was how quickly the death rate from cardiovascular disease shot up after alcohol consumption increased.

Anderson: Yes; this situation is surely an epidemiologist's dream.

Farrell: It's clear that the Russian policy was a disaster from the point of view of future control policies. When we talk to people in central and eastern Europe about control policies, their eyes glaze over and they talk about Gorbachev and this deeply unpopular strategy which may well, in terms of the fall in revenue, have centrally contributed to the collapse of the Soviet Union.

Rehm: The data have now come out: there is a book by the National Academy Press (Bobadilla et al 1997) with a chapter on alcohol in Russia. There has also been a recent publication by the National Center for Health Statistics (1995) in the USA, looking at the mortality rates from Russia. Many of the data released are precise, and so what you can do with those data is make simulations and sensitivity analyses.

When we devised the Ontario low-risk drinking guidelines last year, which is a policy statement based on the current evidence, we found a lot of articles on the different risks for various diseases. We also reviewed what is known about how the public perceives public health messages such as drinking guidelines: overall we found only three articles which were vaguely relevant. At this point what we simply do not know the effects of messages such as 'Do not drink more than two drinks on any occasion', because there has been no systematic research on how those guidelines are perceived. We really need some knowledge in order to better prepare our messages.

Keil: I have always been fascinated by the speed at which changes in cardiovascular diseases take place. In Western Europe we have seen vast declines of 2–3% and even more per year, and in Eastern Europe there is currently this dramatic increase. Thus preventive measures *and* detrimental influences can have very rapid effects. Bobak & Marmot (1996) tried to speculate on the six year life expectancy difference between Eastern and Western Europe: they found that more than half of the life expectancy difference is due to differences in cardiovascular diseases.

Coronary heart disease has a complex aetiology and we shouldn't blame it only on heavy alcohol consumption. There are many factors that are changing rapidly in Russia, including diet, smoking, physical activity and social status: it's a breakdown of society and that obviously has a major impact on the cardiovascular field and not so much on cancer. Cancer has a longer latency period, but in cardiovascular disease the latency periods are short indeed.

Peters: From what we know about the pathophysiology of atherosclerosis, shouldn't there be a greater lag? Here we are seeing cardiovascular mortality shooting up only months after the increase in alcohol consumption.

Gaziano: I would have thought so too, were this excess mortality due to atherosclerosis and light drinking. But I think what we're talking about here is intoxication. I suspect that if we were to do the experiment that Dr Criqui has suggested and watched societies in the lower drinking levels increase or decrease consumption, there will be a lag time for atherosclerotic-related disease. However, when we were talking about sudden death and intoxication I think we are talking about a different mechanism.

Shaper: It is sudden cardiac death that appears to be on the marked increase in the Soviet Union. The one thing about sudden cardiac death, even as it is defined in those studies (under 24 h), is that it is easy to diagnose.

Keil: Again, when we look at the clinical trials for cholesterol we are surprised that already after a year we see the curves branching off. When an individual stops smoking, their risk diminishes after a very short time.

Klatsky: There is increasing evidence and interest in short-term, almost immediate factors having to do with endothelial function and stability of the atherosclerotic plaque. I think Dr Renaud has done some work in this area about Mediterranean diet and its apparently immediate effects.

Renaud: Short-term effects, apparently of diet changes, have been observed during the war in Norway (Stormorken 1973) as well as in France and Germany: within a year there was a drastic decrease of the mortality rate from CHD and after the war there was a similar rapid increase in the mortality from CHD concomitant with dietary changes. With the Mediterranean diet, within two months we see a drastic difference in the cardiovascular mortality and morbidity (Renaud et al 1995). Consequently, the hypothesis is that this effect occurred through reduced thrombosis, and we know that thrombosis is a major event in CHD.

Peters: Skog (1988) has found the same thing for cirrhosis, with rates increasing or decreasing relatively rapidly after overall changes in alcohol consumption.

Anderson: The rapid response in mortality to a dramatic change in aggregate consumption level was illustrated in data from Paris during the 1940s when alcohol was rationed between 1942 and 1947 (Fig. 1 *[Anderson]*).

Rehm: We have time series analysis showing there is an almost acute effect on liver cirrhosis (Skog 1984), and we have intervention effects which relate to prohibition in the USA or to shortage during World War I (Bruun et al 1975) which show an almost immediate reduction in liver cirrhosis. We therefore know that some of the diseases which have a long latency period can be influenced immediately by policy measures. There must be some kind of a threshold effect. What is fascinating about the Russian data is that this is apparently not the case for cancer.

Richardson: Do we know from the Russian data the actual documentation of the underlying coronary disease? Are there any post mortem data correlating with this alteration in apparent death which we're attributing to underlying coronary artery

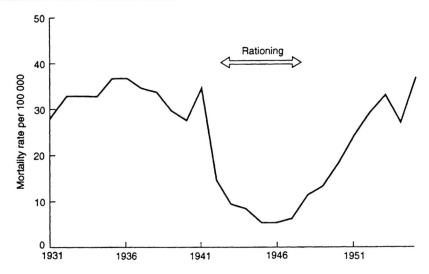

FIG. 1   (*Anderson*) Liver cirrhosis mortality in Paris 1930–1956 (Data from Ledermann 1964, reproduced from Edwards et al 1994).

disease? Intoxication of the level that clearly is present could create considerable electrical instability. We've all seen the effects of binge drinking in terms of sudden onset of ventricular and atrial arrhythmias.

Anderson: According to data from the MONICA project centre in Moscow, 20% of sudden coronary deaths resulted from alcohol intoxication with blood alcohol concentration 3.5 g/l or higher. Another 10–30% of deaths which show post-mortem alcohol concentration of less than 3.5 g/l could also be caused by alcohol intoxication prior to death. Further, the number of sudden cardiovascular deaths which were caused by alcohol poisoning increased during 1992–1993, as compared with previous years.

Peters: I always remember the Brewers' Society telling us that half their profits are generated from people who are drinking well over 50 units a week: can we do anything about that?

Shaper: We keep talking about this optimum level of drinking. We have this assumption that the lowest point of the curve is the optimum level of alcohol consumption. The point that Goya Wannamethee and I have been trying to make during this meeting is that the shape of this curve, irrespective of which group you are using as baseline, is going to depend to a considerable extent on the length of follow-up. A short follow-up will likely render a U-shaped curve for CHD and total mortality, and as you go on using the alcohol classification at entry into the study, in time you get flatter and flatter curves. Once you've got an

L-shaped curve, then any level of alcohol intake at that stage appears beneficial. Sometimes, as in the Health Professionals Study (Rimm et al 1991), the more you drink the better, although they don't have very heavy drinkers. This question of the nadir is an extremely difficult one, because you're using different studies with different follow-up periods in different communities to choose a level. When we say a small amount of alcohol, we are making a judgmental choice of the level we would like to focus on. We focus on one or two drinks a day because that seems to be acceptable in public health terms. If the curve happens to be inverse, we don't talk about it, and if the curve is flat then we don't talk about it.

Peters: But as with politics, advertising public health messages is the art of the possible. We have to try and get across messages that are easily understood. Our previous UK government attempted to shift from weekly limits to daily limits and people just didn't understand the message.

Shaper: I'm concerned about the science, before we get to the public health message.

Peters: In this session we're trying to translate the science into messages that we can put across.

Shaper: But I'm saying that if we don't get the science right then anything else we say is going to be fraught with problems.

Klatsky: When I put on my hat of 'practising physician', I have a big problem with the concept of 'optimum level'. It seems fairly obvious to me that if there is an optimum level, it will be quite different for a 60 year old man who has never had a drinking problem and has high cholesterol, than for the young woman who has no coronary risk factors. Optimum level has to be defined in terms individuals, rather than large groups of people.

Peters: One does this all the time in clinical medicine: giving advice to individuals on the basis of their individual social circumstances.

Shaper: Are you suggesting that confronted with an individual subject, whether it's a 20 year-old woman or a 60 year-old man, there are some circumstances in which you're going to advise taking four or five drinks a day? I really don't believe that.

Rehm: Is this so different from other areas of medicine? We give individual guidance on cholesterol and there are population guidelines on cholesterol. Everybody accepts that a doctor should judge on the individual circumstances and should not cling to some abstract guideline. On the other hand, we are asked constantly for drinking guidelines: this is what society demands of us whether we like it or not.

Klatsky: Guidelines for cholesterol definitely take into account age and other coronary risk factors.

Anderson: I don't think we should use the word 'optimal': instead, we are talking about the level of lower or lowest risk. If you have a J-shaped curve for an individual, what are the implications of this at a population level? The point I was trying to make was that because of the distribution of consumption in a population, the level in the population with the lowest risk is going to be much lower than the level for an individual.

Peters: Susan Bondy gave us a list of about 30 detrimental effects of alcohol but only two or three beneficial effects. Perhaps the alcohol consumption advice for someone who is smoking would be different from someone who doesn't smoke.

Shaper: Nowhere in this meeting have we talked about any model for coronary heart disease and atherosclerosis. If we're concerned with the issue of the underlying factors in coronary heart disease and atherosclerosis, we're concerned with diet as a fundamental issue and the consequent blood cholesterol levels in populations and individuals. Moving on from there, we're concerned with the aggravating and additional factors which are not fundamental, such as blood pressure, cigarette smoking and physical activity. Nowhere in that model does alcohol enter into it. Thus to talk about looking at an individual and trying to assess whether they should be taking one or two drinks a day because of their risk levels seems to be a most unfortunate public health attitude.

Peters: But it's the reality of clinical medicine. It doesn't just apply to alcohol but to all manner of medical practice.

Anderson: There's a difference presumably in approach. If a patient comes in after a heart attack saying that they have stopped smoking and stopped drinking, the physician can suggest that they need not have stopped drinking. However, that is a very different message to actually encouraging people who don't drink to start drinking. Under no circumstances should we begin promoting that message, because of all the dangers and risks of alcohol. But in terms of individual advice, we have new information to discuss with people about what existing drinkers can do.

Gaziano: As doctors there are many recommendations in secondary disease prevention that we make that have risk:benefit ratios similar to that of alcohol. One of these is oestrogen replacement therapy in post-menopausal women. This has measurable risks to patients as well as benefits, and in each case we assess the patient's underlying risk of breast cancer and coronary disease. For a patient who has had a myocardial infarction, there is an 80% chance that they will end up dying of cardiovascular disease. For this patient, the beneficial effects of light alcohol consumption outweigh the risks. For such a patient who doesn't drink, I wonder if we need to be quite so timid about providing this information. To say you would absolutely never recommend a few drinks a week for any patient under any circumstance is a bit of a simplistic message. If we tell the public one message — that we never advocate drinking for anything — but then the scientific literature says in high risk people there is a mortality benefit, we're sending a mixed message. They're then going to have to make a decision on their own in a rather confused way.

Peters: Except that the evidence from a positive intervention with randomized control trials — all the evidence that you'd need before putting people on statins or other drugs — is not there for alcohol.

Gaziano: We happily recommend exercise, weight reduction and oestrogens without randomized trials.

Miller: I am hearing conflicting messages. On the one hand we're talking about a population-based strategy. It seems that on no account could one propose as a public health measure the adoption of light alcohol consumption for the prevention of coronary heart disease from what we know about alcohol as a drug. Then I hear messages about what to do for individual patients, which is an entirely different consideration. Is there ever a case, when faced with a patient at high risk, to prescribe light alcohol consumption? That to me also seems a dangerous strategy. We now understand so much about the pathogenesis of coronary heart disease that our strategies should attack more the primary pathogenic problem itself. If we can't persuade patients to change their lifestyle in ways we think will be of benefit for thrombogenic and the atherogenic components of the disease, we then have drugs which are safer than alcohol. Many cancer drugs put through clinical trials are found to have profound effects on cancer, but nobody would use them in a clinical situation because the complications and the side effects are so profound: alcohol tends to fall into that category. We seem to have found a fortuitous benefit of alcohol, but I don't think alcohol can be recommended for use in ways that some seem to advocate.

Criqui: I agree. As I mentioned in my paper, if alcohol were proposed today to the US Food and Drug Administration for cardioprotection I don't think it would get approval. But I am a little uncomfortable when alcohol is discussed in the broad context of preventive remedies. People do not make decisions about drinking based on health issues. Alcohol until recently wasn't thought to have any health benefits: the majority of people in developed countries make their decisions about drinking based on enjoyment of the beverage. Public health recommendations about alcohol other than to limit excessive drinking seem to me to be a moot point. When an individual comes in as a patient, the first question you ask is whether they drink, how much they drink and whether they have any problems with it: it's a negotiation depending on that particular individual's circumstances. We shouldn't talk about alcohol as though it was some new prophylactic drug that we can use for cardioprotection.

Shaper: If we talk about high risk subjects — people with symptoms and evidence of coronary heart disease — then almost every one of those is going to be put on statins and aspirin and will have their hypertension treated. There is a whole regime of treatment that should be instituted and in almost 50% of cases in this country isn't being instituted properly. The key issue about alcohol is not the question of whether you should be saying to people who are non-drinkers (either lifelong teetotallers or ex-drinkers) that they should start drinking now for health benefit, which I do not think anybody is suggesting. Instead, if light drinkers wish to know whether they should continue drinking, the answer is almost certainly that there appears to be no harm from this level of intake and that you would get much the same benefit in terms of coronary heart disease as you would if you did not have heart disease. If they are heavy drinkers, you are going to give them the kind of advice that you would give to any heavy drinker. What I'm worried about is a positive recommendation for light drinking coming across as a health message.

Puddey: From the 1840s through to the 1870s, alcohol was widely promoted here in Britain for medicinal purposes, so much so that there was a ration of wine for each person who was admitted to a public hospital. And it was not a small ration of wine. More than that, the treatment for pneumonia, typhoid fever and post-partum haemorrhage was with a large shot of alcohol. This promotion led to the widespread use of alcohol, particularly amongst upper-class women, which started to translate into increased alcoholism. There was a wide ranging debate on this over a number of years through the editorial pages of the *British Medical Journal* and the *Lancet* (Anonymous 1861a, 1861b, Hooper 1861). I remember seeing one editorial, entitled 'Alcohol: food or physic?' (Anonymous 1861a, 1861b). It is interesting to me that really we are now re-visiting this whole issue 150 years later, not having made much further progress.

Peters: Except we are talking about orders of magnitude less of alcohol: King's College Hospital was founded by Bentley Todd who advocated the treatment of fevers with litres of brandy a day! One of the first controlled trials compared brandy with milk in treatment of typhus (Hargreaves 1875).

Richardson: As a practising cardiologist I have many patients who come seeking advice regarding alcohol consumption. I commonly see businessmen who after having increased their level of alcohol consumption begin to be aware of palpitations and cardiac dysrhythmias which develop gradually. These patients do ask for a definite health statement regarding safe drinking levels. Should we define a level, as we have done for cholesterol, i.e. a normal range of drinking. The normal range surely is 1–3 drinks a day.

Criqui: Skog (1985) has looked at the distribution of alcohol consumption in populations around the world, and the results have many implications for policy reommendations. The ratio of the mean to the median is fairly constant. The interesting thing here is the proportion of people who are over two times the mean. You'd think there would be many more people two times over the mean in Iceland (mean $\approx$ 3 litres/year) than there would be in France (mean $\approx$ 20 litres/year), but in fact this number is constant; it's about 10–15% of the population. Thus, in countries with high mean intakes of alcohol, alcohol abuse is common and much more likely than in low intake countries. I don't know when you're doing public health policy how you break that link: how do you get everybody to drink lightly, when the distribution is really so constant?

Anderson: The only way you can do it is by rationing alcohol. This was the experience in Sweden. Of course, this is unacceptable to most people.

Keil: This is Geoffrey Rose's message: the mean determines the extremes.

Criqui: Another issue that no one has brought up is what the alcohol industry thinks about these issues. In the USA, the alcohol industry has made several attempts to encourage people to drink less and deal with overconsumption. However, there is a severe disincentive for them to succeed: the top 10–15% of drinkers drink more than half of all the alcohol consumed in the population. Sales are therefore disproportionately to the group that are drinking irresponsibly.

Anderson: We need to look at which policies are effective for reducing which harms. We know that many existing policies, such as taxation, and restriction of advertising and access, probably all impact on harm. The area where we haven't been so effective is in reducing the intoxication harms.

Gaziano: In the USA, drinking and driving has come down considerably with a discrete intervention at a time when the median levels of consumption have not changed dramatically. This suggests that it is possible to uncouple median drinking and certain hazards of heavy drinking, by the use of specific types of messages. I don't think you have to get the entire population to drink less to get rid of drinking and driving.

Farrell: I think in Australia there's a suggestion the measures against drinking and driving have actually brought down the median alcohol consumption level.

One of the issues facing us is not necessarily communicating what might be beneficial, but the level of drinking with the least amount of harm. The figures that seem to have been consistently reported here fall between one and three units. Given the discussions we had earlier about the measurement problem, it is interesting just how consistent that figure is.

Klatsky: In terms of public health policy, what Jürgen Rehm said earlier is very pertinent in that there are no studies about the interaction of the perception of the message and the effect of the message. But we have to keep in mind that any general message to reduce drinking, no matter what the level, will run into a credibility problem with a large proportion of the population in developed countries. This group has heard about the benefits of drinking. Thus any policy which doesn't take into account what people hear from the media could very well be counter-productive: it may lead to scepticism and disbelief, and that certainly would not be desirable in a public health message. This is a real factor that has to be taken into account.

Shaper: The phrase that Dr Farrell used is 'the level of drinking with the least harm'. I think that's one of the best expressions I've heard yet, because it obviates the need to discuss magnitude effects in coronary heart disease, cardiovascular disease or total mortality.

Criqui: Is it less harmful than not drinking, though?

Shaper: I have no idea, except that there is this tremendous problem of the difference between lifelong teetotallers in communities where drinking is the norm, and lifelong teetotallers in communities where it is not.

Keil: We also have to keep away from hypocrisy. There is a saying by the German poet Heinrich Heine: 'They are preaching publicly water and they drink secretly wine'. I saw everyone here drinking and enjoying their glass of wine yesterday night.

References

Anonymous 1861a Alcohol: food or physic? Br Med J 2:360–362

Anonymous 1861b Alcohol: food or physic? Br Med J 2:468–469

Bobadilla JL, Costello CA, Mitchell F 1997 Premature death in the new independent states. National Academy Press, Washington DC

Bobak M, Marmot M 1996 East–West mortality divide and its potential explanations: proposed research agenda. Br Med J 312:421–425

Bruun K, Edwards G, Lumio M et al 1975 Alcohol control policies in public health perspective. Finnish Foundation for Alcohol Studies, Helsinki

Edwards G, Anderson P, Babor TF et al 1994 Alcohol policy and the public good. Oxford Univ Press, Oxford

Hargreaves W 1875 Alcohol: what it is and what it does. In: Alcohol and science. William Nicholson & Sons, London, p 214–215

Hooper D 1861 The alcohol question. Lancet 1:507–509

Ledermann S 1964 Alcool, alcoolism, alcoolisation, vol. 2. Presses Universitaires de France, Paris

National Center for Health Statistics 1995 Vital and health statistics: Russian Federation and United States, selected years 1980–1993. US Department of Health and Human Services, National Center for Health Statistics, Hyattsville

Rimm EB, Giovannucci EL, Willett WC et al 1991 Prospective study of alcohol consumption and risk of coronary heart disease in men. Lancet 338:464–468

Skog O-J 1984 The risk function for liver cirrhosis from lifetime alcohol consumption. J Stud Alcohol 45:199–208

Skog O-J 1985 The collectivity of drinking cultures: a theory of the distribution of alcohol consumption. Br J Addict 80:83–99

Skog O-J 1988 Testing causal hypotheses about correlated trends: pitfalls and remedies. Contemp Drug Prob 15:565–606

Stormorken H 1973 Relation between dietary fat and arterial and venous thrombosis. Haemostasis 2:1–14

Chairman's summing-up

Timothy J. Peters

Department of Clinical Biochemistry, King's College School of Medicine and Dentistry, Bessemer Road, London SE5 9PJ, UK

The meeting achieved the aim of bringing together a wide range of disciplines including sociologists, epidemiologists, cardiologists, biochemists, haematologists, vascular biologists and molecular biologists, to address the principal questions targeted in my introduction. The approach was transdisciplinary rather than a simply interdisciplinary one.

It was particularly valuable to have a historical overview as an introduction to provide a firm platform for the meeting. There are clearly lessons to be learnt from the chequered medical history of cardiovascular science, particularly relevant to the current vogue for evidence-based medical practice. A recurring theme was 'individual susceptibility factors' to the complications of alcohol misuse, an area clinical geneticists and molecular biologists are rather belatedly beginning to address. There is an obvious need for concentrated effort in this area.

The session on metabolic consequences set the biochemical basis for alcohol physiology and toxicity and listed several possible toxic processes. Their relative importance needs urgent attention. Similarly, the unravelling of adaptive responses to chronic alcohol consumption (e.g. mitochondrial and endoplasmic reticulum proliferation) from the toxic effects (e.g. free radical formation) needs to be addressed.

The possible antioxidants in alcohol and alcohol-free beverages was addressed, but the *in vivo* efficacy of these antioxidants needs investigating. Similarly, detailed comparison of the antioxidant activity of ales, beers, lagers, red, white and fortified wines at both the *in vitro* and *in vivo* levels is urgently required.

Alcoholic heart muscle disease is clearly commoner than generally believed, particularly if 'electrical defects' are included. The belief that alcoholic cardiomyopathy is a nutritional deficiency disorder was firmly laid to rest but the basis of individual susceptibility was again raised. Dysrythmias as a cause of sudden death in alcohol misusers was highlighted.

A series of discussion sessions on the lipid, coagulation, thrombolysis and vascular components of alcohol-related benefits and morbidity also provided valuable background. Clearly, more work is needed in the area of thrombosis and fibrinolysis and the pathogenesis of alcohol-related vascular disease, particularly stroke. Similarly, alcohol-induced hypertension, an important clinical problem affecting at least one-quarter of all patients attending alcohol misuse clinics, is ill understood. The pathogenic process(es) of this hypertension remains controversial and its role in the cardiovascular disease of high alcohol consumers needs to be dissected out.

The international spread of speakers ensured that various issues were discussed on a global basis. This was particularly highlighted with the recent remarkable increase in cardiovascular and other causes of death in the former Soviet Union. This provides an interesting 'experiment of nature' on the relationship between alcohol consumption and morbidity.

The J-shaped curve is a highly reproducible epidemiological phenomenon. To date, with the exception of plasma lipid alterations, there is no biochemical basis for it. Can the plasma lipid responses to increasing alcohol intake explain the epidemiological observations? Unfortunately, the jury is still out on this question, especially when certain populations are considered, and we should pursue alternative explanations. It is certainly clear that abstainers are medically and epidemiologically a highly heterogeneous and in many ways an 'unhealthy' group. For example, our own recent studies indicate that they are significant under-users of 'preventive' medical services such as dental and optician consultations, mammography and cervical cytology attendances, but are enhanced users of acute medical services such as Accident and Emergency and General Practitioner consultations, compared with safe-limit drinkers (Cryer et al 1998). The detailed shape of the J-shaped curve varies with factors such as gender, age and ethnicity: that is, the level of drinking associated with reduced/enhanced morbidity is highly variable. An explanation is needed for this variability.

An important issue to emerge from the meeting was the need for biological markers, both state and trait, to be applied to epidemiological studies relating consumption to morbidity/mortality rates. Considerable progress has been made in the area of biological markers and these objective measures should be applied to the epidemiological studies. Similarly, questionnaire development exploring such variables as type of beverage, time of consumption, detailed drink diaries and interrelations with over the counter drugs (e.g. aspirin, tobacco and illicit drug usage) is needed to help refine the epidemiological associations.

The highly specific J-shaped curve relationship between consumption and morbidity poses difficulties from a public health perspective. In young males the curve is flattened but becomes increasingly marked with age. The nadir (trough) is displaced to the left (lower consumption) for females compared with males, and may vary more than fivefold for different populations. These and other profile variations make the health-promoting effects of moderate alcohol consumption extremely difficult, if not impossible, to advocate. In addition, there are competing public health aims, e.g. increasing life expectancy of the middle-aged at the expense of increasing alcohol-related mortality in the young. These are imponderable issues for politicians and public health experts to solve.

The meeting was devised, scripted and held in the best traditions of the Ciba Foundation Symposia, although it is the first of the symposia held under the Novartis Foundation umbrella. Hopefully new avenues of research, including collaborations, joint grants and international studies will emerge yet again from No. 41 Portland Place.

Personally, as a contributor to six symposia over the past 25 years, this meeting continued the objectives of the 'founding fathers' of the Foundation, Robert Käppeli and Max Hartman, and maintained the highest standards of their scientific meetings.

The Novartis Staff, particularly Dr D. Chadwick, the Director, ensured that the meeting was conducted in an apparently effortless manner and are to be again thanked and congratulated on the entire happening. Dr J. Goode, the book editor, is to be thanked with his staff for their high level of professionalism and, in particular, translating the open discussion sessions, an almost unique feature of the Novartis Symposia, into a highly readable text.

A final note is that, because of the commercial implications for the liquor trade of the conclusions of the Meeting, all participants were asked at the outset to declare any financial or other support from drinks or other relevant organizations related to the work presented or discussed at the meeting. Such involvement clearly does not invalidate or tarnish the researches but the reader should be allowed to share this information (Peters 1997).

References

Cryer C, Jenkins L, Cook A et al 1998 The use of acute and preventative medical services by a general population: relationship to alcohol consumption. Addiction, in press
Peters T J 1997 Liquor, tobacco and editorial independence. The Framington Consensus. Addict Biol 2:373–376

Index of contributors

Non-participating co-authors are indicated by asterisks. Entries in bold indicate papers; other entries refer to discussion contributions.

Subject index